Midwifery: Best Practice Volume 3

For Elsevier:

Commissioning Editor: Mary Seager
Development Editor: Kim Benson
Project Manager: Mandy Galloway
Production Manager: Yolanta Motylinska
Layout: INQ Design
Cover photograph: David Fito

Midwifery: Best Practice Volume 3

Edited by

Sara Wickham RM MA BA(Hons) PGCE(A)

Senior Lecturer in Midwifery, Anglia Polytechnic University

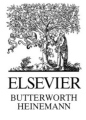

ELSEVIER
BUTTERWORTH
HEINEMANN

EDINBURGH LONDON NEW YORK OXFORD PHILADELPHIA ST LOUIS SYDNEY TORONTO 2005

ELSEVIER

BUTTERWORTH
HEINEMANN

ISBN 0 7506 8846 7

British Library Cataloguing in Publication Data
A catalogue record for this book is available from the British Library

Library of Congress Cataloguing in Publication Data
A catalog record for this book is available from the Library of
Congress

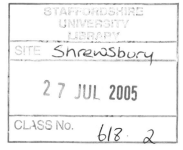

Note
Knowledge and best practice in this field are constantly changing.
As new research and experience broaden our knowledge, changes in
practice, treatment and drug therapy may become necessary or
appropriate. Readers are advised to check the most current
information provided (i) on procedures featured or (ii) by the
manufacturer of each product to be administered, to verify the
recommended dose or formula, the method and duration of
administration, and contraindications. It is the responsibility of the
practitioner, relying on their own experience and knowledge of the
patient, to make diagnoses, to determine dosages and the best
treatment for each individual patient, and to take all appropriate
safety precautions. To the fullest extent of the law, neither the
publisher nor the editors assumes any liability for any injury and/or
damage.

Note
The publisher has made every effort to obtain permission to
reproduce all borrowed material.

The Publisher

Printed in China

Contents

Introduction

Welcome to the third volume of *Midwifery: Best Practice* which, as ever, is a melting pot of the best articles from *The Practising Midwife*, seasoned with a few research articles from *Midwifery* and some original pieces written especially for this volume and topped off with a few thoughts of my own and questions to ponder, perhaps for use in PREP activities, or for reflection. This time around, as well as ideas for personal or group reflection, each "Reflecting On" section includes a suggestion or idea for beginning a piece of writing, and an idea for action.

As ever, this book has a multitude of authors and contributors, listed on page viii, and I would like to begin by thanking them for their work, along with Jenny Hall and Ann Thompson for their editorial work on *The Practising Midwife* and *Midwifery*. It is especially gratifying, in these days where many of us are working long hours under pressure, that so many midwives with full-time jobs are still managing to find the time to write about their practice and their passions.

In the two years that the *Midwifery: Best Practice* series has been published, it has been interesting to note the changes in the kinds of things midwives are writing about. It seems to me that, having talked about social movement and change in the culture of birth for a number of years, we are now seeing an upsurge in the number of articles exploring new ways of thinking and being and projects which are making this a reality for more women. Each of the original articles in this book reframes thinking in a specific area and I would like to thank Deborah Davis, Anna Fielder, Luqman Hayes, Ann Dent, Alison Stewart, Ishvar Sheran and Janice Marsh-Prelesnik for sharing their thoughts and work here.

The four main sections in this volume are 'Women, Midwives and Choice', 'Pregnancy', 'Labour and Birth' and 'Life After Birth'. There are also four 'Focus on...' sections exploring issues around families, spirituality, loss, bereavement and grief, and alternative therapies and, as ever, the final 'Stories and Reflection' section, which celebrates the narrative, experiential kind of writing that is so important to midwives and women.

Finally, I would like to add a big thank you to Kim Benson, Mary Seager, Rita Demetriou-Swanwick and all their colleagues throughout Elsevier who tend not to get thanked by name in books because they work behind the scenes, but who are no less pivotal in their creation.

Sara Wickham

Acknowledgements

We would like to thank all those who have contributed to this volume of *Midwifery: Best Practice*.

Christine Andrew, Shirley Andrews, Barbara Burden, Gill Catron, Jo Coggins, Debra K Creedy, Karin Dahlberg, Lorna Davies, Rosamund Davies, Cathy Davis, Deborah Davis, Ruth Deery, Ann Dent, Sue Deighton, Karen Dunlop, Helen Eatherton, Rosemary Essay, Anna Fielder, Jenny Fraser, Jennifer A Gamble, Jennifer Hall, Anne Hatfield, Luqman Hayes, Rosalind Holland, Amber House, Debbie Howells, Carol Hughes, Deborah Hughes, Sarah Hunt, Liz Jones, Barbara Kavanagh, Graham Kennedy, Linda Kimber, Mavis Kirkham, Chit Ying Lai, Beverley A Lawrence Beech, Lynda Leach, Valerie Levy, Alison Lovatt, Ingela Lundgren, Kim Lyon, Rosemary Mander, Janice Marsh-Prelesnik, Mary Mitchell, Wendy Moyle, Jon Nicholl, Mary Newburn, Alicia O'Caithan, Jill Parker, Belinda Phipps, Xavier Pick, Hilary Pilcher, Joyce Reid, Elizabeth Robinson, Francesca Robinson, Zevia Schneider, Judith Schott, Jancis Shepherd, Ishvar Sheran, Gill Skinner, Andy Spencer, Alison Stewart, P Cynthia Stuart, Karen Taylor, Meg Taylor, Kate Thomas, Charlotte Walker, Denis Walsh, Stephen J Walters, Shirley Webber, Joan Webster, Andrew J Weiner, Jean Wills, Jennifer Wrightson.

Women, Midwives and Choice

It never seems right to me to separate women, midwives and the concept of choice, as these issues are so intertwined in our day-to-day lives and work. Choice is, of course, a relatively recent phenomenon, at least as we understand the word these days; our mothers had much less choice than we do, and our grandmothers had far, far fewer choices again. To use the everyday example of the entertainment (and I use that word in its loosest sense!) that comes into our homes via television, it is only a generation ago that there were barely two channels to choose from; now, if you have the right equipment, there are hundreds. A couple of eighty-year-old women I interviewed recently had just discovered 'reality' television shows, where viewers could cast votes by phone to determine the fate of the contestants. The two women were stunned by this concept, not least because, as young women, they were acutely aware that they had only had the power to vote in political elections for a very short time. It is sometimes easy to forget just how quickly some of the concepts and technologies which we now take for granted have swept over our culture, and changed our everyday experiences in ways we tend not to imagine unless we specifically take time to reflect upon this.

Deborah Davis' article on the concept of choice not only places the current emphasis on choice in our consumer society in an historical context, it also raises some hugely important issues around the politics of choice and the notion of responsibility in holistic midwifery practice – an issue which is also discussed from a slightly different angle by Ishvar Sheran in Section 8. Perhaps it will enable us to consider where we, as midwives, might choose to stand on these issues.

Alicia O'Cathain and colleagues' research adds another dimension to this debate, exploring some important aspects of women's views around informed choice, including whether they felt they made informed choices, and the extent to which they actually wanted to do this. Perhaps most importantly, a significant minority of women in this study did not feel that they were enabled to make informed choices.

The series of articles by Denis Walsh, Rosemary Essay and Carol Hughes, Cathy Davis and Beverley Beech demonstrate that the concept of 'normal' midwifery is just as politically situated and culturally bound as the concept of choice, and further this debate from their different perspectives, while Jean Wills and Sue Deighton outline how midwives are trained to attend instrumental births in an article which raises further questions about definitions of normality and what 'normal' midwifery might be.

There is, quite clearly, a need for this debate to continue. As the concepts of choice and normality are politically situated, there may be a need for more midwives to become politically aware and knowledgeable, in order to further effect the creation and implementation of innovations which improve the experiences of women and the morale of their midwives. Deborah Hughes, Ruth Deery and Alison Lovatt describe their research with midwives, which reveals that there are ways forward. Their work highlights some of the cultural issues that may be standing in the way of the kind of service which some women and midwives would like to see in place. While the researchers themselves note that they felt discouraged by the nature of some of the data, they also demonstrate that, with the right support, midwives can begin to shift the culture towards the kind of service we would like to provide and women would like to experience.

Choice in the Maternity Market

Deborah Davis

The way that we think about people and health is radically different today from how it was just 50 years ago. Today we see responsibility for health resting with the individual and within that construction, the right of individuals to make choices has become an important element. The concepts of choice and individual responsibility are not something that just happened or that have occurred in a vacuum, but products of social, cultural and political forces that have shaped and continue to shape them. This paper will explore the concept of choice in relation to today's health care context and consider some of the implications of the increasing focus on choice for midwifery and women experiencing maternity care. It is hoped that this exploration will make room for further debate within the midwifery community. While this paper was developed within the New Zealand midwifery context I suggest that the issues under discussion are also relevant for midwifery in many other countries.

From patient to empowerment

Throughout the nineteenth century the medical profession rose to a privileged position in society and was afforded a great deal of status and power (Peterson, 2001). Reflecting a patriarchal society, health care was provided in a paternalistic manner where those seeking care handed over responsibility, entrusting the doctor to make decisions and act in their best interests. As the women's movement and anti-government/establishment movements of the 60s gained momentum, women and other health activists began to lobby for change in health care. The medical model of health was accused of being reductionist in its exclusive focus on the biophysical aspects of illness and health activists fought for a more holistic approach. Their lobbying also reflected a concern for individual autonomy, as they demanded 'rights', 'empowerment' and 'self-determination' (Cox-White and Zimbelman, 1998).

We now embrace a more holistic understanding of health and it is no longer appropriate for health professionals to approach the health care encounter in a paternalistic way. Recipients of health care are expected to participate and health professionals are expected to facilitate this. Within this new model of health care those receiving health care are constructed as consumers. As Irvine comments:

With their cognitive competence taken as given, health consumers are understood to be self-actualising, self-activated, autonomous social agents who cannot be subordinated to the professionals, and are capable, with adequate information, of formulating their own intentions, deciding their own preferences and wants, and making rational choices about their fate... (Irvine, 2002).

Patients have become consumers and health care has become a service or commodity that can be bought and sold like any other.

Individual choice and responsibility are central tenets of this new conceptualisation of health care. Recognition of the autonomous, self-responsible, informed consumer of maternity care is something for which many of us have been fighting. Assertive and discerning, armed with a purse full of knowledge – we couldn't wait for her to arrive in the maternity market place with her shopping list and determination to purchase a quality product. Has she arrived and what did we expect of her anyway? I expected her to change the health care landscape, to profoundly alter the power structures of health care relationships. I expected her to choose alternatives to the technocratic, medicalised birth experience. I expected her to choose normal childbirth.

In New Zealand women are choosing midwives. In 2002, 73.1% of women chose a midwife as their lead maternity carer. A lead maternity carer is the person who takes professional responsibility for the woman's care from early pregnancy through to four to six weeks postpartum. Most of these lead maternity carers would be providing maternity care within a continuity model of care (Ministry of Health, 2002). We have worked hard to provide women with choices, to help them be informed, to facilitate their empowerment and we expected that these factors would curtail the steady increase in intervention in childbirth; that midwives and women together would turn the tide on intervention, but this has not been the case. In New Zealand in 2002, 22.7% babies were born by Caesarean section, 20.1 per 100 births were induced and 25% of women had an epidural anaesthetic. Just over two-thirds of women (67.7%), experienced normal birth (Ministry of Health, 2004). On a positive note, midwives faired better than GPs when rates of intervention and normal birth are compared with lead maternity carer type (Ministry of Health, 2004). However, these statistics represent a small but steady increase in intervention and decline in normal birth. Why is that? That's not what we expected to happen. Perhaps we were naïve in not appreciating the myriad of factors that contribute to and shape women's choices and midwifery practice.

The next section of this paper will explore in more detail some of these contextual factors and the implications for choice and midwifery practice. I suggest that on closer inspection the consumer that we had been waiting for is merely a mirage and the choice that was heralded as our liberator, an illusion.

The consumer mirage

The construct of the consumer features prominently in public health policy and health literature. Is health care really a commodity like any other and do we really treat it as such? Irvine suggests that it isn't well established as a practice for recipients of health care.

In the concrete world of living actors, it appears that people continue to think and act in a manner consonant with traditional models of patient-hood... (Irvine 2002).

Lupton's research (1997) suggests that those more likely to engage in consumerist type behaviours are younger, well educated, professionals. Even so, their approach and behaviours are not fully driven by consumer imperatives because health care, unlike other commodities, entails a high level of emotional investment and is not undertaken as a 'purely rationalist response to the perception of a need' (Lupton 1997). While health care choices are constructed in this new environment as an 'outcome of an individualised calculation' (Lupton 1997) they are in fact much more complex.

A number of authors and researchers in health and sociology view the emergence of the consumer construct in health care sceptically. Irvine considers that the concept began as a grass roots resistance to medical authority but has since been appropriated for other ends.

The last decades of the 20th century have witnessed a changing political, social and economic landscape in many Western nations. We have seen a trend to privatisation, deregulation, economic rationalism and the embracing of a new managerialism with a shift to more market driven economies. The medical profession has enjoyed considerable power and status within our society, clinging protectively to what is described as their right as professionals to be autonomous and to make independent clinical decisions. Direct threats to this autonomy are translated as threats to the quality of patient care.

The economic rationalisation of the managerial imperative comes head to head with professional authority and autonomy. Consumer discourses are a convenient ally for the managerial approach, which confronts professional authority while seeming to provide the consumer with an improved service. Irvine states:

...at the level of everyday practice, the language of the health consumer is a vehicle which transports unpopular managerial reforms into health care institutions. It is also a useful instrument which legitimates the penetration of the state into the professional domain; through an appeal to higher principles of 'consumer interests'... (Irvine, 2002)

The notion of the consumer is problematic in that it harbours potential for disorder. So while on the one hand the construct is encouraged, there are processes in place that act to constrain true choice and consumerist behaviours toward health care. Irvine says that health institutions develop strategies to limit the potential for disorder by disciplining subjects in a variety of ways to manage the risk of non-compliance. There is a range of techniques that 'undermine resistance and instil self discipline' (Irvine, 2002).

These techniques include the individualised approach to health, which places both health and responsibility for health at the level of the individual. When health is situated at this individual level, ill health is seen to be a failing of the individual so we see a victim-blaming consciousness accompanying these discourses.

Individualism

The profession of medicine has come to situate ill health or disease at the level of the individual body. With the aid of autopsy and knowledge of anatomy, medicine came to understand that disease as an entity caused real anatomical, observable change in the body. Along with this conceptualisation came the understanding of single pathogenic causative agents. The domination of this way of perceiving disease and ill health has excluded the development of alternative ideas such as those emphasising multiplicity of causation or social determinants of health (Crawford, 1980). Medicine within the dominant medical discourse represents a science of the individual.

The holistic health movement was heralded as a radical break away from the dominant discourses of medicine with its reductionist methods and paternalistic approach. Holistic health philosophy asserts the need to understand health in a more whole and inclusive way, and many proponents of this approach have espoused the importance of claiming responsibility for one's own health. With the popularisation of this movement, the control of individual health has been brought into the realms of individual responsibility. We no longer rely on the authoritative other to fix our health problems. We now claim responsibility for our own health. On the surface this new conceptualisation of health seems like an enlightened one. It is holistic, it acknowledges a connectedness between mind and body, it recognises personal responsibility, but Crawford (1980) considers that it encompasses and so acts to reinforce some of the fundamental elements of medical discourses.

This new approach to health continues to individualise health. It suggests that we can prevent ill health through modifications to our lifestyle, implying that our lifestyle choices are the root of ill health. When the individual is seen as the cause of disease then the cure is also situated in the individual. Personal health is seen to lie within the sphere of personal control. If we make the right choices, eat the right foods and lead the right lifestyle with the right attitude we can experience optimal wellbeing – hence the proliferation of personal health strategies aimed at modifying lifestyles, behaviours and attitudes contributing to health.

This individualised approach to health has been embraced by health policy and health promotion professionals, and by other groups, as we are encouraged and supported in our efforts to embrace healthy living and associated activities (Nettleton, 1997). The problem with this approach to understanding health is that it fails to acknowledge some of the other determinants of health such as genetic, social or economic factors. In this way the discourses of holistic health and personal choice and responsibility depoliticise health by steering focus away from social, cultural, political and economic factors associated with health.

Victim blaming

If health is seen as being determined by the individual through their personal choices regarding such factors as lifestyle and attitude, then ill health is a seen as a failing of the individual or non-compliance with prescribed health behaviours (Crawford, 1980). Health and wellness as concepts in our society have become charged with

moral overtones. We can see the impact of this discourse in attitudes, for example, towards people who are overweight or who smoke. Obesity and smoking are understood as signs of moral weakness, disregard for the self or lack of personal willpower. The genetic propensity toward obesity, the proliferation of fast food, the highly addictive nature of nicotine, the impact of advertising, and other social and economic influences are ignored.

The moral overtones influencing expectations around health behaviour of the pregnant woman are even more pronounced, and so is the propensity toward blame. Women are blamed for any perceived imperfections in their baby whether these are physical or otherwise (Gregg, 1993). Women have begun to censor not just their physical behaviour but their very thoughts and emotions for fear that these may have a negative psychological or emotional impact on the baby (Gregg, 1993). There are so many choices for women to make and it seems everyone is watching and waiting to make judgements.

The illusion of free choice

While the consumer enjoys certain rights within the health policy and social context, these rights are accompanied by a set of responsibilities. We function in a society that has expectations of normal, correct behaviour. These normative discourses establish correct modes of thought and set the standards, boundaries and ground rules of acceptable and competent conduct. They act to ensure that individuals in taking up their rights as consumers

...take charge of their conduct by actively monitoring their behaviour for its acceptability and competence, to ensure that they use their autonomy 'correctly'... (Irvine, 2002).

There have been many examples, both locally and internationally, where women's rights to choice and self-determination have been constrained because they have been seen to be making irresponsible choices. Examples at the extreme end of the spectrum include enforced Caesarean section, and enforced blood transfusions when these have been refused on religious grounds (Ratcliff, 2002). There are some subtle and not so subtle forces shaping our choices. Women are not free to make any choice but only those that are considered to be within the realms of what is normal and responsible. Interestingly, choices that support the dominant medical and scientific discourses such as elective Caesarean section without medical indication, are often not considered irresponsible or irrational. They are rationalised and normalised with recourse to the construction of normal childbirth as a risky event.

Medical discourses on health and childbirth continue to be highly influential, socialising women long before they enter the childbirth services market place. When childbirth is understood as a risky event and medical technology and intervention as key to moderating this risk, then many options will not be considered choices at all. This is evidenced by the fact that so many women choose to give birth in hospitals despite the evidence supporting the safety of homebirth (Leap, 1996).

Within a social and cultural context dominated by medical and scientific discourses, women are pressured to take advantage of an ever-increasing array of technologies associated with childbirth. Many of these technologies are not well understood yet they implicitly promise a safer journey or a more positive outcome for the pregnancy: routine cardiotocographic monitoring or ultrasound-scanning are cases in point. Many of these technologies are not even presented as choices because their use has become routine and part of normal care.

Our medicalised social context and feto-centric medical and legal environment (Gregg, 1993) combine to put women in an invidious position in regard to choice in childbirth. They are pressed to demonstrate that they are being responsible and they are doing everything possible to ensure a healthy outcome for their baby. Often this is understood as taking advantage of medical 'advances' and technologies. Those women declining to take advantage of these services are viewed with suspicion. Women are driven toward medical and technological monitoring and intervention by our social and cultural contexts so many of the choices we suggest that women have, are not really choices at all.

Facilitating informed choice

Where does this leave us as midwives? Within the discourses that emphasise individual choice and responsibility, (those that construct the woman as a consumer), the same process is constructing the health professional or service provider. Health professionals are constructed as neutral conduits for information, facilitating but not influencing the informed choice of the consumer. However, choice is not a neutral event, it is a political concept. Options or services offered as choices and the influences pressing women toward certain choices and not others, are positioned by techniques of power and political manoeuvring. There is no such thing as free choice. In embracing the concept of individual choice and enthusiastically fulfilling our responsibility to facilitate informed choice without bias, I believe we are unwittingly supporting the perpetuation and increase of medical and technological discourses of childbirth. We do have a range of technologies and interventions available for use in pregnancy and childbirth but few of these have been demonstrated to be effective for routine use in normal birth. Why then should they be offered to women as choices?

I also believe that in some situations midwives are abrogating what should be professional midwifery decisions and asking women to choose, for example, to have perineal tears sutured or to have routine admission cardiotocograph monitoring. Has the concept of individual choice gone too far? The following quotation is from the Sydney Morning Herald.

When the highly paid specialist said the decision to have a fancy medical test was up to me, I knew 'empowerment' had gone too far. I was paying for him to make the decisions. But he was acting like the junior partner in my health care. I might have yelled 'power to the people' in some demo 20 years ago when he was clawing his way into the Maquarie Street medical establishment, but I didn't actually mean power to me over every technical decision that would crop up in my life...(Horin 1995, cited in Lupton 1997).

Midwives are specialists with knowledge, skill, experience and important professional values. As Horin suggests, this is what we bring to the woman-midwife relationship. My concern is that in focussing on individual choice and responsibility, and by pushing some practice decisions from midwifery into the consumer arena, we are neglecting some important midwifery input.

I believe that protecting normal birth is an important professional value because we know that normal birth is the safest option for most women (Leap, 1996). In today's health care climate, this role is more challenging than ever before. Our practice context is also complex and there are many factors that act to constrain us and make this difficult to achieve. However, I do believe that we should claim our particular bias toward normal birth unashamedly and actively seek to influence women's choices in this regard. As Leap (1996) suggests, work to "...actively encourage choices that are most likely to optimise safety..." and for most women this is normal birth. I am not suggesting a return to a paternalistic or an authoritative approach to care but within the context of a trusting relationship, that we gently and sensitively work with women to optimise their opportunities for normal birth and a safe experience.

Conclusion

This paper has explored the construction of choice within today's health care environment and has suggested that we are embedded in a context that is dominated by medical and scientific discourses of health and childbirth. While the concept of individual choice and responsibility was heralded as an important strategy of resistance, I have attempted to demonstrate that it may in fact work toward maintaining this dominance.

I have suggested that our focus on individual choice and responsibility has eclipsed interest in what midwifery offers the maternity experience, including our skills in facilitating normal birth. I believe that as midwives we have valuable knowledge, experience, and

professional values and therefore an important active part to play in decision-making processes.

REFERENCES

Cox-White B, Zimbelman J. Abandoning Informed Consent: An Idea Whose Time Has Not Yet Come. Journal of Medicine and Philosophy 1998; 25(5): 477-499

Crawford R. Healthism and the Medicalization of Everyday Life. 1980

Gregg R. "Choice" as a Double-Edged Sword: Information, Guilt and Mother-Blaming in a High-Tech Age. Women and Health 1993; 20(3): 53-73.

Irvine R. "Fabricating health consumers in health care politics" in S. Henderson and A. Peterson (eds). Consuming health. The commodification of health care. London: Routledge; 2002

Leap N. 'Persuading' women to give birth at home - or offering real choice? British Journal of Midwifery 1996; 4(10): 536-538.

Lupton D. Consumerism, Reflexivity and the medical encounter. Social Science and Medicine 1997; 45(3): 373-381.

Ministry of Health. Maternity Services. Notice pursuant to section 88 of the New Zealand public health and disability act 2000. Wellington, New Zealand: Ministry of Health; 2002

Ministry of Health. Report on Maternity 2000 & 2001. Wellington, New Zealand: New Zealand Health Information Service; 2003

Ministry of Health. Report on Maternity 2002. Wellington, New Zealand: New Zealand Health Information Service; 2004

Nettleton S. "Surveillance, health promotion and the formation of a risk identity" in M. Sidell, J. Jones and A. Peberdy Debates and dilemmas in promoting health. Hampshire: McMillan Press; 1998

Peterson, M. (2001). From Trust to Political Power: Interest Group, Public Choice, and Health Care. Journal of Health Politics, Policy and Law, 2001; 26(5): 1145-1163.

Ratcliff K. Women and health, power, technology, inequality and conflict in a gendered world. Boston: Allyn and Bacon; 2002

Midwifery Best Practice Volume 3 (ed. Wickham) 2005; 3-7

Women's perceptions of informed choice in maternity care

Alicia O'Caithan, Kate Thomas, Stephen J Walters, Jon Nicholl, Mavis Kirkham

Objective: to describe the extent to which women using maternity services perceive that they have exercised informed choice.

Design: postal survey of women using maternity services, covering women's views of the extent to which they exercised informed choice overall, and at eight decision points during their care.

Setting: twelve maternity units in Wales.

Participants: 1386 women at approximately 28 weeks gestation (antenatal sample) and 1741 women at approximately 8 weeks post delivery (postnatal sample).

Measurements and findings: 54% of women perceived that they exercised informed choice overall in the antenatal sample (95% CI: 51–57%) and 54% overall in the postnatal sample (95% CI: 52–56%). Perceptions of informed choice differed by decision point, varying between 31% for fetal heart monitoring during labour and 73% for the screening test for Down's syndrome and spina bifida in the baby. There were differences by

maternity unit, even when the characteristics of women attending these units were taken into account. Multiparous women, women from manual occupations and women with lower educational status were more likely to feel that they exercised informed choice during antenatal care. These sub-groups of women were also more likely to report a preference for not sharing decision-making with health professionals.

Conclusions: a large minority of women felt that they had not exercised informed choice overall in their maternity care. The perception of informed choice differed by decision point, maternity unit and characteristics of the woman.

Implications for practice: attaining informed choice is more of a challenge for some decision points in maternity care than others, particularly fetal monitoring. The difference in levels of informed choice between maternity units highlights the importance of maternity unit policy in the promotion of informed choice.

Introduction

Currently in the UK NHS there is a drive to promote partnership between health professionals and clients/patients when making decisions about individual clinical care, basing these decisions on research evidence (Entwistle et al. 1998). Changing Childbirth has acted as a catalyst for this movement in maternity care, promoting care which is women-centred and the provision of information and choice to enable women to feel in control of their care (Department of Health 1993). In response to this, the Midwives' Information and Resource Service (MIDIRS) and NHS Centre for Reviews and Dissemination identified 10 decision points faced by women in pregnancy and childbirth, and produced a set

of 10 evidence-based leaflets – known as the MIDIRS Informed Choice leaflets – designed to encourage women's involvement in these decisions during their individual maternity care (Box 1.2.1). Even though women themselves have identified information, decision-making and control as important aspects of their childbirth experience (Lavender et al. 1999), there is little information available on the extent to which women perceive they have exercised informed choice, whether this differs by the type of decision faced and whether different types of women perceive that they exercise it more than others. This information is needed to help health professionals to identify particular decision points or sub-groups of women to focus efforts upon when attempting to promote informed choice, and possibly help in the design of interventions aimed at improving informed choice. This paper reports the results of a survey of women's perceptions of the extent to which they had exercised informed choice during their maternity care. It was undertaken as part of an evaluation of the MIDIRS Informed Choice leaflets, in maternity units in which these leaflets were not available (Kirkham & Stapleton 2001).

Methods

Of the 15 large maternity units in Wales, three had purchased the MIDIRS Informed Choice leaflets; we approached the 12 which had not and they agreed to participate in the evaluation. A small unit attached to one of these maternity units was also included in the study. For the survey, two six-week cohorts of women were identified in each maternity unit: women at 28 weeks gestation who were receiving antenatal care (antenatal sample) and women who had delivered live babies (postnatal sample). Two questionnaires were developed to cover eight of the decision points addressed by the MIDIRS Informed Choice leaflets (Box 1.2.1), one to be sent to the antenatal sample and one to be sent to the postnatal sample of women.

The antenatal sample

A questionnaire was designed to cover three decisions which women may face during their pregnancy: whether or not to have ultrasound scans; whether or not to have a screening test for Down's syndrome and spina bifida in the baby; and whether to have their baby in hospital or home. It was felt that women would have faced these decisions by 28 weeks gestation. In each maternity unit, women estimated to have reached 28 weeks gestation during a six-week period in early 1998 were identified. Three maternity units had computer systems which could identify the sample and in the other maternity units, midwives and clerks in hospital and community-based antenatal clinics identified women at their booking appointment who would reach 28 weeks gestation during the study period. Women were included if they received antenatal care in any setting from midwives attached to each unit. Attempts were made to exclude women under 16 years old from the sample for ethical reasons. The questionnaire was posted to women as they reached 28 weeks gestation. The intention had been to send only one reminder after three weeks because of the workload involved in checking that women in the sample had not miscarried over the postal period. However, the response rate was not acceptable after the first reminder and a short questionnaire covering four

Box 1.2.1 Decision points addressed by the MIDIRS Informed Choice leaflets

Decision point addressed	Covered in the questionnaires
1 **Support** in **labour**	Y
2 Listening to your baby's **heartbeat** during labour	Y
3 **Ultrasound scans** – should you have one?	Y
4 **Alcohol** and pregnancy	–
5 **Positions** in labour and delivery	Y
6 **Epidurals** for pain relief in labour	Y
7 Feeding your baby – **breast** or **bottle?**	Y
8 Looking for **Down's syndrome** and **spina bifida** in pregnancy	Y
9 Breech baby: What are your choices	–
10 Where will you have your baby – **hospital** or **home?**	

key questions was sent as a second reminder to boost the response rate.

The postnatal sample

A questionnaire was designed to cover five decisions which women may face during labour, delivery and a few weeks later: who to have with them during labour, as well as the midwife; the kind of monitoring to have in labour to listen to the baby's heartbeat; whether or not to have an epidural; what positions to use during labour and delivery; and whether to breast feed or bottle feed. In each maternity unit, women who delivered live babies during a six-week period in late 1997 were identified. Child health computer records were used as a sampling frame for 10 maternity units. Hospital and home delivery registers were used in two maternity units. Women delivering in all settings were included; women who lived in areas outside the catchment area of the maternity unit and women living in areas where antenatal care was provided by midwives from other units were excluded. Attempts were made to exclude women under 16 years old for ethical reasons. The questionnaire was posted to women at eight weeks post delivery and up to two reminders were posted at three-weekly intervals.

Definition of informed choice

We measured women's perceptions of informed choice, where overall informed choice was defined as 'having enough information and discussion with midwives or doctors to make choices together about all the things that happened during maternity care' with the options 'yes', 'partly', 'no', 'there was no choice', 'did not apply'. For analysis, this response was dichotomised into 'yes' versus all other responses. The question was asked for each of the decision points covered in the questionnaire and then for maternity care overall. Standardised instruments were not available for measuring perceptions of informed choice and therefore we devised this question with the help of qualitative research and face-to-face piloting with women using maternity services. We drafted a question about informed choice and asked women attending antenatal clinics at two maternity units to complete the question and offer comments about the question. During this process we added the option 'there is no choice' because some women felt that choices were not available. For example, some women struggled with the concept of choice around ultrasound scans because they considered them to be part of routine maternity care. We then added the option 'did not apply' because some women did not feel that choice was a relevant issue for some decision points. For example, women who did not drink alcohol felt that the issue of choice around drinking alcohol during pregnancy was irrelevant to them. During our piloting we found that women were so frustrated by the concept of informed choice around drinking alcohol during pregnancy that we excluded it from the questionnaire. We undertook a postal pilot of the questionnaires in a maternity unit not involved in the study and made minor amendments based on this pilot.

Preferences

The preferences women hold may affect the extent to which they feel they have exercised informed choice. In particular, women with preferences for unconventional pathways, such as not having an ultrasound scan or wanting a home birth, may be less likely to feel that they have exercised informed choice than women making more conventional choices. Therefore women were asked if they held preferences for specific options available at each decision point, with the options 'yes', 'no' and 'no preference'.

Decision-making style

The extent to which women want to participate in decision-making may affect their perceptions of whether they exercised informed choice. Therefore, women were asked which role they preferred to take when making choices about their care, with the options ranging from making the choice themselves, through three grades of sharing decision-making, to leaving all decisions to health professionals (Degner & Sloan 1992).

Social and demographic variables

Women were asked their age when they left fulltime

education (categorised for analysis into three groups of under 18 years for GCSE-level, 18-19 years for A-level and 20 years and over for further education), the ethnic group they considered they belonged to, their employment status, their occupation (classified into non-manual and manual), their partner's employment status and occupation, and parity.

Ethical approval

Ethics Committee approval was given by the committees covering all the maternity units.

Analysis

Data were entered into a computer and analysed using SPSS. Groups were compared using the chi-squared test for comparison of proportions. Logistic regression was used to adjust differences between maternity units for characteristics of the women using them in terms of woman's age, educational status, partner's occupational status, ethnicity, parity, and preferred decision-making style.

Findings

Response rates

The overall response rate for the surveys was 64% (3127/4851). Of the 2210 questionnaires sent to the antenatal sample, there were 1386 completed responses, 82 'return to senders' and 46 blank questionnaires returned as refusals to participate giving a response rate of 65% (1386/2128). Of the 2762 questionnaires sent to the postnatal sample, there were 1741 completed responses, 39 'return to senders' and 60 blank questionnaires returned as refusals to participate, giving a response rate of 64% (1741/2723).

Description of respondents

The respondents from both the antenatal and postnatal samples were similar in terms of socio-demographic characteristics (Table 1.2.1). A lower proportion of postnatal respondents than antenatal respondents were employed, this may be because some women change employment status to care for their baby.

Informed choice at different decision points

Half of the women (54%) felt that they had made informed choices about all the things that happened during their maternity care in both the antenatal and the

Table 1.2.1 Socio-demographic characteristics of respondents

Characteristic	Antenatal sample	N= 100%	Postnatal sample	N= 100%
Mean age in years (SD)	27.6 (5.50)	1235	28.3 (5.53)	1717
Age left fulltime education		1194		1713
Under18 years	62%		61%	
18-19	23%		23%	
20+	15%		16%	
Employment status		1230		1713
Employed	59%		48%	
Unemployed	36%		46%	
Never employed	5%		5%	
Social class (woman)		1034		1425
Non-manual	68%		68%	
Manual	32%		32%	
Social class (partner)		920		1352
Non-manual	44%		44%	
Manual	56%		56%	
Ethnicity		1234		1720
White	98%		97%	
Other	2%		3%	
Home ownership		1230		1710
Own	68%		67%	
Rent	32%		33%	
Parity		1230		1713
Primiparous	47%		44%	
Multiparous	53%		56%	

postnatal samples (Table 1.2.2). The perception of informed choice differed by decision point, and was lower for fetal heart monitoring at 31% and higher for the screening test for Down's syndrome and spina bifida in the baby (73%) and feeding the baby (70%). A large percentage of women in the postnatal sample ticked 'did not apply' for the decision points of support during labour, having an epidural and positions in labour. When we excluded women undergoing planned and emergency Caesarean sections, 'did not apply' rates remained unchanged except for positions in labour where it reduced to 6% and the percentage ticking 'yes' increased to 48%. The perception of having made an informed choice at any of the decision points was strongly associated with the perception of having made informed choices about all the things that happened during their maternity care. Women who felt that they made informed choices about ultrasound scans were more likely than other women to feel they had made informed choices overall during their antenatal care: 79% (577/735) v 24% (149/611), $\chi^2=393$, df=1, $p<0.001$. This strong relationship was found for each of the decision points: screening for Down's syndrome and spina bifida 68% (675/987) v 14% (52/360), $\chi^2=309$, df=1, $p<0.001$; place of birth 87% (533/610) v 26% (194/737), $\chi^2=501$, df=1, $p<0.001$; support in labour 72% (696/973) v 30% (207/696), $\chi^2=285$, df=1, $p<0.001$; heart monitoring 90% (460/510) v 38% (440/1156), $\chi^2=387$, df=1, $p<0.001$; epidurals 75% (570/763) v 36% (328/901), $\chi^2=244$, df=1, $p<0.001$; positions in labour 82% (591/721) v 32%

Table 1.2.2 Percentage of women perceiving that they exercised informed choice by decision point and overall in antenatal and postnatal samples

Decision	Yes % (n)	Partly % (n)	No% (n)	No choice % (n)	Does not apply % (n)	95%CI for yes	Total
Whether or not to have ultrasound scans	55% (744)	17% (233)	15% (207)	10% (132)	3% (44)	52–58%	1360
Whether or not to have a screening test for Down's syndrome and spina bifida in the baby	73% (996)	15% (201)	7% (99)	2% (34)	2% (31)	71–75%	1361
Whether to have their baby in hospital or home	45% (612)	16% (216)	25% (334)	7% (101)	7% (96)	42–47%	1359
Overall in antenatal sample	54% (730)	31% (413)	12% (162)	1% (18)	2% (29)	51–57%	1352
Who to have with them during labour	58% (985)	11% (190)	12% (199)	4% (66)	15% (250)	56–60%	1690
The kind of monitoring to have in labour to listen to the baby's heartbeat	31% (513)	18% (308)	24% (400)	19% (313)	9% (147)	29–33%	1681
Whether or not to have an epidural	46% (768)	13% (219)	14% (228)	7% (111)	21% (352)	44–48%	1678
What positions to use during labour and delivery	43% (725)	19% (315)	17% (279)	8% (140)	13% (211)	41–45%	1670
Whether to breast feed or bottle feed	70% (1184)	12% (206)	7% (116)	2% (33)	9% (146)	68–72%	1685
Overall in postnatal sample	54% (905)	31% (520)	9% (156)	3% (46)	3% (48)	52–56%	1675

(303/935), $\chi^2=403$, df=1, $p<0.001$; and feeding 67% (783/1174) v 24% (120/497), $\chi^2=255$, df=1, $p<0.001$.

The effect of preferences on informed choice

The majority of women reported preferences for some decision options, and these preferences were associated with whether they felt they had exercised informed choice (Table 1.2.3). Although the numbers of women with no preferences were generally small, it was a fairly consistent finding that they were less likely than women with preferences to feel that they had exercised informed choices. There was some evidence that women making unconventional choices were less likely to feel that they made informed choices than other women, such as women planning home births and preferring not to breast feed. However, differences between conventional and unconventional preferences were small.

Characteristics of women who exercise informed choice

A consistent finding across both the antenatal and postnatal samples was that a higher percentage of multiparous women than primiparous women felt that they had exercised informed choice (Table 1.2.4). In the antenatal sample, women with lower educational status, unemployed women, and women in manual occupations were more likely to perceive that they had exercised informed choice. These differences were not found in the postnatal sample, with the exception of the woman's partner's occupation where the manual group was more likely to perceive that they had exercised informed choice than the nonmanual group (Table 1.2.4). Although statistically significant, the size of the differences between groups tended to be small – less than ten percentage points. Similar differences were found when the full five-category informed choice variable was used rather than the dichotomised version; groups which were less likely to answer 'yes' were more likely to answer both 'partly' and 'no'.

Maternity units

The proportion of women perceiving that they exercised informed choice in the antenatal sample ranged from 41% to 68% in the 12 maternity units ($\chi^2=28.9$, df=11, $p=0.002$) and in the postnatal sample from 49% to 64% ($\chi^2=18.9$, df=11, $p=0.063$). Maternity unit differences persisted in the antenatal sample after the age, educational status, partner's occupational status, ethnicity, parity, and preferred decision-making style of women attending them were taken into account ($\chi^2=36.3$, df=11, $p<0.001$). In the antenatal sample, women using smaller maternity units were more likely to perceive that

Table 1.2.3 Percentage of women perceiving that they exercised informed choice for a specific decision point by their preferences for that decision

Reported preference	%'Yes' informed choice	Total N=100%	Chi-squared	df	p-value
Have an ultrasound scan					Not valid
Yes	56%	(1193)			
No	0%	(2)			
No preference	23%	(10)			
Have a blood test to look for Down's syndrome			18.4	2	<0.001
Yes	75%	(920)			
No	71%	(217)			
No preference	50%	(58)			
Plan to have a home birth			13.5	2	0.001
Yes	39%	(61)			
No	46%	(1044)			
No preference	22%	(59)			
Have support in labour, as well as midwife			5.0	2	0.083
Yes	59%	(1582)			
No	52%	(27)			
No preference	42%	(38)			
Have electronic fetal monitoring (belt around waist)			38.8	2	<0.001
Yes	38%	(598)			
No	35%	(280)			
No preference	22%	(636)			
Have an epidural			52.6	2	<0.001
Yes	64%	(338)			
No	42%	(863)			
No preference	41%	(279)			
Lie in bed throughout labour			0.9	2	0.641
Yes	42%	(341)			
No	44%	(660)			
No preference	41%	(194)			
Breast feed			21.3	2	<0.001
Yes	74%	(942)			
No	65%	(499)			
No preference	59%	(104)			

they had exercised informed choice than those using larger maternity units (Table 1.2.4). However, this was due to two of the largest units having a low percentage of women feeling that they had exercised informed choice. There was no correlation between unit size and percentage of women perceiving that they exercised informed choice in either the antenatal sample (Spearman's rank correlation coeficient $r_s = -0.09$, 95% confidence interval −0.63, 0.51) or the postnatal sample ($r_s = -0.29$, 95% CI −0.74, 0.34).

Decision-making style

Women reported different preferences for the extent to which they wanted to participate in making decisions about their care (Table 1.2.4). Taking the antenatal sample, 83% (998/1201) of women wanted some form of sharing between health professionals and themselves.

Table 1.2.4 Percentage of women perceiving that they exercised informed choice overall by characteristics of women

Characteristic	Antenatal sample					Postnatal sample				
	% 'Yes' informed choice	N=100%	χ^2	df	p-value	% 'Yes' informed choice	N=100%	χ^2	df	p-value
Age of mother, years			0.2	2	0.989			1.8	2	0.412
<21	54%	(144)				49%	(166)			
21–30	54%	(699)				54%	(902)			
31+	54%	(361)				55%	(585)			
Parity			10.5	1	0.001			6.2	1	0.012
Primiparous	49%	(557)				50%	(737)			
Multiparous	58%	(641)				57%	(929)			
Age left fulltime education			18.6	2	<0.001			0.4	2	0.807
Below 18	56%	(717)				54%	(997)			
18–19	58%	(264)				52%	(379)			
20+	39%	(183)				54%	(272)			
Employment status			5.4	1	0.020			0.1	1	0.769
Employed	51%	(707)				54%	(799)			
Unemployed	58%	(492)				54%	(851)			
Occupation (woman)			9.6	1	0.002			0.1	1	0.769
Non-manual	50%	(689)				53%	(943)			
Manual	60%	(324)				54%	(437)			
Occupation (partner)			3.5	1	0.060			8.3	1	0.004
Non-manual	50%	(399)				50%	(566)			
Manual	57%	(503)				58%	(741)			
Ethnicity			0.2	1	0.677			1.7	1	0.190
White	54%	(1177)				54%	(1612)			
Other	50%	(26)				44%	(43)			
Maternity unit			4.3	1	0.042			1.3	1	0.249
Large (2500+deliveries)	52%	(759)				53%	(947)			
Medium (<2500 deliveries)	57%	(593)				57%	(728)			
Decision-making preferences			10.6	4	0.031			7.2	4	0.127
I prefer to make the final choice	61%	(165)				53%	(274)			
I prefer to make the final choice after seriously considering the midwife's and doctor's opinion	51%	(631)				54%	(665)			
I prefer that my midwife and doctor and I share responsibility for making choices	54%	(281)				56%	(415)			
I prefer that my midwife and doctor make the final choice but seriously consider my opinion	55%	(86)				48%	(194)			
I prefer to leave all choices to my midwife and doctor	71%	(38)				65%	(76)			

Most of the remaining women preferred to make the final decision without reference to health professionals (14% [165/1201]) and very few wanted the health professionals to make the decision (3% [38/1201]). The proportion of women perceiving that they exercised informed choices in the antenatal sample was associated with women's decision-style preference. Women who preferred not to participate in decision-making with health professionals were more likely to feel that they had exercised informed choice, particularly if they preferred health professionals

to make choices on their behalf. Caution should be exercised when interpreting this finding due to the small numbers in this group. There was no statistically significant association in the postnatal sample.

Focusing on the antenatal sample only, women from non-manual and manual occupations had different decision-style preferences, $\chi^2=21.6$, df=4, p<0.001 (Table 1.2.5, overleaf). In particular, more women from manual occupations than non-manual occupations preferred not to share decision-making with health professionals. A

Table 1.2.5 Preferences for decision-making held by different groups of women in the antenatal sample, percentages (with numbers in brackets)

	I prefer to make the final choice		I prefer to make the final choice after seriously considering the midwife's and doctor's opinion		I prefer that my midwife and doctor and I share responsibility for making choices		I prefer that my midwife and doctor make the final choice but seriously consider my opinion		I prefer to leave all choices to my midwife and doctor		Total N=100%
	%	(n)	%	(n)	%	(n)	%	(n)	%	(n)	%
Occupation											
Non-manual	11%	(73)	59%	(408)	23%	(156)	6%	(42)	2%	(12)	691
Manual	16%	(54)	45%	(147)	26%	(86)	9%	(29)	4%	(12)	328
Educational status											
<18 years	17%	(120)	47%	(341)	23%	(168)	9%	(63)	4%	(29)	721
18–19	9%	(23)	57%	(151)	28%	(77)	4%	(10)	2%	(5)	266
20+	9%	(16)	67%	(122)	17%	(31)	8%	(14)	0%	(0)	183
Parity											
Primiparous	12%	(65)	57%	(319)	22%	(123)	7%	(39)	2%	(13)	559
Multiparous	15%	(99)	48%	(313)	25%	(160)	8%	(49)	4%	(26)	647

similar relationship existed for educational status (χ^2=47.1, df=8, $p<0.001$) and parity (χ^2=11.1, df=4, p=0.026), with women who left full-time education aged less than 18 years old and multiparous women holding preferences for non-participative decision-making – the very sub-groups of women most likely to feel that they exercised informed choice.

Discussion

In 12 large maternity units in Wales in 1997/1998, approximately half of women perceived that they had exercised informed choice overall in maternity care. This is very similar to findings from elsewhere which have been published since we began this study. In the UK in 1996/1997, 52% of women said they were fully involved in all decisions about their pregnancy, and 54% in decisions during labour and birth (Wyke et al. 2001). In another study undertaken in small maternity units in Wales in 1996/1997, 50% of women delivering in obstetric units felt that they were encouraged to make informed decisions about their care during labour, although a considerably larger percentage (72%) of women felt that they took an active part in decision-making about their antenatal care (Churchill & Benbow 2000). The findings from our study, taken together with those from other studies, indicate that a large minority of maternity care users do not feel that they exercise informed choice. This is no different from health care in general in the UK, where 59% of patients do not feel involved in decisions about their care (Kendall 2001).

The proportion of women perceiving that they had made informed choices differed markedly by decision point. In particular, only one-third of women felt that they made informed choices about fetal heart monitoring. This is similar to the findings from another study where only one-fifth of women felt they had a say in how their baby was monitored during labour (Audit Commission 1998).

So why do more women feel that they have exercised informed choice for screening for Down's syndrome and spina bifida than for fetal monitoring during labour? A pilot study of the introduction into a maternity unit of two of the MIDIRS Informed Choice leaflets, on ultrasound scans and positions in labour, showed differing degrees of resistance on the part of health professionals to each of the leaflets (Oliver et al. 1996) and therefore it is likely that informed choice for different decisions will face different barriers.

Although intuitively we might expect unconventional options to meet more barriers than conventional ones, there was only weak evidence of this in our study. In fact, it was women who reported having no preferences about specific decisions who were less likely to feel that they had exercised informed choice at that decision point. Health professionals who want to promote informed choice may find it helpful to compare decision points with different levels of perceived informed choice in order to identify barriers to informed choice. In particular, it may be important to take an historical view of the introduction of the decision point, looking at whether women are presented with a real decision or are expected to follow routine practice, and considering who is responsible for the consequences of the decision.

Differences in levels of informed choice remained between maternity units after adjustment for women's characteristics, varying between 41 and 68%. This suggests that maternity unit policy may be important in the attainment of informed choice (Anderson & Rosser 1998). Policies may be formal and written, or may simply be determined by health professionals' preferences (Kirkham & Stapleton 2001).

Perceived and actual informed choice

In our study multiparous women, women with lower educational status, and women from manual occupations were more likely to perceive that they exercised informed choice in antenatal care, although actual differences between different groups of women were small. These are somewhat surprising findings in that we might expect less educated women to have difficulties seeking information and articulating choices. This highlights the complexity of making assessments of informed choice. In our study, we chose to measure perceptions of informed choice rather than asking women to report, say, their knowledge, attitude and action about a decision point in order to assess whether they had actually made an informed choice (Marteau et al. 2001), or undertaking a third-party assessment of the interaction between the woman and health professional to determine whether informed choice had actually been exercised. A woman's perceptions may be affected by her awareness of the meaning of informed choice, her expectations of maternity services to offer informed choice, her preferences for informed choice, and her understanding about how decisions were actually made during her maternity care and by whom. For example, health professionals may present women with the risks of a home birth to steer them towards a hospital delivery (Kirkham & Stapleton 2001). A woman giving authority to the health professional might judge that she has made an informed choice because she has been given information, has had a discussion with a health professional, and feels that they have made the decision together to have a hospital delivery. Another woman might ask for further information about both the risks and benefits of home and hospital delivery, feel that the decision is being steered towards the hospital delivery, and therefore feel that she has not exercised informed choice. Thus, different women may assess the same encounter in very different ways, and any woman's assessment of whether informed choice has taken place may be very different from the assessment of a third party witnessing the interaction between the woman and the health professional. One implication is that women's perceptions may overestimate the extent to which informed choice actually occurs and may measure the extent to which 'informed compliance' occurs (Kirkham & Stapleton 2001).

Nonetheless, we feel that it is important to measure women's perceptions of informed choice as well as actual informed choice in the light of evidence that perceived involvement in decision-making is more important to consumers of health care than actual involvement (Edwards et al. 2001).

Preferences for involvement in decision-making

We can see from our study that women have different preferences for the extent to which they want to be involved in making decisions, which is also the case for users of other parts of the health service (McKinstry 2000). The women who preferred a non-participatory style, where either they or the health professional made decisions, were more likely to perceive that they exercised informed choice, and these women were more likely to be multiparous, with lower educational status and from manual social occupations. It is difficult to make judgements about exactly what is happening here until we know more about how women develop their preferences for participating in decision-making. If their views are developed from a position of power and understanding, then their views should be respected and followed. However, if they are developed from a position of resignation or ignorance then we may wish to tackle this from an educational perspective. Until we know more about this, it is important that health professionals at least know how women in their care prefer to be involved in decisions and aim to be sensitive and flexible in meeting women's needs (Levy 1999).

Limitations

This study had some limitations. First, measuring informed choice and women's role in decision-making is far from easy (Entwistle et al. 2000, Marteau et al. 2001), and our simple measure may have failed to fully unpick the complexities of women's decision-making, particularly in a context where choices may not be available or where health professionals may steer women towards specific options (Kirkham & Stapleton 2001). This may be rejected in the usage of the options 'there is no choice' and 'did not apply' when answering our question about informed choice for different decision points. We decided to keep women using the 'did not apply' options in our analyses in this study because we felt that some of them might have answered our question differently if the information about the choices available to them had been presented differently by health professionals. Perceived choice, never mind informed choice, is a complex issue and users of health services may not feel that choice is available even when health professionals (Charles et al. 1998) or researchers feel that it is. Secondly, our antenatal and postnatal samples included different women and we were unable to track women through the maternity system. Nonetheless, we feel that we have been able to contribute important findings on a topic of increasing importance to the health service.

Implications for practice

A large minority of women do not feel that they exercise informed choice in their maternity care. The challenge to promote informed choice is greater for some decision points in maternity care than others, particularly fetal heart monitoring, and in some maternity units more than others. Health professionals who wish to improve this situation could focus on the decision points identified here as having low levels of informed choice and recognise that they may have to change both formal and informal maternity unit policies which work against their goal, whilst taking women's preferred styles of decision-making into account.

Acknowledgements

We would like to thank all the women who completed the questionnaire, and all the staff at participating maternity units who helped with the study. Ceri Rees and Heather Rothwell helped to establish the data collection systems. Helen Stapleton contributed to the design and piloting of the questionnaire. Andrea Shippam and April Dagnall undertook data administration. Donna Mead, Laurence Moseley, Barbara Bale, Gwenan Thomas, and Sandy Kirkman were members of the research team for the wider study, of which this survey was a part.

This work was commissioned by the NHS Centre for Reviews and Dissemination and funded by the Department of Health. The views expressed here are those of the authors and not necessarily those of the Department of Health.

REFERENCES

Anderson T, Rosser J 1998 Informed choice. Was it the wrong choice? Editorial. The Practising Midwife 1:4-5

Audit Commission 1998 First class delivery: a national survey of women's views of maternity care. Audit Commission, London

Charles C, Redko C, Whelan T et al. 1998 Doing nothing is no choice: lay constructions of treatment decision-making among women with early-stage breast cancer. Sociology of Health and Illness 20: 71-95

Churchill H, Benbow A 2000 Informed choice in maternity services. British Journal of Midwifery 8:41-47

Degner LF, Sloan JA 1992 Decision making during serious illness; what role do patients really want to play? Journal of Clinical Epidemiology 45: 941-950

Department of Health 1993 Changing Childbirth. Report of the Expert Maternity Group. HMSO, London

Edwards A, Elwyn G, Smith C et al. 2001 Consumers' views of quality in the consultation and their relevance to 'shared decision-making' approaches. Health Expectations 4: 151-161

Entwistle VA, Sheldon TA, Sowden A et al. 1998 Evidence-informed patient choice. International Journal of Technology Assessment in Health Care 14:212-225

Entwistle VA, Skea ZC, O'Donnell MT 2001 Decisions about treatment: interpretations of two measures of control by women having a hysterectomy. Social Science and Medicine 53: 721-732

Kendall L 2001 The future patient. Institute for Public Policy Research, London

Kirkham M, Stapleton H 2001 Informed choice in maternity care: an evaluation of evidence-based leaflets. Report 20, The University of York, York

Lavender T, Walkinshaw SA, Walton I 1999 A prospective study of women's views of factors contributing to a positive birth experience. Midwifery 15: 40-46

Levy V 1999 Maintaining equilibrium: a grounded theory study of the processes involved when women make informed choices during pregnancy. Midwifery 15:109-119

Marteau TM, Dormandy E, Michie S 2001 A measure of informed choice. Health Expectations 4: 99-108

McKinstry B 2000 Do patients wish to be involved in decision making in the consultation? A cross sectional survey with video vignettes. British Medical Journal 321: 867-871

Oliver S, Rajan L, Turner H et al. 1996 Informed choice for users of health services: views on ultrasonography leaflets of women in early pregnancy, midwives, and ultrasonographers. British Medical Journal 313:1251-1255

Wyke S, Hewison J, Elton R et al. 2001 Does general practitioner involvement in commissioning maternity care make a difference? Journal of Health Services Research and Policy 6: 99-104

Midwifery 2002; 18:136-144

What is a 'Normal' Midwife?

The research midwife's view

Denis Walsh

As a midwife undertaking full-time research and having worked in a research and development post, my reflections on what it means to practise normality are inevitably shaped by my experience in these areas.

My conclusion is that normality is an intensely political phrase where conflict often ensues and where professional boundaries have to be negotiated. It can be a 'discomfort zone' which is a long way from a beautiful, life-affirming birth experience that leaves you in awe of a woman's courage and strength. That is where I would like normal practice to be but...

Is it normal for all women to be screened for gestational diabetes? I didn't think so until I met an obstetrician who did precisely that, based on his postgraduate research. It affected me because I was working with him as linked obstetrician for our team. We were sorting out how antenatal provision would be set up for midwifery-led care and consultant-led care. Our first meeting was amicable and we agreed to exchange research papers on the topic and meet again to work things out. I read his and returned to his office to find he hadn't read mine.

The scales slowly fell from my eyes as I realised he had no intention of reading it, now or in the future. We were to do it his way – the prior amicable meeting was a pretence. Normality for him was what was left after all the screening came back negative and teamwork, to him, meant very definitely being in charge.

Having developed and agreed a job description for a research and development midwife, the remit was clearly midwifery orientated and normality focused. But two years into the post, a senior obstetrician approached me and suggested the post be more generic, so that obstetric-related objectives could be incorporated. For example, sorting out midwifery support for multi-centre, obstetric clinical trials locally and doing a systematic review on hypertension and thrombolic disorders of pregnancy. But there were so many other midwifery priorities, all to do

with developing normal midwifery practice e.g. skill development around postures for birth, physiological third stage, water birth; auditing and increasing the uptake of the midwifery-led birthing unit; supporting a midwifery-led research project into caseload practice among many others.

In addition, my line manager would change to be the clinical director, an obstetrician. I looked for another job, which was just as well because one day, not long after, I came to work and found a job advertised for a research and development officer – its objectives were very similar to what my obstetrician colleague had previously asked me to do.

These are two examples from my past to illustrate that normal midwifery in practice is determined by structures and people, neither of which may view it as a priority. If one works where there are sympathetic obstetricians and midwifery managers, normal birth initiatives can be near the top of the agenda and normal birth practices can develop and prosper, even within a consultant unit.

But if those leading the service are not philosophically committed to the promotion of normal birth, then it needs to be taken out of centralised units and located in its own space where it is free to develop and flourish, unencumbered by medicalisation.

In regard to the relationship between research and normal birth, I believe we should all feel encouraged, as we may be on the threshold of 'something big'. The following factors are creating synergy:

- we are beginning to realise much of the research into normal physiology needs redoing in 'birth friendly' environments
- we are beginning to see a renaissance in the birth centre facility, exactly the kind of environment we need
- we are beginning to examine intuitive and embodied knowledge sources that may teach us much about what facilitates normal birth.

It is of concern that research findings do not have the influence on maternity service strategy that they should have and often decisions are politically motivated. There's nothing new in that phenomena. The history of childbirth reveals similar politically-led decisions, and challenges midwifery to be astute about our use of power and influence.

The Practising Midwife 2002; 5(7): 12

What is a 'Normal' Midwife?

The educationalist's view

Rosemarie Essay, Carol Hughes

Educational programmes shape midwifery practice. Becoming a midwife requires both education and socialisation. We use the term 'education' to refer to the formal requirements and organisation of the midwifery education programme. We use the term 'socialisation' to signify the informal process or hidden curriculum (Illich, 1973) by which the midwife acquires the shared culture of midwifery, its values, beliefs, attitudes, behaviour pattern and social identity.

One of the distinctive aspects of midwifery practice, and what makes it so special, is the potential to specialise in promoting 'normal' birth; but can we call it 'normal' now that the majority of women have some intervention in labour and birth? The truly 'normal' or 'natural' birth is now very rare (Page, 2001).

By examining midwifery education in several different settings we see how the preparation of midwives is influenced by medical and technological advances, new educational ideas, gender relation, state policies and economic and cultural changes (Davis Floyd, 1998).

Midwives, like other NHS staff, are being called upon to work in new ways that are more community-based, and to put women and their families at the centre of care (DOH, 1993; DOH, 2002; RCM, 2000). Choice, continuity and control were the focal points of the Changing Childbirth Report (DOH, 1993) and the maternity services were challenged to provide new schemes of care that were woman-centred, particularly in the area of continuity of care and carer. Many maternity services throughout the United Kingdom introduced the concepts of team midwifery and one-to-one care, but sadly many of these schemes have now been disbanded and we have seen a return to the fragmented traditional maternity care system of hospital midwives and community midwives.

Academic credentials give midwives 'cultural capital', helping them to negotiate attractive work options and to compete on an equal standing with other similar health professionals (Benoit, 1991).

Students trained in the large teaching hospitals associated with universities develop expertise in dealing with individuals of diverse sociocultural and economic backgrounds, and gain experience of a wide range of birth complications with the latest and newest medical technologies (Benoit, 1991). However, this system of training feeds into a pathological position making it almost impossible for the student to remain focused on normality. This system of care provides a backdrop of fear.

To equip the future midwife with a strong faith in themselves, in the birth process and in a woman's ability to give birth without intervention, the education programme must provide experience with a wide range of normal births. Of course, the programme must also include exposure to birth complications, but this exposure should take place against an already established background of trust in the power of women and in the normal process of birth.

Midwifery students have been prepared in many ways and there is no single best way to educate midwives. Knowledge base and socialisation of midwives are arbitrary; academic education can enhance midwives' autonomy, but it can also socialise them into accepting politically-driven models of practice which may not always be in the best interest of the women they serve, or even evidence-based.

Even when midwives are educated to adopt a woman-centred philosophy of care, they often find themselves unable to implement such models inside the technological workplace and under the medical gaze. Midwives who are trained within these institutions find it difficult to think of and treat pregnancy and birth as a normal life event.

To offer a system that provides education programmes where midwives can function in both the home and hospital on a regular basis (like other countries) would be more beneficial to developing and maintaining the focus of normality, thus benefiting the women who access the service. Education programmes must be committed to the preservation of midwifery as a crucial alternative to obstetric-led maternity care. Such developments will assist midwives to provide childbearing women with the best possible care.

The activities of a midwife are defined in the European Union Midwives Directive 80/155 EEC Article 4, (UKCC, 1998) and clearly state the variety of activities which a midwife can pursue. Likewise, there is an international accepted definition of the midwife described in the Midwives Rules and Code of Practice (UKCC, 1998). Despite these very succinct documents, midwives and the midwifery profession struggle at times to define normality and also to define the midwife's role, especially in clinical practice.

Perhaps it is time to consider that there may be two types of midwifery, 'complex' and 'normal'. Perhaps we should consider these two types of care to be as different as obstetrics and general practice? Neither is inferior or superior to the other, they are simply very different roles.

Underpinning all midwifery practices there should always be the importance of honouring and respecting the sacredness of women's bodies and the spiritual experience of pregnancy, birth and the postnatal period.

REFERENCES

Benoit C. 1989. The Professional Socialisation of Midwives; Balancing the Art and Science. Sociology of Health and Illness, 11(2), 160-8

Benoit C. 1991. Midwives in Passage: The Modernisation of Maternity Care. Memorial University of Newfoundland: ISER Press

Davis Floyd R. 1998. The Ups, Downs and Interlinkages of Nurse and Direct Entry Midwifery. Midwifery Today, 67, 118

De Vries R, Benet CER, Van Teijlingen A, Wrede S. 2001. Birth by Design. London: Routledge

DOH. 1993. Changing Childbirth. The Report of the Expert Maternity Group. London: HMSO

DOH. 2002. The NHS Plan. London: HMSO

Illich I. 1973. Deschooling Society. Harmondsworth: Penguin.

Page L. 2001. BMJ, 9(9), 742

RCM. 2000. Vision 2002. London: RCM

The Practising Midwife 2002; 5(7): 13

What is a 'Normal' Midwife?

The practitioner's view

Cathy Davis

One of the ways of practising as a 'normal' midwife, is to work in a midwife-led unit. The focus in my place of work is on the normal. I am aware that it is difficult to get a hold of the concept of what is normal, even in a midwife-led unit! However, in order to give an idea of the possibilities open to midwives, I will discuss normal childbirth within my own practice.

The Penrice midwife-led unit is situated in central Cornwall and is approximately 20 miles away from the nearest obstetric unit. In order to ensure that women have a choice of place of birth, all women in Cornwall without medical or obstetric complications, are offered home care, Penrice midwife-led care or obstetric care in Truro or Plymouth. This means that women frequently travel 40 miles or more to reach a place to give birth.

Steps to keep normality

Parent education sessions are considered to be important for preparing the woman and her birth partner in understanding the process of normal childbirth. In addition, women become familiar with the Penrice unit. For women who travel long distances or do not choose to attend parent education, there are additional days when they can visit the unit and have birth discussions with a midwife. All women are encouraged to visit in order to become familiar with the rooms.

When midwives focus on normal birth they will inevitably create surroundings which have an ambience which will support this aim. Therefore the rooms are equipped in an appropriate way, with fresh clean feminine decoration, being an important but often neglected item! In addition, a TV and music centre are provided for 'diversion therapy'. There are two birth rooms, one with a large corner bath and one with a birthing pool for labour and/or delivery.

Fetal monitoring is by auscultation with Pinnard or Doppler only. Anyone who needs CTG monitoring is considered to be high risk and is therefore transferred for obstetric care. Analgesia provided other than the pool is with TENS, Entonox and sometimes pethidine.

The unit is set in the grounds of a Community Hospital with garden areas and a beach half a mile away.

Women within the 'normal' criteria are accepted for delivery from 37 weeks' gestation onwards.

In the majority of cases the women contact the unit midwife by phone when labour begins. Discussion about the progress of early labour can often prevent unnecessary admissions if the woman feels happy and confident in her own surroundings. From the information given, a plan of action is made with the woman, depending on parity, transport needs and travelling distances. Women who live a long way from the unit usually come sooner than local women. In order to progress labour and reduce restriction to one room, women may choose to go out for a walk or home if not in established labour.

The progress of labour

Once I have admitted a woman to the unit and following palpation I discuss her birth plan. This gives her the opportunity to review any features that she wants to revise or that I need to discuss further. As there are many ways of identifying the progress of labour when a midwife is with the woman, I consider that vaginal examinations are carried out on a need-to-know basis, not 4-hourly. This will limit the procedure to 0-2 examinations. Artificial rupture of membranes is very rarely done and only after much consideration of the pros and cons for that individual woman.

As labour progresses my attendance with the woman increases. At this stage, women usually keep to their birth room and may be in the birthing pool or moving around the room, upright or crouched on the floor. I see it as my role to support her natural instincts, wherever that is. I will try to dissuade women from lying semi-prone on the bed as this does not help descent of the fetal head and can delay rotation of a fetus that is in the posterior or lateral position. However the all-fours position is often instinctively a preferred position for many women and on the bed gives less strain on the knees.

A second midwife is called to the unit for all births. This can be a good opportunity to discuss the progress of a labour if there are delays. Sharing ideas and knowledge with colleagues can help solve any minor problems that may have arisen.

When a woman reaches second stage I wait to see signs of full dilation and only VE to confirm second stage, if there are no obvious signs after a few good pushes. I do not direct pushing unless the woman requires guidance, which is rare.

Women will position themselves for second stage, if they have been moving freely in labour. Auscultation in the second stage when women are in positions other than semi-recumbent can be difficult but the Doppler has proven to be an invaluable tool. Once the baby is born the placenta will deliver physiologically when the woman has no particular preference, or managed when required.

The family are made comfortable and then I usually leave them alone for awhile. When ready, mother and baby are bathed separately or together. Breast feeding support is given when the mother is made comfortable, either immediately after birth or after moving into the postnatal room.

Most of the midwives at the Penrice midwife-led unit have attended the ALSO course, which has proven to have been an essential development in our knowledge base, for the management of obstetric emergencies. In addition, information has been cascaded to midwives still waiting to attend the course and to the healthcare assistants who work within the team.

The Practising Midwife 2002; 5(7): 14

What is a 'Normal' Midwife?

The consumer's view

Beverley A Lawrence Beech

In 1997, the Association for Improvements in the Maternity Services (AIMS) published an article questioning health professionals' perceptions of normal birth (Beech, 1997). The article was provoked by women's accounts of how they often felt abandoned in labour or were attended by midwives who gave them little support or encouragement. One mother described her attendants as 'a flock of vultures standing around and just watching'. Many women felt that the midwives' main priority was to monitor the machines and write their notes.

I became so concerned about the very few examples of un-medicalised birth that I made a point of asking the midwives to indicate what the normal birth rate was in their hospital during my talks to midwifery refresher courses. Jaws dropped when I suggested that the normal birth rate might be 40% (I did not dare suggest that in my view it barely reaches 10%) and the hands began to shoot up once I reached 70% or more. I then asked the midwives to think about the last normal birth they attended and to put their hands down if the woman had any one of the following: artificial rupture of membranes, induction or accelerated labour, a long period of electronic fetal monitoring, epidural anaesthesia or episiotomy. As I progressed through the list so the hands fell, and in the end it was not unusual for there to be only a handful of hands still raised.

Increasingly, AIMS is approached by student midwives who have almost completed their training but have yet to see a normal birth. One teaching hospital prides itself on an 80% epidural rate. How do the midwives in that hospital begin to understand the needs of a woman in normal birth when they do not see it?

Most midwives and doctors have little experience of birth outside the 'laboratory' of centralised hospital birth which does not recognise the negative effects of its routine interventions: semi-recumbent positions, continuous electronic monitoring, regular internal examinations, constantly changing attendants and instructions to hold their breath and push (see Anderson, 2002). We realised that the midwives were not unkind or sadistic, but that many of them appeared to be at a loss at what to do other than offer an epidural or pethidine.

It is an unusual woman who, expecting her first baby, carefully researches the options and tries to find out about how she can give herself the best chance of achieving a normal birth. Most of them express the view that they want a normal birth, in the misguided belief that if the professionals say they support normal birth this will be the case. Few women understand that the chances of experiencing a normal birth in a large centralised obstetric units is less than 1 in 6 (Downe, 2001); and very few antenatal classes will empower them sufficiently to deal with the policies, protocols and practices that militate against a normal birth.

Those midwives who are truly 'women-friendly' are those who accept the right of the woman to make decisions about her care and have an understanding of autonomy that the rhetoric of 'choice' does not have. It means accepting the woman's decision even when it is contrary to what the midwife considers appropriate or what the protocols dictate.

In order to support a woman who wants a normal birth the midwife provides a watchful presence, is confident in her knowledge of normality, knows when to intervene and when to stand back and silently support. It is not uncommon, however, to find that the midwives who have these skills are required to rotate through the labour ward for 're-skilling' with the objective of training them to read the electronic fetal monitors, set up epidurals and comply with the hospital protocols. Their midwifery skills honed and embellished over many years of careful observation and reflection are often ignored or denigrated as unimportant. But a midwife cannot support a woman if she does not have the skills to do so. Instead she may:

- censor information on the grounds that 'it might frighten the woman', or oppose the woman if she makes 'off the menu choices'
- be unaware of how disheartening and disempowering their choice of response can be. For example, a query about the progress of labour is not helped by saying, 'Well you are only x centimetres and you have a long way to go yet' or 'if you think that was painful just wait until your labour really gets going, would you like an epidural?'
- fail to provide support and encouragement especially when the woman is losing heart, and not know when to support and when to step back and let the woman find her own way
- be unaware of the research demonstrating that telling a woman to push once she is fully dilated can result in an exhausted woman and 'failure to progress'
- be unaware that the continuous presence of a supportive midwife can make a significant difference to the progression of the labour for those women who are re-assured by a professional attendant

- but perhaps most important of all she fails to recognise all interventions for what they are – a means of changing the course of labour that should only be suggested when it offers a better alternative to inactivity.

There is no such thing as the ideal midwife, just as there is no such thing as an 'ideal woman' – every woman and every midwife is different. Today, more than ever before, midwives have to face a constant stream of challenges. It is clear, however, that those midwives who are women-friendly and who do respect women's integrity and their rights are the midwives who are respected by women and on whom other midwives can rely for support when facing criticism from more reactionary colleagues.

While AIMS receives a steady stream of complaints about maternity care, it also receives feedback from those women who have found a supportive midwife and whose second birth was a healing experience and one that they could review with happiness. The tragedy is that too many women experience a disempowering and traumatic first birth before they search for a means to ensure that they do not have a repeat experience the second time around.

REFERENCES

Anderson T. 2002. Out of the laboratory: back to the darkened room. MIDIRS Midwifery Digest, 12, 1

Beech BAL. 1997. Normal birth – does it exist? AIMS Journal, 9(2), 4-8

Downe S, McCormick C, Beech BL. 2001. Labour interventions associated with normal birth. British Journal of Midwifery, 9(10), 602-6

The Practising Midwife 2002; 5(7): 14-15

Midwives performing instrumental deliveries

Jean Wills, Sue Deighton

Midwives have been undertaking ventouse deliveries at several units within the UK in recent years. However, the evidence on forceps verses ventouse delivery is inconclusive with no evidence to support the use of one instrument in favour of the other. This article sets out the development and implementation of a pilot training programme for midwives to undertake instrumental deliveries and fetal blood sampling. The article includes the selection criteria, supervision aspect and personal recollections of the midwife involved. The pilot has now been successfully concluded and we are awaiting validation of the 'Instrumental Delivery' module through the University of Leeds. This module will be offered to all midwives within the unit who meet the competency criteria and other interested midwives in the UK.

Traditionally, instrumental deliveries (i.e. ventouse and forceps) have been performed by doctors (Sweet, 1999). However, midwives in at least four UK maternity units have recently started performing low cavity ventouse deliveries (Parslow, 1997; Mulholland, 1997). Some midwives have welcomed this opportunity to extend their scope of professional practice, encouraged by the recent government report, 'Making a Difference' (Department of Health, 1999).

With the introduction of the Calman Report (1993) and the European Working Time Directive (1998) which reduced junior doctors' hours, a gap was created within clinical obstetric cover, giving rise to the question, who will fill that gap and how will it be achieved? The planning and implementation of change in the delivery of care must take into account past events, available evidence and include a proposal for resourcing the planned change.

Preparation for the new policy

In Leeds, senior medical and midwifery staff debated how women could continue to receive high quality care, and following much discussion it was decided that midwives should be trained to perform both ventouse and Neville Barnes forceps deliveries, thereby enabling the best possible evidence-based care to be offered. Several articles have already been published recording midwives' personal experiences at becoming ventouse practitioners (Parslow, 1997; Charles, 1999), but none on forceps practitioners or how their role had been achieved.

On reviewing the literature, many articles were found relating to the relative advantages of the use of ventouse or forceps (Vacca et al, 1993). A recent review of the randomised trials suggested that ventouse deliveries resulted in significantly less maternal trauma than forceps deliveries, but carried an increased risk of neonatal cephalhaematoma and retinal haemorrhage (Johanson & Memon, 2000). However, Johanson et al (1999) in a five-year follow up trial concluded that 'there is no evidence to suggest that at five years after delivery use of either the ventouse or forceps has specific maternal or child benefits or side effects'.

The Supervisor of Midwives set up a working group to plan and monitor the way forward. This group comprised a Consultant Obstetrician, the Head of Midwifery, the Supervisor of Midwives and the Delivery Suite Team Leader. The findings of the literature review, along with the evidence from two midwifery units where midwives were already performing ventouse deliveries, was brought to the working group.

The group set strict guidelines for midwives performing instrumental deliveries and fetal blood sampling, which were presented to the Obstetric and Gynaecology Committee. Following acceptance these were included in the Delivery Suite Guidelines. A training programme was devised which included a comprehensive list of clinical competencies and performance indicators as well as defining the training required and the role of the trainers/mentors. Aims were

Box 1.7.1 Midwives instrumental practitioners competencies for training

Effective Registration on Part 10 of the UKCC Professional Register
Engaged in midwifery practice for a minimum of three years (full-time) within the previous five-year period, with at least two years on delivery suite
Evidence to support the ability to perform perineal suturing, intravenous cannulation and CTG interpretation
Minimum of 30 appropriate credits at Level 2
Access to clinical experience on delivery suite for the duration of the module, 'Instrumental Delivery'

set and the relevant method of recording and assessing progress agreed (Phillips & Bharj, 1996).

Only midwives with recent delivery suite experience of two years or more and who had already attained competencies in cannulation, suturing and CTG interpretation would be considered for training. The midwives would be required to keep a reflective diary of their experiences and a record of deliveries undertaken (a minimum of 10 supervised deliveries with each instrument and 6 fetal blood samples was required before a midwife could be formally assessed for competency). Once a midwife is deemed competent, her skills will be assessed annually by a consultant obstetrician and a Supervisor of Midwives.

The Lead Clinician on the delivery suite gave the training programme his support and ensured that all the Specialist Registrars and consultants were prepared to train midwives.

An audit of each delivery was to be completed by an independent professional on the day following delivery.

This is to assess the woman's feelings on information giving, her understanding of the information, type and efficiency of analgesia, who performed the delivery and any cause for concern.

The flow chart shown in Figure 1.7.1 demonstrates how supervision was pivotal to the implementation and professional collaboration necessary to drive forward this new clinical midwifery initiative.

Personal experience

I undertook two modules at Bradford University at Masters level exploring and offering critical analysis on the background of midwife ventouse practitioners. I also attended a study day of ventouse deliveries, which focused on the practical element of performing a delivery. I was disturbed to discover that a large proportion of the audience (Senior House Officers and Registrars) openly admitted that they had no idea how, or where, to attach the ventouse cup correctly, or perform a ventouse delivery.

I also received formal one-to-one tuition from a consultant on the delivery suite. I revised the anatomy and physiology of the pelvis, fetal skull and respiratory and metabolic acidosis in the fetus. We also discussed the advantages and disadvantages of fetal blood sampling and instrumental deliveries, the complications that might arise for both woman and baby, and when to 'bail out' during instrumental deliveries. Also considered were risk management issues, psychological implications, information giving, informed consent and ethical issues. Finally, practical application of both the

Figure 1.7.1 Midwife instrumental practitioners

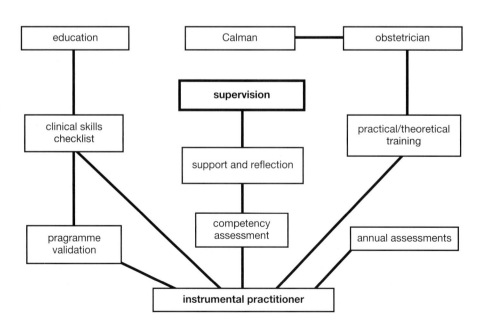

Box 1.7.3 Role of the Supervisor of Midwives in instrumental deliveries

Role

Facilitate safe, evidence-based practice and enhance continuity of care for women.

Support midwives through the training and practice.

Supervisor's Input

Multidisciplinary working

Research knowledge of the subject

Communication and dissemination of information to all stakeholders

Defining safe parameters of practice

Development of evidence-based guidelines

Competency assessment following training

Validation of training programme

Clinical audit for clinical governance

Support for midwives

Box 1.7.4 Criteria for instrumental delivery by midwives

Indications

Maternal exhaustion

Failure to progress in 2nd stage of labour

Fetal distress (when the midwife is competent)

Criteria

Inform Registrar on duty

Term pregnancy (37 weeks and over)

Singleton

Cephalic presentation 0-1fifth palpable abdominally

Vertex at least 1cm below the ischial spines, occipital anterior position

No asynclitism

Cervical os fully dilated

Membranes ruptured

Adequate analgesia

Neville Barnes forceps and ventouse on a demonstration torso was performed.

The Local Supervising Authority Officer was informed, and supported this initiative as an expansion of the midwives' scope of practice. The Trust will be issuing vicarious liability for midwife instrumental practitioners.

As this was a new area of clinical midwifery practice at Leeds, my Supervisor of Midwives was (and still is) my main source of guidance and support during my training. She ensured that the set criteria, guidelines and standards were being adhered to and that all documentation was completed correctly. I had regular meetings with my Supervisor and we both found that my reflective journal helped to generate in-depth discussions on practice issues and tighten up the programme (e.g. the guidelines did not specify the gestational age at which the midwife could perform an instrumental delivery).

The proactive role and ongoing support of the Supervisor of Midwives in the development and implementation of the pilot programme played a crucial part in the successful progress of my training.

During my first three deliveries I was instructed in the use of forceps. The consultant checked the position of the fetal head, and that each blade was applied and positioned correctly. She also performed the episiotomy, until I became more familiar with the timing of the episiotomy when performing a forceps delivery.

None of my initial training and practice on a demonstration torso could have prepared me for that first initial traction on the forceps. It took a lot of encouragement from the consultant to give me the confidence to continue. I was very apprehensive whilst performing the first few deliveries and felt quite clumsy with the instrument. Initially I also had difficulty in applying the forceps blades correctly and I didn't seem to have enough hands to perform the episiotomy, support the baby's head and remove the blades at the same time.

When I was feeling confident with the application and technique required to perform a forceps delivery I was instructed in the application of the ventouse cup and technique required for a ventouse delivery. The Leeds Teaching Hospitals Trust use the 'Kiwi Omnicup', a small hand held device that looks a lot less threatening to the women.

The consultant closely supervised the application of the cup as it is extremely important to place the centre of the cup over the flexion point on the fetal skull. This point is found 3cm anterior of the posterior fontanelle in the midline (Vacca, 1999).

By my eighth delivery with each instrument I was beginning to feel fairly confident. I was now performing deliveries on my own with the consultant observing. During my ninth delivery I had some difficulty applying the forceps blades and therefore removed them to check the position of the fetal head. Eventually I was happy that the forceps were positioned correctly. I applied steady downward traction but this appeared to be ineffective. I waited for the next contraction and again I felt there had been no movement of the baby. At this point I asked the consultant to take over the delivery. The baby was delivered successfully by forceps, but was a large baby and required more expertise than I had acquired at that time. It is of paramount importance to be aware of one's own limitations.

By my tenth delivery with both instruments I felt confident enough to perform a forceps or ventouse delivery within the guidelines on my own. The consultant and Supervisor were present to formally assess my skills. The deliveries went well and I was passed as competent to perform both ventouse and forceps deliveries within the set criteria. I was also formally assessed and passed as competent with fetal blood sampling following six successful procedures.

Conclusion

Whilst waiting for vicarious liability to be formally agreed I am continuing to perform fetal blood samples, forceps and ventouse deliveries under supervision, increasing my skills and expertise.

The Head of Midwifery Studies at Leeds University is awaiting validation of a stand alone Level 3/Masters module, 'Instrumental Deliveries' to allow midwives within the UK to extend their practice. This initiative has generated an extremely encouraging and positive response from both the women and practitioners alike. The most rewarding part for me is that the women perceive they have had a normal delivery as it is the midwife who has been there to help them.

REFERENCES

Charles C. 1999. How it feels to be a midwife ventouse practitioner. BJM, 7, 380-2

Department of Health. 1993. Hospital Doctors: Training for the Future. London: HMSO

Department of Health. 1998. European Working Time Directive. London: HMSO

Department of Health. 1999. Making a Difference. London: HMSO

Johanson R, Heycock E, Carter J et al. 1999. Maternal and Child Health after assisted vaginal delivery: five year follow up of a randomised control study comparing forceps with ventouse. BJOG, 106(6), 544-9

Johanson R and Memon B. 2000. Vacuum extraction verses forceps for assisted vaginal delivery (Cochrane Review). In The Cochrane Library, Issue 1. Oxford: Update Software

Mulholland L. 1997. Midwife Ventouse Practitioners. BJM, 5, 255

Parslow L. 1997. A Midwife Ventouse Practitioner. Midwives, 110, 165-6

Phillips M, Bharj K. 1996. Developing a tool for the assessment of clinical learning. BJM, 4, 471-4

Sweet B. 1999. Mayes Midwifery – Textbook for Midwives (12th ed). London: Balliere Tindall

Vacca A, Grant A, Wyatt G, Chalmers I. 1993. Portmouth operative delivery trial: A comparison of vacuum extraction and forceps delivery. BJOG, 96, 537-44

Vacca A. 1999. Handbook of Vacuum Extraction in Obstetric Practice. Brisbane: Vacca Research

The Practising Midwife 2002; 5(7): 22-25

A critical ethnographic approach to facilitating cultural shift in midwifery

Deborah Hughes, Ruth Deery, Alison Lovatt

Objective: to improve understanding of local midwifery morale, inform development and reorganisation of a maternity unit, and enhance midwifery involvement in strategic planning.

Participants: a randomised stratified sample of 20 midwives working in a UK National Health Service (NHS) hospital and its surrounding community area.

Method: within a critical ethnographic framework, focus groups were tape-recorded and transcribed, and analysed using a thematic content analysis approach.

Findings: key areas affecting midwifery morale were identified, in particular staffing levels, working relationships and organisational issues. One year later, despite many changes having taken place, midwifery morale was still low but participants were more politically analytical of, and actively involved in changing their situation. The findings of the study indicate that there are complex and long-standing cultural inhibitions to the effective development of midwifery care but, if these are made explicit through a planned collaborative process, such as in this study, a process of cultural shift can be seen to begin.

Implications for practice: focus groups can be a useful tool in moving midwifery culture forward within a local context.

Introduction

The publication of 'A Consultation on a Strategy for Nursing Midwifery and Health Visiting' (NHS Executive 1998) which later became 'Making a Difference' (DoH 1999) represented a shift in thinking in England regarding the roles of nurses and midwives. These two documents put the case for clinically-based staff influencing and participating in strategic planning and policy making. However, both documents minimise the cultural and organisational barriers to effecting these proposals in the current UK National Health Service (NHS). Therefore the authors decided to undertake a collaborative study with midwives in a local NHS setting to identify both clinical midwives' vision for the development of their service and the barriers they currently experienced in terms of making their voices heard within the NHS organisation.

NHS strategic planning has rarely been informed by the formal contributions of clinically-based midwives for a wide variety of historical and organisational reasons (Kent 2000). This has traditionally led the process to be management-led with staff sometimes invited to comment on proposals already formulated. The effects of this are two-fold; firstly, there is a lack of expertise regarding strategic planning of maternity care policies amongst an otherwise highly skilled workforce; secondly, the lived experience and practical understanding and insight of that workforce has been underused as a resource at a strategic level.

'The New NHS: Modern, Dependable' (DoH 1997), made it clear that the Department of Health (DoH) wished to see much greater involvement of frontline midwifery and nursing staff in policy development and planning processes. The publication of 'Making a Difference' (DoH 1999) outlines how and why the government proposes to achieve this cultural and organisational shift but does not appear to give due recognition to the long standing and deeply entrenched cultural and organisational barriers to achieving this (Kirkham 1999).

Hunt and Symonds (1995) discuss how midwifery, as a primarily female profession operating in the private sphere, has been culturally excluded from 'the exercising of authority' (p. 35) which restricts its influence in the masculinised, public world of health service management. Hunt and Symonds (1995) argue that whilst midwives might exercise power and authority within the smaller and more private scenarios of their daily work 'the exercising of power and authority outside this sphere' (p. 33) is problematic. Kent (2000) describes how 'patriarchal relations are constituted in the workplace through strategies of exclusion and segregation' (p. 81). Gender and class inequalities continue to exclude the vast majority of workers in the caring professions from strategic planning and policy making. In a paper exploring the culture of midwifery in the UK NHS, Kirkham (1999) draws on the theory of oppressed groups and analyses how powerful forces combine to impede the expression and enactment of midwives' visions and the negative effects this can have, and notes that:

Midwifery insights were muted or denied with damaging effects for those who thereby rejected value in their own traditions and identity (p. 773).

Rather than being coincidental to health service culture, the forces outlined above are in fact key organising factors in the NHS determining its divisions of labour, its career patterns and its pay and management structures. 'Making a Difference' (DoH 1999) underestimates the extent to which health service structures are predicated upon these inequalities and the difficulties that this poses for its stated aim of increasing nursing and midwifery influence.

At the same time that these policy developments were taking place nationally there were other issues that needed addressing in the local Trust maternity service. There was a recognised lowering of morale amongst midwifery staff during 1997 and 1998. Secondly a planned introduction of Labour/Delivery/Recovery/Postnatal (LDRP) rooms to replace the traditional ward layout of the maternity unit was announced. Following discussion between the authors, it was agreed that an evidence-based approach that addressed these various national and local issues should be attempted.

Aim of the study

The aim of this study was therefore to inform local developments in maternity care and enhance midwifery involvement in strategic planning, through better understanding of the culture of midwifery locally, particularly midwifery morale.

Methodology

The investigation of ideas and feelings requires a qualitative research design (Hammersley & Atkinson 1995, Morse & Field 1996). As the inquiry would focus on important cultural aspects of the maternity service, namely current midwifery morale and the organisational and cultural impediments to hearing midwives' voices, the authors decided that an ethnographical approach best suited the study. Ethnography is the study of culture and can focus, for example, on the study of institutions or a professional group, both of which are cultural phenomena (Morse & Field 1996, Grbich 1999).

Ethnography can itself be sub-divided into various approaches according to research theorists (Hammersley & Atkinson 1995), and critical ethnography best describes the method employed in this project. Critical ethnography focuses on power and how it is distributed within a cultural setting (Grbich 1999) and is based on the following assumptions:

False consciousness exists among people regarding the hierarchies of power. Society is in a state of crisis and people are dissatisfied. Society is inequitably structured and dominated by powerful hegemonic practices that create and maintain the continuance of a particular world view (Grbich 1999, p. 159).

In this, critical ethnography shares much in common with both feminist ethnography and action research (Jordan & Yeomans 1995, Maguire 2001), but a discussion of the similarities and differences of the three approaches is beyond the scope of this paper. The purpose of critical ethnography is to understand the origins of the power structures that exist within institutions or social groups. The aim of critical ethnographic research is to 'enhance collective action, improve societies, and foster the emancipation and empowerment of individuals and groups' (Grbich 1999, p. 160). In terms of the aims of understanding and addressing issues of low morale within the context of the changes proposed in 'Making a Difference' (DoH 1999) this approach is apt. It allows for the researchers to become actively involved in the critical analysis of the cultural hegemony of the maternity unit and its working relationships.

Methods

Within this broader critical ethnographic approach, a data collecting method needed to be chosen. Due to the, then, imminent relocation of the maternity unit, there were time limits on the project as well as considerations relating to staffing difficulties. Focus groups therefore provided time-efficient means of gathering information from a number of people (Morse & Field 1996, Grbich 1999). They are also a rich source of views on cultural behaviour and enable the degree of consensus on a topic to emerge (Morse & Field 1996, Grbich 1999). Focus groups are a pertinent method for qualitative data collection on midwifery views and working practices as they mirror the social organisation of midwifery practice that is dependent on a team approach and verbal communication. The literature on focus groups describes the facilitation of these as more participative than in many other methods of data collection (Twinn 2000).

Two of the authors undertook the facilitation of the initial focus groups during September and October 1998, and follow-up focus groups one year later in autumn 1999. The sessions were tape recorded and later transcribed. In addition detailed notes were made during the focus group sessions by one of the facilitators. Whilst there was a list of questions (see Figs. 1.8.1 and 1.8.2) to be explored it is necessary to recognise that these needed to be supplemented by the facilitators in order to maximise response and insight and to move discussion from the general to the specific (Hammersley & Atkinson 1995, Grbich 1999).

The reactions of the facilitators themselves to the emerging data can influence what they throw into the discussion in terms of probing questions or ideas. However, with reflexivity, this can lead to the enrichment rather than the undermining of the data collected (Hammersley & Atkinson 1995). By reflexivity the authors mean the researchers' active engagement with their own self-awareness to identify the impact of their personal values and positions on the research process and the data collected (Reed 1995). Grbich (1999) describes how in critical ethnography 'the researcher's position is one of active involvement in the critical, theoretical analysis of inscribed power' (p. 160). Post focus group reflective meetings enabled the researchers to discuss their experiences and make field notes. In addition it is important to remember that this influence is not one way and the participants are not passive recipients of the facilitator's viewpoint. Grbich (1999) points out that the group itself strengthens the reliability of the data 'because of the inbuilt checks and balances of a variety of viewpoints' (p. 114).

Therefore focus groups as a method of data collection accord well with the chosen paradigm of critical ethnography in which 'the researcher's position is one of active involvement in the critical, theoretical analysis of inscribed power' (Grbich 1999, p. 160). In this instance, the facilitator's probing questioning was consciously seeking out participants' experiences and feelings about their work culture and the power relationships operating in it. In addition, the researchers were also able to directly observe something of these phenomena within the focus group dynamics. This was important to the aim of the study, of gaining insight into the midwives' lived experience and the issue of low morale. Wilkinson (1999)

Box 1.8.1 The Interview Schedule (first round of focus groups)

1	What is it like being a midwife in this organisation?
2	What makes you feel positive about the service you offer?
3	What disappoints you about being a midwife in this organisation?
4	What difficulties do you encounter that prevent you from being the sort of midwife you want to be? [Supplementary probing questions to 1–4 to establish current feelings about the hospital units.]
5	Describe your ideal maternity service.
6	What changes would you like to see to maternity care locally? [Supplementary probing question to 6 to seek ideas on how the new unit should be structured and staffed.]
7	What sort of education do you need to support this?
8	What would you like to see happen as a priority?

Box 1.8.2 The Interview Schedule (follow up focus groups)

1	What were your reactions to the report of last year's focus groups?
2	What was it like to participate in the groups?
3	Reading through the report, what struck you as having changed for the better about being a midwife in this organisation?
4	What is the same or even worse?
5	What do you think are the immediate priorities?
6	What should the service look like in two to three years?

likens the focus group experience to consciousness raising, which has been recognised as a vital precursor to cultural shift. The focus group can be a method that fits the critical ethnography paradigm because: [Focus] group work can help individuals to develop a perspective which transcends their individual context and thus may transform 'personal troubles' into 'public issues' (Kitzinger & Barbour 1999, p. 19).

This reinforces the conscious raising potential of the critical ethnographic approach within current midwifery culture.

The sample

A sample of 30 midwives was randomly selected from the total population of local midwives. The sample was stratified to reflect the number of midwives employed on each grade (salary points) and the percentage of full- and part-time midwives. Through a process of randomisation, involving envelopes containing all the names of midwives employed on each grade, 10 midwives were allocated to each of the three focus groups, again in a stratified way to reflect the staffing make-up of the unit. The number 10 was chosen as the upper limit of participants for an effective focus group (Morse and Field 1996) and time constraints allowed for three such groups hence the total sample size. It was agreed not to facilitate any of the groups with fewer than four participants, as this may not be authentic in terms of data obtained (Green & Hart 1999). Twenty of the 30 randomised midwives attended one or both sessions to which they were invited, this 20 being 21% of the total local population of midwives.

The study was commissioned by the hospital management and was supported by the University in terms of researcher time and resources. All participants were invited to attend by letter from the Head of Midwifery and were informed that focus group attendance would be counted as part of the working week. Ground rules were established within each group to emphasise the collaborative, anonymous and democratic nature of the focus groups (Kitzinger & Barbour 1999).

Data collection and analysis

Three focus groups were held, each meeting on three occasions. The first two meetings of each group were held in the autumn of 1998 with a third meeting for each held in autumn 1999 (Deery et al. 1999). The first meeting of each group took two hours and focused on data collection in accordance with the aims of the study. The second meeting was concerned with confirming the data. The third meeting, held one year later, sought to investigate what, if any cultural shift had occurred and whether the midwives felt that the data collected the year previously had influenced the development of the service in terms of practice development, strategic change and midwifery morale. Of the 20 participants who attended the focus group meetings in autumn 1998, 12 accepted the invitation to attend these follow up sessions one year later. Two focus groups met on one occasion each, in November 1999. The researchers were disappointed that the response rate to the 1999 follow-up groups was not higher; however, this reflected the fact that there had been movement of the sample due to maternity leave and some participants leaving their jobs.

Semi-structured interview schedules were developed to address the aims of the project (Figs. 1.8.1 and 1.8.2). The questions in Fig. 1.8.1 were put to all three focus groups in the first of the three sessions held with each. These first sessions with each group involved a structured discussion on midwives' current feelings about their working lives and their vision for the future of the maternity service.

The second session with each group was held three weeks after the first, following the distribution of the initial analysis of those first sessions to all participants. The purpose of the second session was to assess the resonance and strength of the data and its thematic analysis (Reed & Biott 1995). This was done by inviting feedback and comments from participants and asking

Box 1.8.3 Categorical and thematic headings identified

Categories	Themes
Staffing levels and skill mix	Staffing levels Grading Hospital maternity care Community maternity care Midwifery skills
Organisational issues	Communication Working overtime Change Working effectively Stress, morale and job satisfaction Pay Midwives' roles and boundaries Organisation of the hospital unit Organisation of the community service
Working relationships	Relationships with clients Relationships with each other Relationships with medical staff Relationships with managers
The working environment	The hospital environment The community environment
Educational needs of midwives	Current education Educational priorities

them to agree any alterations, deletions or additions. Each group reached a consensus about what should go forward into the report. Following this process, the data from the three groups were merged into one document and distributed to all participants asking them to read through it and comment on how reliably it reflected their experiences and vision as expressed during the focus groups. Feedback confirmed that the data presented were a true and accurate reflection of everything that had been said in the groups. There were also many statements made about how closely the data from all three groups echoed each other. The midwives chose the order of the themes in the final report. This collective process of confirming the data attempted to decrease hierarchical relationships and increase collaborative relationships between the researchers and the participants in keeping with the aims and rationale of the study and its chosen methodology (Ely et al. 1991, Reed & Biott 1995).

Thematic content analysis (Burnard 1991) took place following the first focus group meetings and emergent themes were coded and then clustered into categories and sub categories, until all data were exhausted (Twinn 2000). Following transcription, the two group facilitators looked at the responses to each question and identified the major themes. These were staffing levels and skill mix, organisational issues, working relationships, working environment and educational needs. The facilitators then went through each transcript and coded the data according to the five main themes identified (Fig.1.8.3). These themes were then further sub divided into categories, for example 'organisational issues' was sub-grouped into nine categories. Thematic analysis was considered complete when all data were categorised into these sub-groups.

The follow up focus groups (Deery et al. 2000), one year later, also had a semi structured interview schedule (see Fig.1.8.2) which invited participants not only to review their working situations but also to comment on their experiences of participating in the earlier focus groups.

Ethical issues

Confidentiality and anonymity were the key ethical considerations identified. It was emphasised by the researchers to the participating midwives that confidentiality was important but could only be limited due to the nature of the project, that is, what the group said would be written up and presented in other forums. The participants were also asked not to discuss what had gone on in the focus groups with anyone other than members of their own focus group. Local Research Ethics Committee approval was granted during the planning stages.

The midwives were reassured that all data would be anonymised so that it could not be traced back to any individual or indeed any specific focus group. The transcripts of each first session were distributed to all participants of the relevant group in a sealed envelope marked 'private and confidential' and the midwives were asked their permission for the content of the transcript to be included in the final report. Some deletions of material that was felt to be too personalised or recognisable were made. Conflating the data collected from the three focus groups meant that nothing could be attributed to, or traced back to any single group. It was only after this process had been completed that the report was distributed outside the focus group participants, including to the Head of Midwifery. This same process was followed one year later for the follow up focus groups.

The major ethical dilemma was that the researchers, in the first instance, found the negative nature of the data that emerged from the groups overwhelming. Whilst this had been foreseen to some extent it had been hoped that this would be counter balanced by more positive views and opinions in the midwives' vision for the future. However, despite probing by the facilitator, more positive views were not forthcoming. Further discussion therefore took place on how to ensure that the data were viewed and dealt with constructively within the organisation. These concerns were largely dissipated by the collaborative nature of the project, the commitment of the midwifery manager and the more positive data which emerged a year later in the follow up focus groups.

Findings

A summary of the key findings of the initial focus groups is presented below and represents the dominant themes that emerged.

Staffing levels and skills mix

All three focus groups unanimously agreed and talked at length about inadequate staffing levels and talked a lot about how these had deteriorated during the course of their working lives:

We've all been fools to ourselves. We've accepted now that, if it's busy, you don't have a break, you just carry on working. (Focus group B)

Staffing problems were described as 'the biggest bugbear' with midwifery establishment levels being derided as woefully inadequate given the changing working practices of midwives and the increasing medicalisation of pregnancy and birth:

I'm not the midwife I want to be because of lack of time... we seem to be losing something somewhere. (Focus group C)

A national reorganisation of nursing and midwifery career structures known as 'clinical grading' (Demilew 1996) was viewed as 'the worst thing that ever happened' with participants expressing resentment at a lack of recognition of their ever extending role:

We've taken on more and more, we've got an extended role and it's being extended all the time and we just have to do it. (Focus group B)

Alongside this many midwives talked about the barriers to promotion and career development, such as on-calls and the scarcity of promotion opportunities. It became apparent that in addition to the clinical grading criteria there had developed internal unit criteria for promotion to a higher grade, examples being a requirement to be on call or to scrub for Caesarean sections for promotion:

A clear career structure for midwives would come into it [vision for the future] with some guarantee that when they've worked hard there is a good chance of promotion. (Focus group A)

Hospital maternity care was felt to have steadily deteriorated due to workload and an all pervasive climate of risk management. Alongside this, the culture of midwifery was also felt to be less friendly and supportive than it had been previously, with midwives expressing a desire for 'a bit of joviality but you just don't get that any more... there aren't many smiles around'.

Whilst midwives who worked in the community were more positive about their working lives the issue of workload was also prominent here:

I can't envisage how to do anything more, as we can't do what we're doing now... two and a half people are going to be doing the work of five. (Focus group A)

It was felt that the rising expectations and expressed needs of women had increased the workload but that this had not been adequately recognised with regard to staffing levels.

Organisational issues

Participants experienced a wide range of problems relating to the organisational culture, structure and policies of their employing organisation. It is unlikely that these are unique or unusual. Many of these problems relate to deficiencies in communication, for example, the imposition of policies without consultation was thought by the midwives to be due to the mistaken belief that staff 'do not need to know'.

An example given related to the organisation's plans for the future of the maternity services in this and a neighbouring area:

Lack of information is almost total. I found out more by reading [the local paper] or even from watching the [regional TV news] than I have from the hospital. (Focus group C)

The midwives felt disadvantaged by various policies and practices particularly in terms of gender and their roles as carers. Restrictions on claiming overtime were seen as discriminatory:

It wouldn't happen in industry. It's because we're women. (Focus group A)

Both hospital and community midwives felt that their work seriously affected the quality of their home lives. It was seen as becoming increasingly impossible to combine midwifery and motherhood:

Every night that I am working next week, I won't see my children at bedtime because every one is a late shift. (Focus group B)

This was compounded by a continual pressure to work extra shifts which left midwives often feeling bullied by comments such as:

Oh I'll remember this when it comes to the half-term requests. (Focus group A)

Participants were keen to see maternity service develop in more woman-centred ways but there were a number of tensions around this. The hospital had recently introduced midwifery-led care and, whilst this was generally seen as a positive development, high client expectations were potentially threatening:

They want that intimate one-to-one... it's psychologically draining... they want you there all the time... it's just as stressful as some of the extreme situations on the labour ward. (Focus group B)

However, midwives wanted to provide more continuity of care and influence service development if they had the resources and opportunities to do so:

We can provide holistic care, we are equipped and we can do it if we have the time. We know what happens, we know about the inequality... we should be a voice to be heard... we are at ground root level and we know the problems that there are... we should all be collaborating together and working together... there may be a chance, for once, that we can improve and make some changes. (Focus group C)

The midwives' inability to develop care and to give care in the way that they aspired to was reported to be due to lack of time. Reasons for this were diverse including ever-increasing amounts of paper work, increasing client expectations, early transfer of postnatal women and the rising Caesarean section rate. Morale was unanimously perceived to be low as a result and there was some evidence of burnout:

Everyone's depressive really. People don't want to come to work and take days sick. The more apathetic everyone gets, the worse it is going to get. Just when you think morale can't get worse it does. Everyone is talking about leaving. (Focus group B)

Working relationships

Working relationships provide the core of both the positive and the negative aspects of midwives' working lives and are central to their experience of midwifery. Relationships with clients were identified as particularly rewarding, as were their relationships with each other, although they felt that they did not support each other enough. However, not all midwifery relationships were seen as positive:

We've all been with the midwives from hell and hoped they would go, and things get better. (Focus group C)

It was, however, relationships with doctors and managers which posed the greatest problems for participants:

I mean, the doctors close shop if anything does go wrong, and they always say the onus is on the midwife. (Focus group A)

In particular, midwives talked about a culture of blame compounded by a lack of support at times of crisis:

If something goes wrong, how many people are going to jump on your back? Everybody. (Focus group B)

One year on . . . the follow up focus groups

During the year between the second and third meetings, one of the authors, as Head of Midwifery, made a number of management interventions based on the data that emerged from the first round of focus group meetings. More senior posts were created and skill mix improved, a midwifery forum was inaugurated to give midwives more opportunity to put forward ideas formally, the National Maternity Record was introduced and the leadership of one of the wards was strengthened. In addition, the participating midwives sought a meeting with doctors at which they raised a number of the issues identified during the focus group sessions.

Participants were generally positive about having taken part in the focus groups a year earlier:

The opportunity to say things and get it off my chest. It felt a bit easier because we knew the people who were in the group that we hadn't had a lot of contact with were saying exactly the same thing. (Focus group D)

Some evidence of a cultural shift began to emerge. The midwives were using more political terms and describing their working situation in terms of being oppressive rather than simply unfortunate. This reflects what Weitz (1987) found in her study of English midwives, which compared politically active midwives with those who accepted the status quo. The focus group midwives were demonstrating more of the characteristics that Weitz (1987) identified with 'radical' midwives, namely awareness of power relationships and their impact on working lives. This development may represent the beginnings of a cultural shift:

I think it [focus group participation] is better than a course, it made me really look at things. I was having a major dilemma about talking about key politics within my team, so I read an awful lot of books and I'm trying to empower my colleagues. (Focus group E)

This was most clearly expressed when participants talked about their relationships with doctors, which remained problematic:

We've got the classical gender domination... medics are still largely male dominated and they wanted to amalgamate, we are largely female dominated, we want to keep the two units going, guess who won? (Focus group E)

...we ought to say to consultants 'as a human being I can't accept that behaviour from my five year old never mind a grown adult'. They don't seem to accept that they can learn from us as much as we can learn from them...(Focus group D)

However, the participants had also been very disturbed by what had emerged during the focus group sessions and whether any change would result:

It scared me that it was so clear and that's really how everybody felt. I thought it was really frightening that it's got so bad, it really worried me because it was so negative. (Focus group E)

When asked for an overall assessment of how things had changed over the intervening year, the midwives listed a number of changes for the better. Examples given included an increase in promotions, progress towards a higher minimum clinical grade for midwives, the organisation of the antenatal/postnatal ward, communication with doctors and the new maternity records:

As a result of that we did eventually have a meeting with the consultants... that went down very well and the consultants did say that they were glad that we had approached them... we should really have more of the meetings. (Focus group D)

Most things, however, were felt not to have changed or not to have changed significantly. The midwives had a lot to say about some of these issues, the main one being, once again, staffing levels and the pressure they felt to work extra shifts and the dilemmas this posed for them as mothers and carers:

It is unfair and I particularly remember one quote that I read time and time out of there, 'what's it going to take?'... what's going to have to go wrong before they, whoever they are, whoever makes the decisions, realise that no we can't cope, we can't do this anymore. (Focus group E)

I was on maternity leave... I was sat breastfeeding my baby and they said 'can you come to work?' I said 'when?' they said 'tonight' and they wanted me to work an hour later. It's that bad. (Focus group D)

Participating midwives were acutely aware of continuing problems around communication and support and had experienced mixed success in addressing these during the year. They talked about some improvements but made many comments regarding the anxieties they continued to experience. They suggested that a regular peer support group, 'a bit like a focus group', would be beneficial to talk issues through and to support each other. This accords with a growing amount of evidence of midwives' needs for better supportive structures in clinical practice (Deery 1999, Kirkham & Stapleton 2000):

There's no support there, the mental support is there, people say 'yes, brilliant idea', but the practical support isn't there because one person goes off sick and the whole system falls apart. (Focus group E)

It was apparent that some midwives were having difficulty in adapting to a change of culture in which management structures had been flattened and midwives were being given more opportunity to make changes themselves:

If you've got something that you want to be done she [the midwifery manager] throws the ball back at you and says 'well go ahead and do it, or go and approach your team leader' and then it is up to us to sort it out from there. (Focus group D)

Discussion

This discussion will focus on the study as a whole, that is its aim and methodological approach, as well as the data and findings. The aim of the study was met with the exception of detailed midwifery contribution to strategic planning, inasmuch as an overall vision for the future was not clearly articulated. Despite careful but consistent probing by the researchers, the midwives were not able to articulate any clear vision for future service development during the focus group sessions. This closely parallels Kirkham's (1999) findings about the muting of midwives and the difficulties they encounter in expressing or achieving change. Kirkham (1999) also discusses the negative effects that a long subservience to doctors and other forms of perceived authority has on the ability of midwives to move beyond the status quo and articulate their hopes and expectations. Despite the new midwifery manager's commitment to change it was obvious that the prevailing culture was inhibiting midwives from being able to capitalise on this. The pace and nature of change in the local maternity service was therefore going to have to take the above factors into account. The oppressive culture of midwifery (Stapleton et al. 1998) may not only inhibit change locally but may also explain some of the difficulties in realising change broadly, such as that envisaged in 'Changing Childbirth' (DoH 1993) and 'Making a Difference' (DoH 1999).

The aims of critical ethnography in terms of consciousness raising and empowerment were realised to some extent. In the 1999 follow up focus groups, the midwives articulated their situation in more clearly political terms, for example, participants were much more critical about the behaviour of doctors and described medical behaviour much more in terms of power and gender than they had done previously. Whilst their attempts to improve communication and support structures had been of limited success, they nonetheless were more acutely aware of their needs in this area and remained proactive around these issues. The midwives made a number of links between their experience of participating in the focus groups and their current attempts to make changes. In the follow-up focus groups the midwives talked about concepts such as empowerment and exchange of ideas, which they had not done a year earlier.

The overwhelmingly negative tone of the data obtained from the first focus groups in 1998 posed problems for all three authors. Firstly, the experiences and culture described by the midwives were both saddening and angering. Whilst the authors' long experience of midwifery told them that these findings were not uncommon, the intensity of the data-collecting process and the emotions expressed by the midwives were deeply upsetting and frustrating. Their stories were very much part of our own histories and, whilst we are now teachers, researchers and managers, as midwives and as women, we are essentially still oppressed by the same forces that oppress them, albeit in different ways. Oakley (1981) describes the intense emotions that can be generated in interviewers when enquiring into experiences that have personal resonance. The two interviewers felt that the midwives had projected some of their emotional distress onto them and it was difficult to discharge the feelings this gave rise to appropriately. This was dealt with through a process of reflexivity whereby both researchers were able to take a more dispassionate view of the data. This involved not only discussion with each other but also with other researchers not involved in the project.

The initial reaction of the Head of Midwifery was one of disappointment and frustration in terms of the midwives' difficulty in expressing a clear vision for the future of the maternity services and their many criticisms of the then current service. Midwifery managers involved in these types of study, where morale is known to be low, need to recognise and work with the emerging themes and not feel despondent. There needs to be a genuine managerial commitment to continuing the process and not to regard listening as an isolated exercise but as a springboard for change.

It is evident that many of these issues are deep seated and of long standing, giving rise to a work culture which will take time to reform and change. The maternity service that was the focus of this study is not unique: these cultural problems are widespread in UK midwifery (Kirkham 1999). Nonetheless, how the midwives in the groups expressed themselves showed some personal growth and increased insight and objectivity. It was also apparent that many participants had experienced material change in their work situation through promotion and role development.

In this study one specific British maternity unit was examined and whilst the data it generated clearly resonate with other descriptions of midwifery culture, the findings of this study should not be generalised to other maternity units without careful consideration of the culture and organisation of those units. Nonetheless the research processes involved during the study are transferable and would be useful as a means of data collection in other units and, together, such data would shed further light on the culture of midwifery.

Conclusion

There are many cultural impediments to the realisation of the UK Government's aim of giving nurses and midwives a greater role and involvement in health service development. These impediments are not addressed in the key documents such as 'Making a Difference' (DoH 1999) despite an increasing body of work (e.g. Hunt & Symonds 1995, Leap 1997, Kirkham 1999) which is beginning to describe the deeply entrenched and problematic culture of midwifery.

In this study, culture within one maternity unit was examined with the aim of positively developing and changing the midwifery service. A cultural ethnographic approach was best suited to the consciousness raising and analysis of power relationships that is pre-requisite for the cultural shift that is necessary if midwives are to be empowered in the way that is envisaged within current UK government policy. The researchers chose focus groups as a method of data collection because these parallel the social organisation of current midwifery care and can broaden the perspective of participants by enabling them to see their private concerns as public issues.

The findings of the study indicate that there are complex and long-standing cultural inhibitions to the effective development of midwifery care. If these are made explicit and then actively addressed through management strategies, as outlined in this study, the process of cultural shift may be seen to begin. However, once cultural shift has begun and organisational changes made, improvements in morale may not occur at the same pace. This year-long study suggests that morale in the study unit lagged behind organisational and individual material change in this maternity unit.

Participants were largely unable to articulate their vision for the future of their service although they were very clearly able to enumerate and describe a variety of problems with the, then, current service. The opportunity to articulate and discuss their current problems may constitute an important gateway for midwives to pass through in order to enable them to develop a vision for the future. Had we been able to continue this study over a longer period of time, this phenomenon may have been better understood. Whilst the researchers were discouraged by the negativity of the data, a conscious and concerted process of reflexivity meant that they were able to take a more detached view.

Data analysis of the second focus groups, a year after the first ones, revealed an element of positive cultural shift. Participants used a different sort of language when discussing their situation and they analysed this using more frankly political terms. Despite the fact that they had many criticisms of their working environment there was evidence of a degree of altered consciousness. This leads us to conclude that focus groups can be a useful tool in moving midwifery culture forward within a local context.

Acknowledgements

The authors thank Tricia Anderson and Dr Nigel King for their helpful and constructive comments during the writing of this paper.

REFERENCES

Burnard P 1991 A method of analysing interview transcripts in qualitative research. Nurse Education Today 11: 464-466

Deery R 1999 Improving relationships through clinical supervision: 2. British Journal of Midwifery 7(4):160-163

Deery R, Hughes D, Lovatt A et al. 1999 'Hearing midwives' views': focus groups on maternity care in Calderdale NHS Trust. Unpublished report, Primary Care Research Group, University of Huddersfield

Deery R, Hughes D, Lovatt A 2000 'Quite a healthy exercise': follow-up focus groups on maternity care in Calderdale NHS Trust. Unpublished report, Primary Care Research Group, University of Huddersfield

Demilew J 1996 'Independent midwives' views of supervision. In: Kirkham M (Ed) Supervision of Midwives. Books for Midwives Press, Hale

DoH 1993 Changing Childbirth: report of the expert maternity group. Department of Health, London

DoH 1997 The new NHS: modern, dependable. Department of Health, London

DoH 1999 Making a difference. Department of Health, London

Ely M, Anzul M, Friedman T et al. 1991 Doing qualitative research: circles within circles. The Falmer Press, London

Grbich C 1999 Qualitative research in health. Sage Publications, London

Green J, Hart L 1999 The impact of context on data. In: Barbour R.S, Kitzinger J (Eds) Developing focus group research: politics, theory and practice. Sage Publications, London

Hammersley M, Atkinson P 1995 Ethnography: principles in practice, second edition. Routledge, London

Hunt S, Symonds A 1995 The social meaning of midwifery. Macmillan Press, Basingstoke

Jordan S, Yeomans D 1995 Critical ethnography: problems in contemporary theory and practice. British Journal of Sociology and Education 16(3):389-408

Kent J 2000 Social perspectives on pregnancy and childbirth for midwives, nurses and the caring professions. Open University Press, Buckingham

Kirkham M 1999 The culture of midwifery in the National Health Service in England. Journal of Advanced Nursing 30(3):732-739

Kirkham M, Stapleton H 2000 Midwives' support needs as childbirth changes. Journal of Advanced Nursing 32(2):465-472

Kitzinger J Barbour RS 1999 Introduction: the challenge and promise of focus group. In: Developing focus group research: politics, theory and practice. Barbour R S Kitzinger J (Eds) Sage Publications, London

Leap N 1997 Making sense of 'horizontal violence' in midwifery. British Journal of Midwifery 5(11): 698

Maguire P 2001 Uneven ground: feminisms and action research. In: Reason P Bradbury H (Eds) Handbook of action research: participative inquiry and practice. Sage Publications, London

Marcus G 1994 What comes (just) after 'post'? The case of ethnography. In: Denzin N Lincoln Y (Eds) Handbook of qualitative research. Sage Publications, London.

Morse JM Field PA 1996 Nursing research: the application of qualitative approaches, Stanley Thornes (Publishers) Ltd., Cheltenham

NHSE (1998) A consultation on a strategy for nursing, midwifery & health visiting. NHS Executive, Leeds

Oakley A 1981 Interviewing women: a contradiction in terms. In: Roberts H (Ed) Doing feminist research. Routledge & Kegan Paul, London

Reed J 1995 Practitioner knowledge in practitioner research. In: Reed J,

Proctor S (Eds) Practitioner research in health care: the inside story. Chapman & Hall, London

Reed J, Biott C 1995 Evaluating and developing practitioner research. In: Reed J, Proctor S (Eds) Practitioner research in health care: the inside story. Chapman & Hall, London

Stapleton H, Duerden J, Kirkham M 1998 Evaluation of the impact of the supervision of midwives on professional practice and the quality of midwifery care. An ENB and UKCC commissioned project. University of Sheffield

Twinn S 2000 The analysis of focus group data: a challenge to the rigour of qualitative research. Nursing Times Research 3(2):140-147

Weitz R 1987 English midwives and the association of radical midwives. Women & Health 12(1):79-89

Wilkinson S 1999 How useful are focus group in feminist research? In: Barbour RS, Kitzinger J (Eds) Developing focus group research: politics, theory and practice. Sage Publications, London

Midwifery 2002; 18: 43-52

Reflecting on Women, Midwives and Choice

- In relation to the issue of choice, what cultural changes have taken place in your lifetime, or during the time you have been involved in midwifery? Have any of these had an impact on you, or your practice? How do your experiences compare with those of your colleagues, especially those who are of a different generation from you?

- What are your personal beliefs about choice, and how might these affect your practice? Of the issues discussed in the articles here, which do you feel most strongly about? Of the choices that women face during childbirth, which do you feel are the most important, or have the most potential impact on their lives? Does this affect the way you practise, or offer information to women and their families?

- Do you agree with Deborah that we should stop offering women the 'choice' of receiving untested or poorly evaluated interventions? Do you agree that there is a danger in abdicating professional midwifery decisions by offering women too much choice, as in her example of perineal suturing? Where would you draw the line here?

If you feel like writing…

- What would you have written about if you had submitted an article (or poem or story) in the "What is a normal midwife?" series?

If you feel like taking action…

- Do women in your area have enough information on which to base their choices? Is there a local resource centre where women can access information for themselves, or a local arm of an organisation that supports women? If there is an existing organisation, how might you be able to help them get information to women? If there is not already an organisation, how could one be helped to get going?

Focus on:
Families

SECTION CONTENTS

A disposable culture?

Supporting parents to make real choices about nappies

Anna Fielder, Luqman Hayes

At some point after the initial ecstasy of meeting Aaron, of feeling his warm soft skin next to ours, and of him taking his first breastfeed, somebody put him in a disposable nappy. Neither of us are quite sure who it was, or why they did it, but they did. In the context of the birth itself and in relation to issues such as whether we wanted him to have vitamin K and how we were going to feed him, his first nappy perhaps fades into insignificance. Or does it?

As parents, we really wish we had been given the choice. It is such a simple one – a cloth nappy or a disposable – yet the implications are huge, on a personal, social and environmental level.

In this article, we will present some of those implications as we perceive them as parents and discuss how informed choices about nappies are as important as any other in the precious steps of having and caring for a baby. What are the real issues that parents need to be aware of if they are to make informed choices regarding their use of nappies? And how can midwives help women in the decision making process?

Freedom of choice?

We were given 'choices' (some of them more real than others) at every step of the pregnancy. And yet which type of nappy we were thinking of using was hardly touched upon, certainly not in the context of our antenatal care. This is interesting because nine months later, opting to use cloth nappies (which we did as soon as we left hospital) seems like one of the most real and enduring decisions that we made during those nine months. The others came and went (choices over screening tests, place of birth etc.) and yet it is the nappies that we are left facing 8 or 10 times a day. We don't intend to flippantly dismiss the other choices – of course they are very important. However, on a mundane level, it is the day-to-day things such as nappies that

continually impact upon a family's life 6, 12, 24 months down the line.

Due to our backgrounds and belief systems, we were aware of the options we had in relation to nappies. This is not the case for everyone. Put simply, there is far more awareness and more presence of disposable nappies than there is of cloth nappies. When we turn on the television we are bombarded with advertisements of cute babies apparently wearing the latest, softest, most absorbent brand of disposable; there are numerous sources of free samples for pregnant women; the pregnancy literature is filled with adverts and special offers for disposable nappies, the Bounty packs contain free samples... and so it goes on.

By contrast, information about cloth nappies is less easy to come by. Despite there now being a wide range of cloth nappies and accessories, they are far less visible (if they are there at all) in supermarkets, high street chemists and baby stores. Often it is through the internet, or a small scale locally based specialist supplier, that cloth nappies are purchased. This makes them less accessible to a whole range of people, including those who are not computer literate, those who prefer not to do internet shopping, and those who simply do not have the time to spend shopping around. What busy pregnant mother doesn't fit into at least one of those categories?

And so perhaps 'choice' as a word is inappropriate to describe the process by which many parents end up using particular kinds of nappies. Due to a lack of awareness, information and access to reusable nappies, it is almost a *fait accompli* that many parents use disposables.

Convenient excuses

Some parents are aware of the choice, but base decisions on misperceptions or inadequate information. For example, we have heard disposable users talk a lot about convenience. In some respects this is understandable. When we travelled with Aaron for six weeks we used disposables (we hold our hands up here – we are not quite militant cloth nappyists). Neither of us was totally comfortable with this, but it was easier as we were on the move.

However, generally speaking we have not found cloth nappies inconvenient. Many cloth nappies are now as easy as disposables to put on, with Velcro and popper fasteners. And perhaps much of the argument that reusable nappies are inconvenient derives from something of an image problem, stemming from the days when our grandmothers and great grandmothers spent hours bent-double hand-washing soiled cotton squares in a tin bathtub. Reusable nappies have moved on – although the perception of them as time-consuming, cumbersome and hideously messy and smelly has not. Like mud, it has stuck, and perhaps has even been inadvertently reinforced by the marketing messages of the disposable nappy manufacturers, which convey 'hygiene', 'cleanliness', 'comfort' and 'ease'.

And yet many cloth nappy users don't experience their nappies in such a negative way. A friend of ours thinks they're 'cute and cuddly', 'they smell so lovely, they feel so soft.' And yes, they need washing. But overall it only takes a matter of minutes to fill up the washing machine, hang the nappies up to dry and put them away again. Personally, we get great pleasure from our washing line of terries. It looks kind of aesthetically pleasing, and invariably invites encouraging comments from elderly neighbours. Believe it or not, we enjoy using cloth nappies. And we are not alone in this.

The nappy market

The marketing of nappies in itself is an odd thing; whether it is from the disposable market where styles are frequently improved upon offering more dryness or more efficiency, or from the reusable market where concepts of naturalness prevail, both are guilty of generating twee, jovial names, albeit appealing to different sets of consumers. From the cartoon motifs on the fasteners of disposables, to the leopard-skin prints of some cloth nappy wraps, the nappy industry in general seems to want to convince us that the whole process of going to the toilet is more fashion than function.

Yet it's a mark of the power of marketing and the strength of the companies behind the disposable nappy industry that within a generation, disposables have been transformed from being a marginal product to one so omnipresent. The first disposables were developed in the 50s and 60s, but only hit the High Street in the 80s. Once the big supermarket chains had got wind of their popularity, their mass proliferation was inevitable.

As parents and consumers, we see this as something of a sleight of hand; not only is the full choice partially concealed, but the most visible product is also the most costly. Disposables were never cheap and they remain more expensive than reusable nappies. The average cost of a disposable nappy is, to quote figures from the Women's Environmental Network, 12.7p. Over 2.5 years, this makes for an average cost of £700 per baby.[1] Reusable nappies vary in cost depending on style or system. Terries are the cheapest and major retailers such as Boots and Mothercare do stock them at around £10 for six. Plastic pants are around £2.60 for six. Nappy pins are £1.10.[1]

Based on these prices, and bringing laundry costs, including washing machine depreciation, detergent and energy into the equation, WEN has calculated that using home laundered cloth nappies could save you £500 over 2.5 years.[1] For people on low incomes, this is hugely significant. And if families use the same nappies for two or more children, the savings are increased for subsequent babies.

However, the cost difference is not widely publicised. Instead, disposable companies publicise the latest designs, the latest ranges and the latest technological developments in disposable nappy manufacturing. The fact is that every parent wants the absolute best for their baby. Those in the business of making money out of nappies know this.

Environment

In addition to cost, it was also the environmental impact of a plastic-based product such as disposable nappies that affected the nappy choices we made.

In the UK, as in 'developed' countries generally, it is easy to dispose of things. So easy, that we habitually do it without asking where it is going and what will happen to it once it has been removed from our bins and thrown into the back of the rubbish truck. We have become such an individualised society, which thinks in terms of personal rather than community responsibility, that it is often only when issues such as waste affect us directly that we finally consider the effects elsewhere.

The issue of nappy waste in the UK has developed more topical relevance of late because of the Government's need to adhere to the strict targets set by the European Union's Landfill Directive. While much more substantial contributions to landfill may come from elsewhere, for example, the industrial and construction sectors, household waste is still a big factor, and within that disposable nappies figure significantly.

The statistics vary but the contribution to household waste which disposable nappies make is enormous when you consider the small proportion of the population which nappy-wearing babies make up. Some 600,000 babies are born in the UK each year. It is considered that around 90 per cent will use disposable nappies.[1] Between them and those already in nappies, they contribute up to 4% of all household waste sent to landfill, according to the Department of the Environment, Farming and Rural Affairs (DEFRA).[1] Put another way, the Women's Environmental Network estimates that 8 million disposables are thrown away every day or 3 billion a year. That's approximately 450,000 tonnes or the total municipal waste of a city the size of Birmingham.[2]

We found it quite staggering how much rubbish could be accumulated in the few times we reverted to using disposables, such as when travelling long distances. It is not simply that landfill is a problematic form of waste management. The plastics in nappies will take hundreds of years to decompose. In addition, the process of decomposition itself is not ideal because it releases methane into the atmosphere, a gas that contributes to global warming. So when people talk of finding a more bio-degradable disposable nappy, this is not a solution to a pollution problem.

While landfill is the main process of disposal for disposables (the Government's Waste Not Want Not report cites that 90% are disposed of this way),[1] nappies are also incinerated in those municipalities where such methods continue to be used and in hospitals and nurseries along with clinical waste. This is also a poor option as the incineration of mixed waste creates toxic substances in air emissions and ash.

The issue of disposables blocking up toilets and being sent to sewerage systems has decreased, but it doesn't stop the odd package of baby-dos washing up on the beach. Depressingly, like any other litter, disposables will feature in the park, on the street, by the hedge. More often than not the baby's excreta are wrapped up in the disposable rather than being flushed down the toilet. The disposable by its very design - the sticky flaps allowing you to seal the soiled nappy as well as tie the clean one on the baby – encourages you to throw the whole thing away. There have been health concerns over such contents not only being dangerous in a public setting, but also to workers on landfill sites. As such there is no available data stating whether vaccines such as polio, which live in the faeces some time after immunisation, pose a significant threat.

Cloth nappies do have environmental impacts of their own, which are significant, but perhaps not, as the disposable manufacturers might have you believe, as significant as those of disposables. Washing nappies takes water and energy, and the majority of us continue to get our energy from non-renewable fossil fuel sources. In an ideal world, a local wind farm, supported by solar and methane generators would power our washing machines. But for now we have to accept that coal or nuclear powered electricity is what drives our spin cycles. Water is a massive concern of global proportions, but in both cases, there is no gain in comparing one negative environmental impact with another. Positive alternatives that reduce or remove the environmental impact are always preferable, and in the case of cloth nappies, the issue of waste is all but prevented (save for a paper-based liner, if that's what you use). Methods of disposal, health and hygiene and atmospheric implications are all avoided because the product is durable and re-usable – you can use them on subsequent children or if you're not having any more, pass them on to a friend or relative who is. What could be more environmentally – and – socially friendly?

What can midwives do?

However natural cloth nappies may be, how to use them did not come naturally to us as parents. How to fold them, fasten them, soak them, wash them... it was all quite bamboozling at first. By a process of trial and error, and some invaluable input from two very special midwives, we gradually grew in confidence and found our own way. Midwives are ideally placed to provide women and their partners with that help in the first few days. After all, who else is there with reassuring words and suggestions when new parents tentatively change their baby's nappy for the first time?

And who is there through the trials, traumas and joys of those first few postnatal days when everything, from the enormity of motherhood to the mundanity of washing a nappy, is totally and utterly new. Midwives can make all the difference to people's experience of adapting to parenthood, and supporting them in their choice of nappies and providing straightforward practical advice about how to use them, is just one aspect of that.

We would have found it useful to have thought more about nappies during the antenatal period. As it happened, we left nappy shopping until the last minute, and then found it difficult to find what we wanted. In fact we were genuinely surprised by the lack of cloth nappies in many chemists and baby shops. Again, it seems to us that midwives, especially community midwives, are well placed to talk to women about nappies at some point during their pregnancy, and to point them in the direction that is right for them. Something simple like 'When it comes to changing your baby's nappy, you have a number of choices...' would be a start. An awareness of what's available locally in terms of retail outlets, nappy laundering services, real nappy support groups etc. would be useful, perhaps in leaflet form. And maybe such a leaflet could be put in the

Bounty packs? In some parts of the country, local authorities subsidise low-income families to use real nappy laundering services. Midwives need to be aware of, and to support, such initiatives if they are to help women make the best choices for their own social and economic circumstances.

Some hospitals have display boards depicting the variety of cloth nappies available to parents. Providing information about local nappy networks and initiatives is a great way of helping women to get the support they need to make the choices that are right for them.

Maybe antenatal classes could be adapted to incorporate a talk from a local parent who uses cloth nappies? Perhaps a parent would be willing to come along to the group and show them how s/he does a cloth nappy change. After all, there's nothing more likely to get an antenatal group enthused than the sight of a real baby – and a real baby doing a wee is bound to get some laughs!

Hospital provision of cloth nappies is also an effective way of introducing everyone to the idea of cloth nappies. What better time than in those first few days when parental habits have not yet been formed, and when midwifery staff are readily available to help?

Support groups

Finally, our own experience has been that real nappy groups and networks provide excellent and ongoing postnatal support for families in a more general sense. A friend of ours went to a whole host of 'mother and baby' groups before she found the local 'real nappy group', where she felt immediately more at home and comfortable. She puts this down to having something more in common with the other mothers than 'simply the fact that we are mothers'. From sharing tips on how to fold or wash nappies, to helping one another through the multitude of challenges that the first few years of parenthood bring, such groups are far more than just arenas to talk about cloth nappies. They are ongoing sources of support, information and friendship. Given the isolation that many women experience during those first few months and years of motherhood, what ideal resources for midwives and health visitors to be aware of.

Conclusion

A friend of ours, whose birth and postnatal period were difficult and traumatic, now feels that choosing to use cloth nappies was the only choice around birth that she made herself. Other decisions she feels were made by doctors, midwives, or were taken out of her hands due to medical circumstance. That feeling of having control over something, when all other choices were taken away, has kept her going when many other aspects of her life perhaps felt out of control. Decision making about nappies was therefore important to her for reasons of control and choice. For other parents, it will be about cost, convenience or environmental factors. As with any aspect of the birth and postnatal experience, parents make particular choices for a whole variety of reasons. But what is important is that they are actively involved in the decision making process - that it is their choice, and that it is an informed one. Midwives are uniquely placed to provide unbiased information to parents, and to support them in decision-making regarding the use of nappies. In doing so, they will be supporting parents to make decisions with long term social, personal, financial and environmental impacts.

REFERENCES

1. Women's Environmental Network. Nappies. Available at www.wen.org.uk/facts.htm

2. Waste & Resources Action Programme (WRAP). www.wrap.org.uk

Midwifery Best Practice Volume 3 (ed. Wickham) 2005; 42-45

Pregnancy, birth and feeding:
what do picture books tell our children?

Sarah Hunt

Mandy Robotham in her article in the September 2001 edition of MIDIRS, 'Fast and furious: childbirth on TV', wonders why birth on TV is still in the dark ages, with its round of life-threatening scenarios with the doctor as the hero. The portrayal of birth in picture books for young children also seems to need a little nudge to edge it into the 21st century, where not every baby is born in hospital, and even when in hospital many women are cared for by midwives.

With over 5000 picture books published every year, children's books can have significant influence over the information around pregnancy, childbirth and breastfeeding that the very young receive and perceive to be 'normal'.

At the conference on Home Birth in September 2001 organised by Caroline Flint at St George's Hospital, I browsed through the books for sale on the ACE Graphics stall. I came across a picture book for children showing a home birth. This led me to think about how the youngest members of our society gain their knowledge of pregnancy, birth and breastfeeding through words and pictures.

I collected 13 books which dealt with these topics, all but three published within the last 3 years, and did a little light reading...

Portrayal of pregnancy

Overall, the portrayal of pregnancy in the picture books I looked at is fairly positive, although there are some notable exceptions. As the majority of books on the topic of pregnancy and birth are intended to help young children prepare for the birth of a sibling, they cover the same areas of concern for the young child.

Without exception, the picture books prepare children for a period of separation from one or both parents while the mother goes into hospital to give birth. I had hoped to be able to describe the picture book illustrating a home

birth that I saw at the Home Birth conference, however it is now unavailable from ACE Graphics or from all the internet bookshops that I tried.

The pregnant mother in *Topsy and Tim and The New Baby* by Jean and Gareth Adamson, wears normal clothes and although is obviously pregnant, continues with her normal activities, having children to tea and preparing for the baby's birth by sorting baby clothes and equipment.

Jan Ormerod's *Mum and Me* shows a pregnant mother playing with her still crawling baby, illustrating pregnancy as neither incapacitating, as she is shown doing lots of bends and stretches, nor as overwhelmingly tiring as it is portrayed in many books for children on this subject. For example, in Rebecca Hunter's *My New Sister*, we are told that 'Mum is often tired and can't always play with me'.

Compare Jan Ormerod's positive and attractive portrayal of the changing body in pregnancy with Bob Graham's *Brand New Baby*, where we are told the pregnant Mrs Arnold 'wore dresses as big as tents', and similarly in the Usborne book on the subject, *The New Baby*, where the pregnant woman, Mrs Bunn, (has she got one in the oven I ask myself), wears a sack-like garment which reaches down to her ankles.

For many firstborn children, the birth of a sibling is their first experience of separation from their mothers, and many mothers report that this first separation from their firstborns is one of the most distressing parts of giving birth in hospital.

Most of the books prepare children for the disappearance of the mother in a sensitive or matter of fact way. For example, in *I'm Still Important* by Jen Green and Mike Gordon, the older sibling reports that: 'When Mum and Dad went to hospital to have the baby, Gran came to look after me.'

However, one book describes the disappearance of the mother from the viewpoint of the child who wakes in the night to find her mother gone. In *A Baby for Grace* by Ian Whybrow and Christian Birmingham, Grace wakes in the dark of the night and goes to find her father in bed. '...Grace was worried about Mummy. Where had she gone?' Grace is told that her parents went to 'fetch the baby' and that her mother would be home tomorrow, and that she should wait a little longer before seeing her. Not a very comforting image for a young child.

Labour

Many of the books I looked at did not attempt to describe labour, either through words or pictures – perhaps understandable as the vast majority assume that the woman will labour in hospital and will not be seen by other children. The Usborne book on the subject, *The New Baby*, does attempt what all the others avoid. Mrs Bunn, the reader is told, 'feels the baby coming', and this is backed up with a picture of a somewhat bemused looking Mrs Bunn holding her bump and her back. I misinterpreted the next illustration, which shows the phone call to the hospital being made, and is illustrated by a female hanging over the banisters, which seemed to me a very positive and helpful picture of active labour. On closer scrutiny, I realised that it is not Mrs Bunn in the picture, but Lucy Bunn, the older sister, who has been woken by the commotion of getting Mrs Bunn to hospital – shame! Apart from this brief mention of labour, most babies are just born with no mention of the process of labour.

Birth

All the babies are born in hospital, with the new mother firmly tucked up in a hospital bed. Three of the books I looked at had very clinical looking hospital settings, with the Usborne book showing both mother and father in hospital gowns. Mothers are always semi-recumbent if shown giving birth (very discreetly), and are on raised hospital beds.

Kathy Henderson and Tony Kerrins in *The Baby Dances*, open with a view into the tower block hospital room with the mother on a hospital bed, and father wearing theatre greens, holding the new baby. In the background are shadowy medical figures with charts and machines. Similarly, the clinically very accurate *Happy Birth Day* by Robie Harris and Michael Emberley, has the mother semi-recumbent in hospital gown, and this time she has a venflon in her hand – just in case?!

Generally though, hospitals are shown fairly realistically, with wards containing beds and bedside cupboards, typical fishbowl hospital cots, and flowers and congratulatory cards.

Midwives feature only twice in my sample – full marks to Pat Thomas in *My Amazing Journey* which tells the reader that 'During labour, a midwife was there to check that you and your mum were all right'. This is illustrated by a woman being supported from behind by a male partner, and by her side the midwife, who is not wearing uniform and is from a multicultural background. It's a real pity that the midwife did not support the mother to breastfeed, as there is no mention of this in this otherwise very good book.

Otherwise, birth attendants are nurses wearing hats, and one with a stethoscope around her neck, (*The New Baby* – Usborne First Experiences), or shadowy medical figures in hospital gowns.

Feeding

Feeding new babies either features very prominently in these books or not at all! It appears from these books that most babies don't feed at all, as there is no mention of it, but reassuringly the ones that do feed are usually breastfed. and perhaps the increased rates of breastfeeding noted by the Infant Feeding Survey 2000 can be partly attributed by the generally positive images of breastfeeding shown in picture books for children.

Brand New Baby by Bob Graham, features beginning and end papers which have a recurring pattern of things to do with babies. One of these is a feeding bottle, which means that there are 38 feeding bottles on the front papers alone. Having got that out of the way, the new baby is breastfed, and baby-led feeding seems to be practised as the reader is told, 'Mum was always feeding the baby'. Similarly in *My New Sister*, by Rebecca Hunter and Chris Fairclough: although photographs are used predominantly as illustrations, there is a background of baby motifs which again includes a feeding bottle, so there is a subtle reminder on every page of this book. Strangely, this baby is never fed, or so we are led to imagine by the lack of references to feeding in the actual text or photographs. Perhaps this is why this baby 'sleeps at lot and cries a lot' – as does baby Harry in *I'm Still Important* – he never seems to be fed and 'mostly cried or slept'.

The Usborne baby, Susie Bunn, seems a much more satisfied customer who is breastfed when hungry and 'will need to be fed many times each day'. No crying baby for the Bunn family, but while older sister Lucy watches Mrs Bunn breastfeed the baby, Lucy bottle feeds her doll.

Topsy and Tim see their friend's baby breastfed, with the baby on its side and held close to its mother. Other illustrations of breastfeeding leave something to be desired concerning the positioning of the baby at the breast, but probably I'm being over-critical here. And since I'm in critical mode, why is it that all but one breastfeeding mother breastfeeds with her dress or blouse fully unbuttoned? Gold star to Mick Manning and Brita Granstrom in *The world is full of BABIES* who show a mother breastfeeding standing up with the baby feeding under her T-shirt.

Generally, where breastfeeding is portrayed, it is shown as natural and normal. In Jan Ormerod's *101 Things To Do With A Baby*, the frontispiece shows a mother breastfeeding her baby in bed while reading with her older child and looking very comfortable. The baby is not new-born and is being breastfed in conjunction with some mixed feeding, which is encouraging.

As midwives, we know that women have often decided how to feed their babies even before they are pregnant, and that decisions are influenced by the social and family messages that they grow up with. It seems likely therefore, that people's views of the pregnancy, labour and birth could be influenced by similar factors, and these must include the visual images that young children are shown. So, next time you buy a book about this topic to give to a child, have a good read first.

Postscript

An Australian friend has sent me a copy of *Hello Baby*, the picture book by Jenni Overend and illustrated by Julie Vivas that I had seen at the Home Birth conference. The book describes a home birth from the point of view of a child who looks about 7 years old. The mother has an active labour, going for a walk in the woods to 'help the baby along', and the midwife is a familiar figure to the family. The birth of the baby is depicted with the mother standing, being supported by the father, the midwife kneeling to receive the baby, and two children and two adults watching. We see the baby's head emerge on one spread, followed by the baby still attached to its umbilical cord on the following spread. The placenta is also shown in a bowl and its arrival is described: 'Anna gently pulls on the cord between Mum's legs and out comes a big purple shape.' The final pages of the book show the whole family in a makeshift bed together, the mother close to the new baby and the displaced youngest sibling secure in his father's arms.

REFERENCES

Infant Feeding Survey 2000 www.doh.gov.uk
Robotham M. 2001. Fast and furious: childbirth on TV. MIDIRS Midwifery Digest, 1(10), 77-8
Weston R. 2001. How to keep baby friendly. The Practising Midwife, 4(8)

Overend J and Vivas J. 1999. Hello Baby. Sidney: Australia Broadcasting Corporation

The Practising Midwife 2002; 5(5): 17-19

Birth of a midwife?

Sara Wickham

Several months ago, I attended my friend Megan's home birth in what was a new role for me; as the support person for her 3-year-old daughter, Eleanor. Eleanor and I had a marvellous time; we played in the garden, shared chocolate, visited Megan from time to time to see how she was doing in the water pool, and spent so long choosing the video we were going to watch that, by the time we had chosen '*The Tweenies*', Megan was nearing the second stage of her labour.

At Eleanor's request, we went to sit next to the pool and watch the baby being born.

The reason I am writing about Megan's birth (with her blessing) is that I was so amazed by Eleanor's instinctual behaviour. As a midwife, I have always welcomed children to their sibling's births, on the understanding that, like Eleanor, they have a support person who can meet their needs without removing attention or energy from the labouring woman.

During my time as a midwife, there has been debate about whether or not it is appropriate for small children to attend births; for the majority of women who give birth in hospital this has not yet become a realistic option. After this experience, I am convinced that we are missing the point; by focusing on the debate about whether they should be there or not, we are not attending to the things we can learn by watching children at birth.

Megan had warned me that she tended to have a very fast and intense second stage. When she started reacting verbally to a few massive and intense contractions, I tried to make this okay for Eleanor by chattering softly in her ear, letting her know that Megan was fine, and that having a baby was hard work. James, her dad, joined in this reassurance. Megan was getting no relief between contractions and for a while was unable to reassure Eleanor herself. Eleanor was a little scared initially – and what three-year-old wouldn't be? – but soon turned around to me and confirmed, 'It's hard work having a

baby, isn't it?' This having been established, she then snuggled into my lap and reached out her hand to pat Megan, in a gesture of support.

She reminded me of Joshua, the four-year-old son of another woman I attended a few years ago, who spent over three hours leaning over the side of a pool pouring water over his mother's back from a paper cup because she found it soothing. This woman's husband and I both felt there was no way we could have kept the monotonous movement up for that long!

As baby Rachel began to emerge, I asked Eleanor if she would like to see. She nodded, and we moved to the other end of the water pool. As Megan was on all-fours, we could see baby Rachel's face. 'Oh, it's a bit scrunchy,' Eleanor said. 'Let's go see mummy again now.' So we went back to Megan's 'head-end', where, as baby Rachel was born and passed under Megan's legs, Eleanor leaned over to give Megan a kiss 'well done'.

The intensity of Megan's second stage meant that we were all concerned afterwards that Eleanor might have been affected by it. Our desire to ensure that she understood birth to be a normal, natural event was tempered with our need to help her understand that it wasn't always a silent time, and that the feelings Megan experienced were intense.

We worry about the effect that watching the intensity of a woman verbalising her labour and birth experience will have on children. Yet Eleanor seemed to take it all in her stride and, despite their bringing the subject up on a few occasions, Megan and James have never seen any evidence that she was worried or disturbed by her experience.

Of course, all children are different, but I keep asking myself how much our concern about having children at birth is about our fear rather than the fear of our children?

As we waited for Megan's placenta to be born, Eleanor stayed on my lap and we all chatted as we admired baby Rachel. I was a bit surprised that Eleanor was so matter-of-fact about the whole thing, especially after seeing Megan experience such an intense labour.

At one point, I leaned over the pool side to hold Rachel next to Megan's skin while she reached down to catch her placenta. Eleanor was still on my lap. A few minutes later, after James had taken a series of photos of Megan, Rachel and the placenta, I realised I was no longer holding on to Eleanor. She was still on my lap, transfixed by the scene in front of her, holding on to my clothing like a baby monkey holds its mother's fur!

Eleanor is one of those children who is sometimes described as an 'old soul'. We surmise that babies and young children are much more in touch with ancient, 'otherworldly' things than we who have reached adulthood and forgotten what we knew then. I wouldn't be at all surprised if Eleanor knew more about what was going on than anyone else in the room.

She might not have had the words in our language, but she seemed to have an instinctual knowledge about birth, and about being with her mother in labour. She was infinitely patient with the journey of birth, primal in her responses.

I'm sure we have more to learn from watching our children at birth than we could ever imagine.

The Practising Midwife 2002; 5(6): 27

Midwives urged to make room for dads in the maternity unit

Francesca Robinson

New dads are to be invited to stay over night after the birth of their babies in some NHS hospitals in a move to make maternity services more father-friendly. The initiative is reported in a major study, How To Build New Dads, published by Fathers Direct, the national information centre on fatherhood. The change is being hailed as one of the biggest culture shifts in maternity practice in 30 years. It will come into effect next year, just after the introduction of statutory paid paternity leave.

In July 2003, Grimsby Maternity Hospital opened a pioneering new unit with purpose-built double bedrooms and en suite facilities in which both parents can stay throughout the mother's admission to hospital.

Karen Robinson, head of midwifery, gynaecology and sexual health for North Lincolnshire and Goole hospitals, responsible for the Grimsby initiative, said: 'Fathers will be brought into caring for their partners and infants and we expect that this will have a knock-on effect for our midwives, reducing their workload by fathers performing practical tasks such as running baths, helping their partner to move about and get comfortable, lifting the baby and helping the mother to feed.'

Tom Beardshaw, campaign manager for Fathers Direct, said: 'Dads can be a vital support to mothers and new babies after the birth, cutting the workload for over-stretched midwives and learning important baby care skills. Research shows that involving dads early on can be crucial to long-term child development and for bonding families particularly when the relationship between mother and father is fragile.'

The £11.5m Grimsby rebuilding programme is part of a £100m NHS-funded maternity unit refurbishment programme announced by Alan Milburn, then Secretary of State for Health. In a recent interview, Mr Milburn urged maternity units that allow fathers to stay over to publicise the facility as a mark of their excellence.

At Grimsby, the purpose-built rooms have tea-making facilities and domestic-style built in wardrobe and cupboard space in which all the equipment for baby delivery can be stored. The scheme design is based on the latest advice on new hospital building from the Department of Health.

How To Build New Dads also highlights other NHS 'father-friendly' initiatives such as a policy to encourage fathers to take off their shirts and have skin-to-skin contact with their babies at Forth Park Maternity Hospital, Fife. Some hospitals have begun routinely bathing new-born babies in the evenings rather than during the day so that fathers can attend.

At the Queen Mother Hospital, Glasgow, midwives have introduced a scheme for auditing the satisfaction of fathers with the services on offer to them and many hospitals have in recent years have relaxed their visiting hours to allow fathers to remain with their new families for most of the day. Nottingham City Hospital now allows the entire family, including siblings, to stay over in its 'Patients' Hotel'.

For further information visit www.fathersdirect.com

Table 2.4.1 How midwives can include fathers

Make couples aware that they are free to choose whether the father attends the birth or not and that there is a range of roles he can play during labour
Let the father-to-be know that his presence can be very reassuring and helpful to his partner
Learn his name, make eye contact and smile at him. Where appropriate make suggestions to him about how he can offer practical help such as with massage, lifting or touch
Keep him involved in conversations about the progress of labour and any decisions on interventions and pain relief
If his partner is taken into surgery for an emergency Caesarean make sure someone can reassure him and make sure he is OK
Remember to congratulate the father as well as the mother when the baby is born. If he has a camera, offer to take a photo of mum and dad together with the baby.

The Practising Midwife 2002; 5(7): 9

Balancing work and babies

Mary Newburn

The National Childbirth Trust and midwives often pay a great deal of attention to the details of clinical care and its management during pregnancy, labour and afterwards. These matters are highly important, yet for women the significance of the transition to motherhood – or to becoming a bigger family – is much broader. This is increasingly recognised, with the growing focus on improving public health and tackling health inequalities (DOH, 1999).

Yet for women at these key transition points in their lives, and throughout their years of childbearing and looking after dependent children, an important issue that is often neglected is whether, or how, to attempt to combine paid work with being a mother. This issue is important for midwives as providers of individualised, woman-centred care, and as working mothers and fathers themselves.

More women with a young family work outside the home now than was the case in the immediate post-war period, though in earlier centuries and in all but the most privileged classes, mothers have generally contributed to the family income (Anderson, 1994). One key change has been the opportunity for women, including those in professional and managerial occupations, to continue in employment after starting a family. In this article, I will present and discuss findings from a survey the NCT conducted with Practical Parenting magazine, which suggests that employers can make a difference in terms of women feeling that paid work and caring for babies and young children can be combined in a positive, life-affirming way.

Background

In the 17th, 18th and 19th centuries many women in the UK earned an independent livelihood. Women's economic activity outside the home was extended by a significant proportion remaining single or postponing motherhood through late marriage, but many mothers also earned (Goldthorpe, 1987). Many of the forms of families we see today, including lone parent families, separated families, stepfamilies and babies born outside marriage, were just as prevalent, though the causes and consequences may have been different (Bradshaw, 1996). During the second half of the 20th century, there was a steady rise in the number of married women going out to work in Western societies. However, this trend in the UK lagged behind a number of other European countries, particularly for women with pre-school age children. In the 1980s, women aged 25-35 years old, those most likely to have a baby or young children, were less likely to be in employment than similar women in Denmark or France (Goldthorpe, 1987).

In a 1996 discussion paper on parenting, the Shadow Home Secretary acknowledged that 'despite the great increase in the proportion of mothers in paid employment, many British fathers are still functioning as the main or only breadwinner, working very long hours away from their family' which many men believed put their relationships with their children and family at risk (Straw & Anderson, 1996). In March 2000 the Prime Minister launched the Government's Work-Life Balance campaign in England and Scotland with the aims of encouraging employers to give workers more choice and control over their working hours and tackling the long hours culture (www.dti.gov.uk/ work-lifebalance). There has been particular emphasis on improving the work-life balance for parents with young children.

Transition to parenthood

'Silence helps to perpetuate the myths of motherhood being 'natural' and therefore easy... The lived experience of being a mother, in contrast to anticipating motherhood, throws lives into confusion.' (Miller, 2002)

It isn't possible to consider how women balance work

and babies without considering first what the transition to parenthood means to them. Never mind 'work-life balance', what about 'motherhood-life balance'. Are women's lives thrown into confusion when they have a baby?

Women's lives have changed radically over the last fifty years, with opportunities opening up in education and employment. Women have much greater control over their fertility and extended legal rights. Technological changes have revolutionised housework, shopping, socialising and communicating. In contrast to so many features of a post-modern, virtual reality world, the needs and demands of babies and young children have changed relatively little.

Research on first-time motherhood suggests that the transition for women is a struggle. Tina Millar proposes that there is a gap – maybe a gulf – between expectations and reality. By this stage in their lives, women have strong internalised beliefs about what is good or bad mothering and they judge their own behaviour in terms of these beliefs (Miller, 2002). Their assessment of themselves as mothers is not neutral; they judge their own behaviour and often find it doesn't fit their idealised notion of the good mother. As a result, they are often emotionally isolated and unable to confide in other mothers about their feelings (Miller, 2002).

Looking after a baby involves a repetitive but unpredictable round of feeding, crying, sleeping, and nappy changing, tidying and entertaining (Oakley, 1979) which some women find exhausting, isolating or infuriating, especially those used to jobs involving diversity, creativity and considerable autonomy (Gavron, 1976; Boulton, 1983). As well as the hard work and monotony, the emotional upheaval can be gigantic and unprecedented. Paid work is not a good preparation for the demands of motherhood.

Yet, Miller (2002) says:

'Women's accounts are constructed in relation to their previous experiences, especially in relation to the world of paid work outside the home, and are contingent upon their perceptions of appropriate, and 'normal' transition to motherhood.'

Childcare

In practical terms, although the Government recognises the importance of children's safety and development in the early years (Sure Start, 2001), there is little evidence that provision of high quality childcare is a policy priority. Most families get little financial help or support in finding a suitable person or institution to look after their children while they go out to work. Attempting to combine work and motherhood is not therefore a simple challenge. There are practical, social and emotional

barriers to overcome in some way. Women who plan to continue working must provide for their baby's needs in their absence and they need to feel that they are good enough mother. Arguably, changing patterns of work, together with high levels of poverty, an increase in divorce and pressures on relationships, mean that the outside world impinges more on family life than ever before (National Family and Parenting Institute, 2001). Recent longitudinal research concludes that although there has been a near doubling in the number of mothers with children under the age of five in paid work, women are still reluctant or unable to mix full-time jobs with motherhood:

'a complete understanding of women's labour market choices after childbirth depend as much on understanding the constraints which affect women as it does on understanding their preferences' (McRae, 2001).

Our investigation came two years after the Government first launched its campaign on Work-Life Balance. The Green Paper emphasised the need for both competitiveness and choices. New rights have already been introduced for working parents. Notably, from December 1999, the right for mothers and fathers (including adoptive parents) to take 13 weeks unpaid parental leave up to their child's fifth birthday, or for parents with a disabled child up to the 18th birthday. But what is happening in practice and how do parents feel about their family and working lives?

NCT/Practical Parenting Survey

Earlier this year, the NCT and Practical Parenting magazine carried out an in-depth survey sponsored by the Ford Motor Company, with statistical analysis conducted by NOP Media. The survey was designed to explore:

- the 'work-life balance' during the transition to parenthood
- women's attitudes towards work and babies
- access to family-friendly employment including parental leave
- problems parents experience, and their preferences.

Altogether, 1281 women responded: 93% already parents of pre-school children and 7% expecting their first baby. The sample was not nationally representative; it reflected the readership of the magazine, with most respondents (83%) having professional or skilled occupations (ABC1). However, its size provided clear indicators of important themes for new parents in terms of work-life balance. The survey was open to all parents but analysis has been carried out on the women only as so few of the respondents were men. The 24 dads who responded had an unusual profile: two thirds were either at home full-time or worked part-time, and three were currently on parental leave.

Results

More than half of the women (58%) who already had a child said their ideas about a good work-home balance had changed since they had had their baby. Certainly for those trying to balance having a baby and a paid job it wasn't easy reconciling the two. The women tended to say that they wanted to spend more time with their baby than they had anticipated, or that they found the demands of juggling work and family life too much of a strain to maintain over time (see Table 2.5.1). However, as in other studies, some women also said they found being at home looking after babies full-time left them feeling isolated and dissatisfied.

Initially I didn't want to return to work at all but I soon realized I needed to return 'for myself'. I was 'bored' and 'stressed' being a full-time carer. I soon 'craved' adult company – without children!

At the time of the survey, around two thirds of women were going out to work and a third of the women were either currently on maternity leave or 'at home full-time'. Almost three quarters of women (70%) were concerned about missing out on their child growing up, and many felt that they could provide the best quality childcare (42%). These factors, and a sense that their child needed them, were most commonly cited as motivating women to want to be their child's main carer. The factors that most motivated a return to work were:

- needing the money (61%)
- needing to get out and spend time with other adults (51%)
- needing to keep up to date in the job (33%).

We asked all the employed women who were currently pregnant (n=215) 'what work arrangements would you ideally like to have in place for when the baby is born?' Forty five percent said they would like to be their 'child's main carer' for at least the first few years. Another third said that ideally they wanted to be their child's main carer for a minimum of 12 months. So, around four out of five pregnant women feel they would prefer to be home with their baby for at least the first year.

Women in employment

Of those in employment, twice as many worked part-time compared with those working full-time. While almost a third said their ideal would be to work only 1-2 days a week, only one in six women had this arrangement in practice. A third wanted to work 3-4 days; the same proportion was working this length of

Table 2.5.1

Before my daughter Jessica arrived I thought I would return to work full-time without any doubt or fears. Jessica is now the most important part of my life. I have extended my time off to the maximum possible and will return when she is 7 months. I can't bear to think about leaving her – I would like to spend much more time with her than working will allow.

I thought working part time would help me to keep my 'hand in' at work and keep up to date so I can return full-time. (But) I am often tired and feel I do not devote enough time to the child or my job, or indeed my husband.

I had always thought that the right balance was for me to work 3 days a week and to be home with my baby for the other 2. I went back to work on this basis when he was about 7 months old. Everything was fine for a few months. Before I decided to leave work, I was finding that I would get very stressed at times and was often tearful for no particular reason. Daniel was not sleeping through the night. I was finding it difficult to enjoy anything!

I face 1.5 hours of commuting each way, picking up baby and settling her for the night, then eat, sort out bills, mail, etc, all the housework, all on my own. I never thought about these things before.

Table 2.5.2 Actual and preferred working arrangements for employed women with children

	Ideal (%)	Actual (%)
Maternity leave	12	19
Home f/t	13	-
Work f/t	1	16
Work f/t flexibility with no extended hours	6	4
Work 3-4 days	31	33
Work 1-2 days	29	17
Evenings	2	3
Weekends	2	1
Not stated	4	6
Total	100	100

n = 897

week, but not necessarily at the status of their choosing or competence. Only 7% said working full-time would be their ideal arrangement and most of these supported a suggested 'package' of more 'flexibility and no extended hours'. In practice only a fifth of the full-time workers said they had 'flexibility and no extended hours' (see Table 2.5.2).

Leave packages and flexible working

Maternity and paternity leave

Results from this predominantly ABC1 sample, show that a third of women were getting more paid maternity leave than the statutory minimum of 18 weeks. However, 30% said that their partner was given no paid paternity leave and 20% received just 1-3 days paid paternity leave. Only 13% said that their partner's employer provided over five days paid paternity leave.

Parental leave

Since December 1999, both parents have been entitled to 13 weeks unpaid parental leave up to their child's fifth birthday, but 45% of the women said either there were no arrangements in place at their work for the leave to be taken or they didn't know of any such arrangements. Just 11% said that they knew they could arrange to take unpaid leave if they booked it in advance in blocks of 1-4 weeks. However, 20% said they could work flexible hours from time to time, such as when their child was sick, and 12% worked flexibly in other circumstances, including working from home. Seven per cent said their employer provided some additional paid leave when needed for those with dependents.

Family-friendly employers

Only 20% of women went so far as to say that their employer lacked family-friendly policies or failed to be flexible and supportive in practice. But the responses to open-ended questions illustrate some of the problems working mothers encounter.

I worked for a US based multinational organization, fantastic policies for childcare breaks but when it comes down to it the reality is oh so different. On my return after my second child I persuaded them to allow me to return on a part-time basis (4 days/week) but I paid the price in terms of the type of job I was given... I accepted this for about 9 months and then asked to return to a full-time assignment in order to get back on track with my career. They made sure they gave me the most inappropriate job for a mother of 2 young children. I had to travel to the US for at least 1 week a month and I only got that after many arguments. Initially they wanted me to go for a 6-week stint!

I never realized how difficult things can be with my husband working between 10-14 hours a day. I was really hoping to obtain a part-time job as I work for a very large company that in theory has a lot of family-friendly policies. But it's always at the discretion of your manager, so no one has to respect it.

It was not just managers who posed a problem for parents of young children trying to juggle their family and work commitments:

My husband and I both work shifts in the same department. It has been fairly easy to fit my 2 x 5 hour shifts in around my husband's 37.5 hour week. But it hasn't been all plain sailing, as we get comments from older working mums. The older mums feel unfairly treated, as there was no paid maternity leave, or flexible shift patterns when they were pregnant.

And in terms of facilities, even large employers were offering little help.

I am very disappointed. My employer, an NHS Trust (6,000 employees), has no crèche; they like us to take antenatal appointments in our own time and offer no private room for breastfeeding mums to express milk.

And childcare was a problem, particularly for parents working long shifts on jobs requiring 24-hour cover:

I love my job and will be sad to give up a profession I have enjoyed and spent years training for. It's hard to believe that hospitals and police services cannot arrange flexible childcare for their staff. They consider it easier to lose staff than to support parents. Paid childcare is impossible to find to cover shifts that end at 1am, or last 7am to 7pm.

Although few women criticised their employer, a clear relationship emerged between employers' attitudes and the quality of women's lives. Three quarters of those who felt that their employer was family friendly were happy with the balance they were able to achieve between work and family responsibilities and time for themselves. This compares dramatically with just one third of mums who said that their employer wasn't flexible and supportive in practice saying they felt they had the balance right. Looked at from the other perspective, two thirds of those in our study who felt their employer was not family-friendly and supportive were not happy with the balance in their lives.

Effects on family and health

Over half of the women said it was stressful (42%) or very stressful (13%) trying to work out arrangements that were right for all the family. As well as not seeing enough of their children, or not having enough time for themselves, a number of women commented on wanting more time with their partner. High numbers reported feelings of anxiety or depression during the last twelve months that they coped with on their own (33%) or with support from their partner, family or friends (35%). A further 13% said they had sought professional help.

Discussion

There is a wide variety of experience among mothers of young children. For some the positive aspects of going out to work, a pay packet, social contact with other adults, and the opportunity to keep up to date in the workplace outweighs the stresses of long hours, constant juggling and the potential for feeling neither job is being done well enough. Having a supportive employer clearly makes a very significant difference.

McRea has constructed a typology based on the varying work histories of different groups of women (McRae, 2001). The 'I want a career and child' type typically returned to work within a year of their first child's birth and stayed in full-time jobs. Many of these, mainly professional women, experienced marital disruption. Ten years on, 73% of those who had a partner when they became a mother were still together. The second group, described as 'I want children and a job', also returned to work within a year of having their first child and stayed employed subsequently, but they worked part-time in order to balance their work and family lives. Their marital relationships were significantly more stable, with 92% still with their child's father ten years on. The third group of 'my family comes first' mothers went back to employment later and had a more intermittent employment history, mixing periods at home with part-time and full-time work. Some of the youngest mothers were included in this group and those who achieved less in the labour market. The final group, for whom 'my family is my job', gave up paid employment when they became a mother, though often not by choice but because of difficulties finding work or affordable childcare.

Given the tendency among women to attempt to cover up the evidence that they are finding it difficult to cope, midwives seeking to provide individualised care may find it useful to ask women in employment about what support or difficulties they encounter at work. This may be a way into uncovering how much stress a woman is under without asking the woman directly to reveal things about herself she finds it painful and exposing to admit. Miller emphasised that for women in her study 'presentation of self as a coping and competent mother to those perceived to be experts became an over riding concern' (Miller, 2002). Women finding it difficult to cope often feel angry with themselves, inclined to low self-esteem and guilt. They crave kindness and understanding but fear others will judge them harshly. Ironically, the more vulnerable a mother feels the more she fears she has to lose by admitting her feelings.

All those working with parents can help them in their efforts to achieve a balance in their lives by ensuring they know about their employment rights and opportunities, and the changes being introduced in April 2003. These include two weeks paid paternity leave, 26 weeks paid maternity leave plus the right to take a further 26 weeks unpaid extended maternity leave. In addition, employers will be encouraged to increase flexible working arrangements, with a legal obligation to consider requests for flexible working from employees who are parents of children under the age of six or of a disabled child under 18 years old (Maternity Alliance, 2002).

Conclusion

Despite the increased numbers of women combining employment and motherhood, doing so poses challenges and creates stress that can have a negative effect on their health and relationships. There is clear evidence that employers who are flexible and supportive enable more mothers to achieve a better balance between their work and their young children. Enabling parents to achieving a sense of balance is good for mums and dads, good for children, and good for workforce morale and retention. The NCT welcomes the legislative changes that will improve leave and pay around childbirth and encourage flexible working.

REFERENCES

Anderson M. 1994. Today's families in historical context. Family and Parenthood: Seminar Papers. York: Joseph Rowntree Foundation
Boulton MG. 1983. On being a mother. London: Tavistock Publications
Bradshaw J. 1996. Family policy and family poverty. Policy Studies, 17(2), 93-106
Department of Health. 1999. Our Healthier Nation. London: DOH
Gavron H. 1976. The Captive Wife – conflicts of housebound mothers. Middlesex: Pelican
Goldthorpe JE. 1987. Family life in Western societies: A historical sociology of family relationships in Britain and America. Cambridge: Cambridge University Press
Maternity Alliance. 2002. New maternity rights in 2003. Maternity Action, 90, 10-11

McRae S. 2001. Mothers' employment and family life in a changing Britain. Final report to the ESRC. www.regard.ac.uk/cgi-bin/regarding/showreports.pl?ref=R000223137
Miller T. 2002. Adapting to motherhood: care in the postnatal period. Community Practitioner, 75(1), 16-18
National Family and Parenting Institute. Listening to ethnic minority parents. London: 2001
Oakley A. 1979. Becoming a Mother. Oxford: Martin Robertson
Straw J, Anderson J. 1996. Parenting. London: Labour Party
Sure Start. 2001. Making a difference for children and families. Nottingham: DfES Publications www.dti.gov.uk/work-lifebalance

The Practising Midwife 2002; 5(9): 22-25

Give dads a chance!

Baby massage for fathers

Lynda Leach, Karen Taylor

As part time midwives at the Birth Unit of the Hospital of St John and St Elizabeth in North London, we hold weekly sessions for babies born at the Birth Unit. We alternate facilitating the sessions. One of us leads the class whilst the other observes and helps with any baby who is unhappy. We find that this works well and gives the parents individual attention, when appropriate.

Fathers, although welcome, rarely attend the weekly sessions held on Wednesday mornings due to work commitments. The inability of fathers to attend was felt to be a disadvantage and therefore we started monthly Saturday morning sessions a year ago. The Fathers sessions have now become a regular activity, with requests for more Saturday sessions. On average, ten fathers and babies attend the monthly Saturday sessions. As with the Wednesday classes, there is no obligation to pre-book.

The format for both the weekday and Fathers classes is similar. Cards are put in front of each father to assist both us and the other fathers. The cards show the father's name, the baby's name and the baby's age. The fathers sit in a semi-circle on the floor on cushions with their babies in front of them. To provide a relaxing atmosphere, candles and aromatherapy oils are used and classical or new age music is played. Fathers are given an opportunity to introduce themselves and their babies, say where they live and say whether or not they are familiar with baby massage techniques. New friendships are often formed when people discover that they live quite close to one another. Five minutes are spent on relaxation and releasing tension.

During the massage, each father is encouraged to focus on his baby and observe their cues. Towards the end of the session each father is involved in his own activity with his baby. It is lovely to see them all interacting in different ways. After the massage, which lasts about twenty minutes, an hour is devoted to refreshments and informal chat. On rare occasions where there is not much interaction, we introduce discussion topics such as 'How do you feel when your baby cries?' or 'How did you feel returning to work?'

Fathers are encouraged to attend the sessions without their partners if:

- their baby has attended at least one mid-week session
- it is not the first time they have been left in sole charge of their baby
- their baby has recently been fed or will accept expressed breast milk or formula.

If the baby is fully breast-fed and may require a feed, the mothers are encouraged to sit at the back of the room and to become involved if needed. These criteria, formulated on the basis of practical experience, are designed to help fathers who dislike appearing incompetent in front of their peers. In practice, many mothers arrive with their baby and partner and then leave to have a chat and coffee with the other mothers.

Massage helps fathers to bond with their babies and to understand when their baby wants to be touched or wants to be left. Massage also helps with communication. One father was heard to say, 'It's a long time since I spoke your language but I am listening to you'. In addition, the massage sessions give fathers an opportunity to meet other fathers, to see other babies of similar age, to observe their baby's development and to see how their baby interacts with other babies and with adults. Also, the sessions incorporate practical advice on dealing with crying, colic and constipation. The massage sessions provide fathers with an enjoyable activity apart from changing and bathing their babies. It gives fathers more confidence in handling their babies. It particular, first-time fathers can see how this confidence develops with second and third time-fathers.

Fathers are still regarded primarily as providers. They are not expected to be carers. Instead, fathers are 'assigned the more tertiary tasks' (Cook, 1995). Mothers see themselves as the primary caretaker of their babies and this can cause the fathers to feel less competent in this area, leading to ill feeling on the part of both (Watson et al 1995). At this early stage, a pattern of non-involvement by fathers can be set for the whole of the baby's life (Jafarzadeh, 1999). Fathers at massage sessions are not, for once, merely in a supporting role. 'Visitors to the hospital briefly shake your hand before bombarding mother and baby with attention' (Howard, 1995). At the Fathers massage sessions, the fathers and their babies are the focus of attention for one and a half hours. One father said that he couldn't remember the last time somebody made him a cup of tea. 'If midwives want to provide holistic care for women and their newborn infants they must extend their practice to include men' (Lester &

Moorsom, 1997). Fathers have been acknowledged as sufferers of postnatal depression, as well as women (Sullivan-Lyons, 1998). Baby massage and postnatal support groups have both been seen to help ease this condition. (Cooke 1995; Watson et al 1995; Lester & Moorsom 1997; Sullivan-Lyons 1998; New Generation 1999; Brooker 1994; Adamson 1996). Fathers should therefore have access to both baby massage and postnatal support. If the needs of the father are not met, how can we expect him to meet the needs of the baby?

We have derived great satisfaction in facilitating both the weekly and weekend baby massage sessions. Having often met both parents antenatally and during labour, it has been rewarding to meet them postnatally as a family.

REFERENCES

Adamson S. 1996. Teaching baby massage to new parents. Complimentary Therapy in Nursing and Midwifery, 2, 151-9

Brooker E. 1994 One bump or two? The Guardian, 12 April, 16

Cooke E, 1995. Tears before bedtime – from dad. The Independent,1 February, 23

Howard I, 1995. A neglected role? New Generation, 14(2), 10

Jafarzadech J. 1999. Turning men into fathers: boot camp for new Dads. Childbirth Instructor, March/April, 20-1

Lester A, Moorsom S. 1997. Do men need midwives: facilitating a

greater involvement in parenting. British Journal of Midwifery, 5(11), 678-81

Need a hand, Dad? 1999, New Generation, January, 19

Sullivan-Lyons J. 1998. Men becoming fathers: "Sometimes I wonder how I'll cope". In: Clement S (ed). Psychological perspectives on pregnancy and childbirth. Edinburgh: Churchill Livingstone

Watson WJ, Watson L, Wetzel W et al. 1995. Transition to parenthood: What about fathers? Canadian Family Physician, 41, 807-12

The Practising Midwife 2002; 5(3): 26-27

Parent education:
meeting the needs of fathers
Judith Schott

Whilst acknowledging that some women have female partners and labour companions, this article focuses on how antenatal classes can meet the needs of expectant fathers. Good antenatal classes can offer men a unique opportunity to prepare for birth and fatherhood. However classes do not always meet fathers' needs (Nolan, 1994; Donovan, 1995; Smith, 1999a), and some classes are 'endured and not enjoyed' (Barclay et al, 1996). Some men are keen to come to support their partners and to learn alongside them (Smith 1999a). However, some may be genuinely worried about what might be expected of them. One father said coming to classes 'was like entering a women's Masonic lodge'.

Men expecting babies

Expectant fathers have real and legitimate needs. These need to be addressed, not only because the wellbeing of fathers is essential for the wellbeing of the mother and the baby, but also because the father too is facing one of the biggest life changes he is ever likely to experience. Everything is shifting: his relationship with his partner, his perceptions of himself, his lifestyle, his relationships with his parents, her parents and with his peers. He may be concerned about restricted freedom, increased responsibility and earning capacity. He may be worried about his partner's wellbeing, the health of the baby and his own ability to offer support.

Some men may not have any contact with men of their own age who are already fathers. Media images do not help, as positive role models are few and far between. Portrayals of fathers are often mocking, their concerns tend to be ridiculed, and they are often depicted as absent, unsupportive, inadequate or abusive (Burgess, 1997). It is not surprising therefore that some men feel uncertain about their new role.

Gender conditioning can affect men's ability to acknowledge their concerns and their willingness to seek support. Like women, men are strongly influenced by the expectations that society and their peers have of them. The stereotypical man is tough, strong, decisive, knowledgeable, competitive, and in control. He may equate masculinity with dominance and resort to aggression when he feels threatened or powerless. He downplays and disguises any feelings of helplessness, uncertainty, weakness, or sensitivity, does not admit to anxiety or fear and does not cry (Clare, 2000).

Of course the male stereotype is a generalisation. Personalities and attitudes vary from person to person. In addition, society's expectations of men are constantly changing and many men adapt accordingly. Most men want to be supportive because they love their partner and want them and the baby to be safe. However, many men are likely to be confused and uncertain about their role (Lewis, 1999). They are more likely than women to be isolated, and less likely to talk about relationships, feelings and fears. Yet a great deal is expected of expectant and new fathers. They are required to be gentle, sensitive, intuitive and aware, qualities that in other settings might be labelled 'unmanly'. In the labour ward he is expected to be a 'hand maiden' and to cope, with little or no preparation or support, with unpredictability, powerlessness and the stress of seeing his partner in pain and difficulty without being unable to do much about it (Hallgren at al, 1999). Men may feel better if they can provide practical help in labour but many women prefer 'quiet support' which can be harder to give (Somersmith, 1999). Despite these demands, men often receive little input. They are seldom encouraged to express their needs and feelings, and may not be offered the support skills and information they need. In short the father is 'the most neglected member of the family' (Bennet, 1998).

Like the women they accompany to classes, men bring with them their own feelings and needs as a well as a lifetime of experience. Class leaders are much more likely to be aware of the practical and emotional needs of pregnant women than of expectant fathers. The key to discovering men's needs is to listen to them when their partners are not there. When women are present, their perspective tends to take over. Men tend to censor what they say in order to protect their partner and may keep quiet about their concerns because they do not want to seem selfish (Szeverènyi et al, 1998; Somers-Smith, 1999).

Class leaders can improve their skills by taking every opportunity to listen to men. This can be done by dividing the class into single sex groups or by inviting only men from a class back to talk together after their babies have been born. Listening to male friends, relatives, colleagues and new fathers can elicit useful information. At home visits even a brief 'How are you?', while the mother is busy elsewhere can be enlightening. One new father burst into tears when asked this, and said, 'nobody else has asked me that. Not even my own mother'.

There are a whole range of questions that could elicit useful insight into the needs of fathers. For example:

- How did you feel during your partner's pregnancy? What changes did you notice yourself?
- What was it like for you coming to classes? What was good? What was hard?
- What was it like for you being at the labour and at your baby's birth? What did you feel prepared for? What would you have liked to have known more about?
- What was it like leaving your partner and baby in hospital after the birth? How did you get home? How did you feel?
- What was it like bringing your partner and baby home? What did you feel prepared for? What would you have liked to have known more about?
- What has been good and what has been hard about life with a new baby? What did you feel prepared for? What would you have liked to have known more about?
- What else do you think we should be saying to fathers in antenatal classes?

The class leader who takes time to listen to men will, over time, hear about a wide range of experiences and can adapt classes accordingly. It also enables the class leader to be conduit between new fathers and expectant fathers. A useful phrase is 'What many fathers say is...' Hearing what other men have said may be, for many men, a more acceptable way of taking on new ideas than being told what to expect by a health official.

Welcoming and involving fathers

Men can't just be tacked on to a women's course. They have to be included, from planning and publicity, to the actual work done in classes. Include a specific welcome to fathers in all written and verbal invitations to couples classes and to fathers' evenings. Consider every topic and activity from the father's point of view. Traditionally, classes, books and written material have focused mainly on the women's perspectives (Singh and Newburn, 2000) and perhaps on ways in which fathers can offer support. Men who come to classes are usually keen to know what they can do to help, but helping strategies alone are unlikely to prepare them for what they will experience. Although there are some practical things he can do to support his partner during labour, there are likely to be periods when all he can do is just 'be there'. This is the hardest role of all for many people, regardless of gender.

It is important to include the father's perspective not only as supporter, but also as a person who is experiencing life changing events. What will he see, hear, smell or touch? What feelings might the experience trigger in him? What information will he need to make sense of what is happening? What can he do to take care of his own needs and feelings? Try doing this for every single topic and issue that might arise during an antenatal course. Start by deciding what you would say to a men-only group. Then consider if you would change what you would say if women were present.

Having decided what to say to fathers, it is important to develop ways of conveying different perspectives to the women and the men in your class. Both need to know what might happen and why. Women need to know what it might feel like and how to help themselves. Men, on the other hand, need to know what they can expect to witness and how they might feel, as well as what support and comfort they could offer.

As well as topics common to both men and women, include the things that only fathers may experience. For example:

- arranging to leave work at a moment's notice when labour starts
- being a labour supporter and the feelings that this can evoke
- taking care of himself
- seeing his partner in pain or difficulty
- witnessing the birth of their baby
- being left abruptly outside the theatre during an emergency Caesarean birth
- being separated from his partner and baby when he leaves the hospital
- juggling the demands of a job, visiting hospital, keeping the home in order and fielding calls from relatives
- negotiating paternity leave or days off work to be with his partner and baby when they come home from hospital

- having to go to work after sleepless nights
- managing the conflicting demands of work and family life

One issue that is often not tackled in class is whether men want to be present at the birth. Although many men say that they would not have missed it for the world, and both men and women can benefit from being there together, it is important not to assume that his being there is the best thing for everyone. Some men may be terrified and squeamish. For some men, witnessing the birth has a profoundly negative effect on their emotional and sexual relationships with their partners (O'Driscoll, 1994). Class leaders can help couples to decide what is best for them by giving clear information about the physical and emotional realities of being a labour supporter, by offering the men practical suggestions about giving support and about caring for themselves, and by giving them space to reflect (Bartels, 1999).

Another neglected topic is what men do after the birth, especially at night. Most men will have missed at least one and possibly two or three nights' sleep. They will not have eaten properly for many hours and will have been through an extremely demanding and emotional experience. In the absence of rooming-in facilities, fathers are often encouraged to 'go home and sleep'. So they need to think about how they will get home and what support they might need. Public transport may not be available. Driving is not the safest option. Several midwives have spoken of sleep-deprived fathers having accidents on the way home and, tragically, of one fatality. Some fathers may welcome the opportunity to return to the peace and quiet of home, but others find it hard to be alone after such a momentous experience. Antenatal classes can offer fathers time to reflect on various options – having cash for a taxi, calling a friend to pick them up, staying with family or friends and so on – and to decide what they would prefer to do.

Involve fathers in everything

Everything the leader says should be inclusive. 'Your baby' applies to men and women; 'pressure on your back passage...' does not. Even the occasional use of 'you' or 'your' in a way that excludes the partners will cancel out all your assertions about this class being for them too. One way of avoiding this is to direct information to the women first and then to the partners. For example: 'At this stage women often feel pressure on their back passage, while their partners often notice that she catches her breath and seems to want to push at the height of contraction.'

Always involve men in practical work. Some may be very reluctant to join in, but with gentle encouragement most can be persuaded that this will be less awkward than sitting on the sidelines as a spectator. Invite them to try out relaxation and breathing for themselves and to receive a massage before they give it. During these activities, ensure that men look after themselves. Watch posture and positioning so that they avoid straining their backs when they support or massage their partners. Acknowledge how tiring it can be helping a woman in labour. Look at ways to ease the harder bits, and identify the things that men can do to take care of themselves and conserve their energy.

Fathers are expected to take an active part in caring for their babies and therefore have the same needs for information and skills as new mothers. Couples who learn together start off on an equal basis, while fathers who are left to learn from their partners can be at a disadvantage (Burgess, 1997: 131-5). Whether you are working with groups or individuals, antenatally and postnatally, involve men whenever you discuss or demonstrate practical aspects of infant care.

Opportunities for peer support

Antenatal classes can offer expectant fathers a unique opportunity to talk to each other. This is more likely to happen in single sex groups. This can be done by holding a fathers-only evening or, when the group is well established, by dividing the class into single sex groups. If there is a mixture of male and female partners, it may appropriate for male and female supporters to be together, or they may prefer separate groups. The best way to decide is to ask the participants what they would prefer.

If you want men to talk really freely, it is important to start by setting some ground-rules about feedback. Sometimes, simply giving people time and safety in which to talk and listen is enough. Not reporting back to the whole class often spurs couples into talking together after the class. If this is the plan, say so when you set up the groups and remind people that anything that is said in their group must remain confidential or be shared in a way that respects others' anonymity. Here are some suggested questions to trigger discussions in single sex groups:

- 'How do you feel about the prospect of labour?'
- 'What do you think will be good about being a parent? What will be hard?'

Because men have few models and few positive images of fatherhood, they can benefit from realistic and practical insights into the father's perspective. One way of doing this is to start a discussion on what men have heard from their male friends and relatives about being at the birth and becoming a father. Another way is to invite a new father to talk about his experience of labour, birth and the early days of parenting.

Visual aids, including slides and videos, should be inclusive. Anything shown to a mixed group should depict an involved and active man rather than an anxious-looking one sitting awkwardly in the corner. The focus on mothers could be balanced by displaying a collage of fathers holding, changing, soothing, bathing, or playing with their babies.

Fathers may come to classes willingly or unwillingly. Smith (1999b) describes three attitudes amongst the fathers in her study - 'totally committed, passive acceptor or reluctant attender'. Satisfyingly, she found that when class content and structure were relevant to a man's needs, reluctant attenders became committed. The implications are clear. What class leaders do to include men's needs makes all the difference.

REFERENCES

Barclay L, Donovan J, Genovese A. 1996. Men's experiences during their partner's first pregnancy: a grounded theory analysis. Australian Journal of Advanced Nursing, 13(3), 12-24

Bartels R. 1999. Experience of childbirth from the father's perspective. British Journal of Midwifery, 7(11), 861-3

Bennet HJ. 1998. Apgar scores for dads. British Medical Journal, 317, 1712

Burgess A. 1997. Fatherhood Reclaimed: The Making of the Modern Father: London: Vermilion, an imprint of Ebury Press

Clare A. 2000. On Men: Masculinity in Crisis. London: Chatto and Windus

Donovan J. 1995. The process of analysis during a grounded theory study of men during their partners' pregnancies. Journal of Advanced Nursing, 21, 708-15

Hallgren A, Kihlgren M, Forslin L. 1999. Swedish fathers' involvement in experiences of childbirth preparation and childbirth. Midwifery, 15, 6-15

Lewis C.1999 Transition into fatherhood, In: Transition to Parenting: an open learning resource for midwives. London: The Royal College of Midwives Trust

Nolan M. 1994. Caring for Fathers in Antenatal Classes. Modern Midwife, 4 (2), 25-8

O'Driscoll M. 1994. Midwives, childbirth and sexuality: men and sex. British Journal of Midwifery, 2(2),74-6

Singh D, Newburn M. 2000. Becoming a father: men's access to information and support about pregnancy, birth and life with a new baby. London: The National Childbirth Trust

Smith N. 1999a. antenatal classes and the transition to fatherhood: a study of some fathers' views. MIDIRS Midwifery Digest, 9(4). 463-8

Smith N. 1999b. antenatal classes and the transition to fatherhood: a study of some fathers' views. MIDIRS Midwifery Digest, 9(3), 327-30

Somers-Smith MJ. 1999. A place for the partner? Expectations and experience of support during childbirth. Midwifery,15, 101-8

Szeverènyi P, Póka R, Hetey M. and Török Z. 1998. Contents of birth-related fear among couples wishing the partners presence at delivery. Journal of Psychosomatic Obstetrics and Gynaecology, 19(1), 38-4

The Practising Midwife 2002; 5(4): 36-38

Pregnancy

I have already mentioned in section 1 that I have recently been interviewing women about their experiences of pregnancy, childbirth and mothering, and something one of them said to me has stayed with me ever since. 'Emma' is in her thirties and she gave birth last year. She was a fairly small woman who had experienced quite a lot of intervention during her pregnancy because her baby was perceived to be 'small for dates'. Only afterwards did it dawn on her that all the technology had provided was a measure of what was perceived as 'the problem' – there was nothing that the midwives, doctors or their machines could do to make her baby grow more. Her baby had no problems when she was born and appeared to me to be 'just the right size' for the woman and her partner. The words she used that stayed with me were that she had previously thought pregnancy would be a time where she could 'sit in the garden and bloom'; instead, she was faced with constant worry and invasion from professionals and machines.

One of the great things about the kind of research that we term qualitative is that, while it might only explore the experiences of a few people (a fact which is sometimes challenging to those of us who have been raised to believe that, when it comes to research, larger samples are better), it does explore those experiences in depth. And, when it comes to our attempts to appreciate what pregnancy in this ever changing, information-filled, medicalised world is like for women, there is a great need for more depth in our understanding. In this section, Zevia Schneider's research article both highlights the diversity of women's experiences and pulls out some of the issues that remain key to women, such as control, information and support.

Several of the articles in this section go on to explore aspects of information and support in more depth. Early pregnancy care is one relatively recent initiative, and Jo Coggins' article explores this area, asking why some women are dissatisfied with some forms of early pregnancy care and considering what they would prefer. Debbie Howells then offers information and research findings in one specific area: that of exercise in pregnancy, while Hilary Pilcher and Kim Lyon look at the needs of one particular group – teenage mothers – and how we can effectively support and be with these women.

Another mini-theme concerns preparing for parenting during pregnancy, and two articles discuss the eternal dilemma, often discussed by midwives, of enabling pregnant women to see beyond birth. Judith Schott and Judy Priest look at how we can put 'life after birth' on the agenda during parent preparation sessions and Andrew Julian Wiener writes about his experience of observing midwives running such sessions and makes some suggestions for change. Judith Schott and Judy Priest also argue that, although it has disappeared from the agenda of some sessions (perhaps because of constraints on midwives' time) teaching relaxation and breathing are still an essential part of parent education.

A lot of attention has been placed on CTGs recently, although the focus has tended to be on CTGs in labour. It is important not to forget that many women encounter this technology during pregnancy as well, and Shirley Andrews' article looks at some of this issues raised by the use of this intervention. As she notes, technology has certainly changed the midwives' role, but I'd like to think that we could still help women find a space, amongst the mass of things we offer them (in the name of informed choice) in which, if they would like to, they could sit and bloom.

An Australian study of women's experiences of their first pregnancy

Zevia Schneider

Objective: to describe women's experiences and perceptions of their first pregnancy.

Design, setting and participants: a qualitative study, using grounded theory. Data were obtained from 13 women whose interviews were tape-recorded and transcribed. Interviews were conducted in the women's homes on three occasions during pregnancy.

Findings: the women's experiences were varied and diverse. Most had difficulty coping with the physical and emotional symptoms of pregnancy. Loss of control caused anxiety. Need for support emerged as important. Antenatal education classes were favourably commented upon, however, the women wanted more information on breast feeding, baby feeding/sleeping patterns and behaviour, and self-care.

Key conclusions and implications for practice: midwives committed to a wellness, woman-centred model of care and willing to provide continuity of care should endeavour to implement this model in the hospital environment. Teaching in the ward or childbirth/parenting programmes should not be compromised by midwives who believe that pregnant women cannot learn. A comprehensive review of the philosophy, content, delivery and evaluation of current childbirth/parenthood programmes should be undertaken, together with a review of the qualifications and aptitude of educators conducting the programmes.

Introduction

Pregnancy has the distinction of being an event that is culturally, socially, and physically transformative (Davis-Floyd 1988), and, must therefore, of necessity be viewed in the context in which it occurs. The conventions and mores surrounding a birth in any particular culture play a major role in prescribing for the woman and her family appropriate behaviours and how the birth will be conducted. The meaning and interpretation a woman gives to events in her pregnancy are uniquely hers and become a source of discovery, of new information, rather than verifying other women's experiences.

Pregnancy and birth have cultural and biological definitions (Davis-Floyd 1992). Herein lies the paradox. A pregnant or labouring woman must negotiate many alternatives. Firstly, the medical model espouses, indeed prescribes, behaviours for the health-care system (Glikison 1991). The medical model of care is an illness model; it focuses on standards and outcomes (Brodie 1999), and views birth as potential pathology where anything can go wrong at any time (Lazarus 1994). This is a doctor-dominated model. The woman is thus viewed as a patient dependent upon the health professionals. In the patient role, the woman is 'habituated to the idea that others know better and she is dependent on being told' (Duden 1993, p. 29).

Secondly, there is much evidence that midwives perpetuate the prescriptions while often encouraging the women in antenatal classes to question these same prescriptions (Hancock 1994). The women are likely to experience confusion and conflict in situations where the midwives themselves are entrenched in the medical model of care and in such situations it is probably less stressful for the women to accept the dependent patient role (Callaghan 1993). Indeed, it appears that many midwives 'are content to function as obstetric nurses and do not have alternative professional ambition' (ACMI 1999, p. 17).

Thirdly, feminists and some midwives, champion a woman-centered, holistic approach to pregnancy and childbirth (Gregg 1995). This approach is congruent with a wellness model of care, where the woman feels in control of her pregnancy and labour and in a position to exercise choice and options. In this model, women are encouraged to ask questions and to participate in making decisions about their care.

In Victoria, Australia, the women wanted to 'have more information and resources to help them make informed choices about their health care' (Women's Health Resource Collective, Victoria 1993 p. 14). Further, it appears that Australians are demanding less intervention in childbirth (Summers 1998). However, the messages received during her antenatal visits and antenatal education programme have engendered a list of acceptable behaviours; the community, and often her own preference, may be urging her to behave otherwise (Victoria Women's Council 1995).

The midwifery models of care attempt to address the women's demands for a midwife primary carer (Goer 1995, Johnston 1998), and increased choice and control over their pregnancy (Davies & Evans 1991, Campbell & MacFarlane 1994, Rowley 1995, National Health & Medical Research Council 1996). Also, there is a notable paucity of published research on, and evaluation of, preparation for childbirth and parenthood programmes in Australia during the past 20 years considering the importance placed on antenatal education classes (O'Meara 1993). There have only been five published studies on the operation of antenatal education programmes in Australia and New Zealand despite obstetricians supporting the concept and recommending attendance to women in their care (Redman et al. 1991). This small study attempts to gain a comprehensive appreciation of the women's experiences and perceptions of pregnancy and the meanings they attach to those experiences.

Methods

Two qualitative research approaches were used in this study, namely the grounded theory method of data collection and analysis and a feminist, phenomenological interviewing technique, sometimes called 'phenomenological interviewing'. This interviewing technique refers to 'an interviewee-guided investigation of a lived experience that asks almost no prepared questions' (Reinharz 1992, p. 21). Feminist approaches 'have in common a focus on the everyday world of women, work with methods appropriate for understanding the very lives and situations of women, and understanding is a

means for changing the conditions studied' (Kvale 1996, p. 72).

In this study an *emic* or insider's point of view (Spradley 1979) was adopted. It is important to gain an inside perspective of the women's experiences of pregnancy, because the researcher needs to see and understand the women's experiences during their pregnancy, and the meanings they attach to those experiences, as they themselves see them.

Sampling

Following approval by the universities and hospital Ethics Committees, flyers advertising the study were placed on the appropriate notice boards. Women interested in participating in the study phoned the researcher. The nature and purpose of the study were explained, and, in addition, an information sheet was posted to each woman who met the criteria for the study, namely, in her first pregnancy, being able to read, speak and understand English, and living in Melbourne, Australia. A consent form was signed and witnessed at the first interview.

Sample size was not pre-determined and interviewing continued until saturation occurred, that is, no new data emerged regarding a category and categories are well developed (Strauss 1987, Rice & Ezzy 1999). Thirteen women participated in the study. Tape-recorded interviews were conducted with 13 women at the end of each trimester of pregnancy. The interviews were conducted between June 1998 and August 1999 in the women's own homes by the principal investigator and lasted about 60 minutes. Face-to-face interviews in a familiar and comfortable environment facilitated the process. In order to ensure confidentiality and anonymity, each woman's real name was changed to a pseudonym.

One or two broad questions, such as 'How would you describe being pregnant to a friend?' and 'Describe your feelings and the events surrounding your most positive/negative interactions during your pregnancy with family or friends' were used initially as a prompt to begin the conversation. Additional explanation and clarification were sought when needed.

Data were analysed from the transcribed tape recordings. Thirty-nine interviews were transcribed. Open coding was used to reduce the data into concepts and develop categories (Strauss & Corbin 1990). The units of analysis, words, phrases and sentences were compared for similarities and differences. Data were broken down, interpreted and given conceptual labels. The concepts were related by means of statements of relationship and a conceptual scheme developed (Strauss & Corbin 1990). Significant meanings and interpretations of these units were then coded and categorised into groups. A major feature of the grounded theory method is that data collection and analysis occur simultaneously; this is called *the constant comparative method* and *the asking of questions* (Strauss & Corbin 1990). Concurrent with these analytic processes is reference to the literature, *theoretical sensitivity*, all of which facilitate the development of 'a theory that accounts for much of the relevant behaviour' (Glaser & Strauss 1967, p. 30).

The following steps were taken to satisfy the requirements of credibility, fittingness, confirmability and auditability. Colleagues skilled in the paradigm listened to a few tapes, read the verbatim transcripts and compared their interpretations with those of the investigator's category scheme. In addition, each woman received a hard copy of her transcript by post within a few days following each interview. This strategy was important because it provided the opportunity for the women to read the transcript and make any corrections. It also provided the occasion to note modifications to the transcript and seek additional clarification when required. Finally, it helped verify what the women said and meant in a way that would satisfy me that I had understood them. A stamped addressed envelope was enclosed for the return of the transcript. Audit trails were created for each of the three interviews to demonstrate how categories were formed. These were confirmed by colleagues.

Limitations associated with this study are self-selection of the sample. Given the demands of the study, the length of the study (about seven months) and three interviews, it is likely that the women were highly motivated to participate. Also, the study provided the occasion to share the entire experience with someone, outside their social circle, interested in hearing about their experiences, and having some knowledge in the area. An advantage of having highly motivated women in a study is that they are more likely to fully share and disclose information about their experiences because they want to. Also, the women were, generally, well educated and one could assume this group would be more articulate. The aim of qualitative research is not to produce generalisable findings but 'the sample units are typically representative of a class or group of phenomena' (Sarantakis 1994, p. 15). However, the findings provide the opportunity for practising midwives to compare them with the situation in their clinical area.

Findings

The participants were 13 women, aged between 25 and 42 years experiencing a first pregnancy. Ethnic family background for one woman was Australian Chinese, and Anglo-Saxon for the remaining 12. All were Australian born. The women were well educated in the main: all but one woman had a degree or diploma. Eleven women were employed full time until the 34th week of gestation, one woman was engaged in part-time teaching, the other was unemployed.

The women shared their experiences and perceptions of pregnancy and any events which related to their condition. All the women had 'booked' into a hospital for birth. Inducted from their accounts of antenatal visits, were the models of care the women experienced. Analysis of the data occurred by trimester. Subcategories were identified for the physical, emotional, and cognitive symptoms, interaction with family and friends, and interaction with the health-care system. Most of the women had difficulty coping with the physical and emotional changes. The concept of control, need for support, and the antenatal education classes emerged as important issues. The women wanted more information on breast feeding, infant feeding/sleeping patterns and behaviour, and self-care.

The women's quotations appear verbatim. It will be noted that the women experienced and reported on the symptoms in many instances in similar vein. Perhaps an awareness, on the part of the health professionals, of the intensity and unexpectedness of the women's experiences and their apparent lack of knowledge, may dispose health professionals to review the information they provide at antenatal visits and the kind of information they impart at childbirth/parenthood classes. A summary of the findings including some verbatim comments the women made follow according to trimester.

Portrait of the first trimester – 'a world turned upside down'

Subcategories identified were: physical, emotional, cognitive, interaction with family and friends, and interaction with the health-care system. A core category was developed and labelled Adaptation to pregnancy. This label was subsequently changed to Adjustment to pregnancy. The reason for the change was that adapting to a situation implied an active process requiring some action on the part of a woman, whereas adjusting to a situation appeared more passive. The data show that most of the women were indeed passive and somewhat incapacitated. It was difficult for them to adapt to a situation so transitory and unpredictable in nature.

The physical symptomatology was categorised as 'dis-ease' because it best describes the discomfort the women experienced. The emotional symptoms were categorised as 'ambivalence' to describe the sometimes conflicting attitudes they had towards their pregnancy, and the cognitive symptoms as 'disorientation', a word which encompasses a lack of focus, feeling vague, difficulty concentrating, and loss of memory. The remaining two subcategories related to interaction with family/friends/colleagues labelled 'support', and interactions with the healthcare system labelled 'information seeking'.

Dis-ease – the physical subcategory

The division of pregnancy into trimesters was maintained because this is the model the women encountered during antenatal visits. The women experienced in varying degrees the dis-ease of the physical symptoms and ambivalence which resulted from feeling out of control. They were concerned by these feelings because they believed that pregnancy should be a source of great joy and a time of well-being:

I feel a bit like a vessel, it's all just happening to me. (Grace)

There was no pattern to the nausea and vomiting. Each day was different. I couldn't anticipate how I would be feeling. The nausea was indescribable – it just came over in waves. (Beth)

I felt an emptiness in my stomach all the time – I had to eat and then I would feel nauseated and sometimes vomit – then I had to eat again. I felt I needed to eat through the nausea. (Amy)

Ambivalence – the emotional subcategory

Ambivalence was experienced because the women's expectations were not congruent with reality. All the women, with one exception, had planned their pregnancy and all were very happy to have their pregnancy confirmed:

I was quite delighted because I'd always been of the belief that this would not be something that comes easily. I was keeping myself back a little bit from it, so that I wouldn't be disappointed if it wasn't true. (Merryl)

It's almost like there's something taking place in my body that just takes over – it's filled me with joy. (Maureen)

Two women experienced only breast tenderness, the others who experienced more than one symptom were surprised by the suddenness and discomfort of the symptoms, and just how incapacitating they were. They said: 'Why didn't anyone tell us we would feel this bad?' There were other reactions too:

I did experience ambivalence, there were definitely some 'buts' – a lot of reflection, a lot of questioning of my life and my relationship, things that I hadn't really questioned before. (Beth)

I expected to feel excited, beautiful and radiant – I wish someone had told me about the emotional roller coaster of it. I'm still excited but oh! this isn't what I thought it would be like. (Penny)

Six women believed that they had become more emotionally labile, however, no woman reported experiencing mood swings.

I just find I cry so easily, I mean... watching the news or hearing a sad story, the tears just well up in my eyes. (Merryl)

I cried one night watching a 10-minute segment of trashy Bay Watch. When this happened my husband said: 'Oh God, you're going peculiar!' – but it was after all a funeral scene! (Margie)

Most of the women experienced anxiety about labour; some about the possibility of having a miscarriage or fetal abnormalities.

Disorientation – the cognitive subcategory

Six of the women believed that they had become forgetful, or vague, or had difficulty concentrating:

I have forgotten a few things at work. My boss pointed out a few mistakes and said: 'Oh! Of course, you're pregnant!' (Merryl)

Concentrating has been hard but I don't think it's affected my ability to think. (Grace)

I'm generally prone to forgetfulness, but since I'm pregnant it's increased. I had been told by other women that this would happen and I also read about it. (Maureen)

Some women who were working said they felt very tired and lethargic but did not feel cognitively impaired in any way:

I have a lot of responsibility at work. I've worked above and beyond my normal role so I don't expect to become dull-witted which people tell me you do. (Jane)

I haven't become vague. I see about 15 patients a day and I can give you information about these people without having to go back to the files. (Margie)

I'm not vague, or forgetful, or confused. I'm just very tired. (Penny)

Support – interactions with family, friends, and work colleagues subcategory

The need for support became obvious for most of the women when their dis-ease caused by the symptoms of pregnancy began. The women's feelings of loss of control, reinforced by their lack of ability to alleviate the symptoms, made some of them feel fearful and uncertain. They were unashamedly forthright about their need for support from family and friends, and also from the health professionals.

All the women said that their family, friends, and colleagues were supportive and interested in their pregnancy. Work colleagues were notably more protective: they gave them a lighter workload and assisted with some activities like carrying files or moving patients:

I get advice from everyone. I'm feeling special. I feel very cared for. (Margie)

My family and everyone at work are happy for me – they have become more protective, more concerned. (Susan)

Seeking information – the interactions with the health care system subcategory

All the women were seeking information of some kind or another during the first trimester. First, confirmation of their pregnancy, then advice on the nature of the symptoms and how to cope with them. Most of the women had one consultation with the doctor, or their general practitioner, or for those women having 'shared care', the doctor and the midwife. All had at least one ultrasound. In general, the visits were spoken about positively, however, three women found their appointment with the doctor frustrating. They felt they were 'herded' in and out of the doctor's room, not given the opportunity to ask questions, and one woman said the doctor did not even look at her during the consultation. The women's interactions with the midwives were spoken about in very positive terms. Some positive and negative comments about their interactions follow:

I like the environment at the birthing centre, and I found the midwives very caring, knowledgeable, and calming. They've been great! (Beth)

The person who did the ultrasound didn't give me a chance to look at the baby – he was moving the probe around so quickly. He was so business-like. Then I met the midwife. She was wonderful, warm, open and very approachable. (Susan)

I had some spotting early on and went to hospital. The midwives gave me incorrect information about abortions but I didn't know any better at that stage, so I went home and waited for the miscarriage to happen. (Maureen)

Most of the women had heard about 'birth plans' from the midwives, but only one woman considered writing one. In general, the women felt it would be inappropriate to write a birth plan because they said they had no idea what to expect.

Control

Control was a concept that appeared in all five subcategories. Various questions occurred to me during the analysis of these data, for example: Is there a link between feeling a loss of control and anxiety? Is anxiety related to fear of not knowing what physiological or psychological changes to expect? Is anxiety related to not knowing if and how they will cope with the changes? Does ambivalence about the pregnancy result when a woman experiences loss of control? What does the woman mean when she says: 'I need to be in control?' Does she mean in control of her behaviour? In control of any procedures and decisions related to her pregnancy, labour, and delivery? In control of the direction and course her pregnancy, labour, and delivery might take? Or does she mean something else?

The women were asked to clarify what they meant by needing to be 'in control'. Their answers were not self-explanatory and an example of how they felt when they were not in control was asked for. The following examples, together with my interpretation of what I understood was being said, follow:

I was remembering saying to my mother that it's the first time in my life that I haven't felt in control. I'm not in control any more and it's made me aware of… I've never thought about it before – of almost what a control person I am in a way, and that's not necessarily a good thing, but I've always thought I support myself and basically I'm in control of myself. Now it's just all happening to me and I really don't have any control. (Beth)

Here Beth demonstrates awareness of the changes that are occurring and recognises the difference between her self-perception of herself as being in control and discomfort with the present situation where things are 'just all happening to me'.

I get panicky. I get childlike. I lose my centre and I get panicky. I cry. I just dissolve into tears. So I lose my centre. I lose my adult and that's the danger for me. (Maureen)

Maureen recognised her anxiety and became dysfunctional when she was not in control. She needed to be in control in order to manage her emotions.

The feeling of 'loss of control' has properties (frequency, degree, extent, intensity, and duration) and dimensions (often-never; more-less; high-low): dimensionalising provides specificity to the feeling (Strauss & Corbin, 1990).

The following examples from this study demonstrate that 'control' is a matter of degree and intensity:

Researcher: *How would you react if you didn't have the control that you wanted?*

Susan: *I suppose I would get quite frustrated.*

Researcher: *How do you show your frustration?*

Susan: *I'm usually pretty vocal about it. I hope the hospital walls are sound proof!*

and,

Researcher: *How did you react to the situation with the health professional at hospital X when you had some spotting during the first few weeks of your pregnancy?*

Maureen: *I cried. I mean I came back home and lay on the sofa and just dissolved into tears.*

The women interpreted the concept of 'needing to be in control' in a variety of ways. Two women hoped they would be in control of their bodies again once the symptoms in the first trimester had passed; four women wanted to have the opportunity to discuss alternatives with the health professionals and be part of the decision-making process; one woman wanted to make the decision about whether students would be permitted to view the birth; four women wanted to make the decision about intervention; one woman wanted total control over the process and progress of her labour and delivery, and one woman said she would dictate the intervention.

Portrait of the second trimester – 'Getting back on track'

All the women experienced a return of energy in varying degrees. Generally, they felt well physically and were once more able to eat the foods they liked. Only one woman said she felt 'high', but no one reported feeling euphoric at any time. Similar questions to those asked in the first trimester interview were asked.

Well-being – the physical subcategory

Generally, the women were feeling well. Those who had previously undertaken some form of exercise such as walking, swimming, yoga, and aerobics, resumed these activities. The high points during the second trimester were the cessation of fatigue, nausea, and vomiting, although three women continued to feel nauseated for six to nine weeks into the second trimester. Half the women spoke about having a return of energy, others only that they felt much better. The only low point was the discomfort when sleeping caused by an enlarging abdomen.

At the second interview (26-28 weeks gestation), each woman was invited to respond to some of the comments she had made about her pregnancy at the end of the first trimester. This was done in an attempt to discover the extent of the disparity, if there was one, between how they felt then and how they were feeling now. Two women said they felt like frauds because they had not experienced nausea or vomiting or other discomforts of pregnancy (apart from some breast tenderness); a third woman, while not experiencing nausea or vomiting complained of feeling bloated, and of soreness in her abdomen and legs. These women reported that their pregnancy had made no difference to their lifestyle; indeed, apart from tiredness, they were asymptomatic. Other women had different experiences:

My energy levels have returned. I still feel tired now and then but it's a reasonable sort of tiredness. The last 12 weeks have been much better. I feel as though I'm coping again. (Jane)

When they talk about the minor disorders of pregnancy, sometimes I think some of them aren't so minor. The word 'minor' makes you feel almost, well, I'm not coping with this very well. I've noticed that I don't tend to talk about the discomfort or awful aspects – I guess it's because I don't want to sound like a failure. (Beth)

At the end of the second trimester other discomforts had arisen:

The centre of gravity has shifted forward with this huge stomach and that's quite strange. It's quite awkward to sleep. I didn't realise how awkward you would feel. (Susan)

I've noticed now that when I get up in the night to go to the toilet I've sort of got to roll out of bed – I can't just get up. And I can't do up my shoes or bend over easily. (Barbara)

I've had to change my lifestyle a lot. I've become more confined to home. It's an effort now even to walk for 10 minutes. (Maureen)

Feeling better – the emotional subcategory

At the first interview (11-14 weeks gestation), all but one woman said that they were normally inclined to be emotional, and six women believed they had become more emotional. Of these women, one was feeling 'high', four remained emotional, and one woman said she still sometimes felt angry with her partner:

I must admit I still am emotional, and I wonder if it's the pregnancy or the problems at work. (Merryl)

I normally cope very well with my husband away, but this time I felt devastated and the day he left I bawled my eyes out without really knowing why – I just felt sort of detached. (Diane)

I still get a bit upset at times but I think it's because my husband doesn't understand me or what I'm going through. (Maria)

Forgetful – the cognitive subcategory

The seven women who reported no cognitive changes (ability to think clearly, vagueness, loss of concentration, memory loss) during the first trimester, experienced no changes during the second trimester. Two women who had experienced cognitive problems reported that their difficulties had passed, and four women reported still experiencing some problems:

It's not like it was in the first trimester – now it's just silly things that I would be doing and saying – things that I should have known. My colleagues say: 'Ah yes, it's the pregnancy'. (Maria)

I often think: What was I doing? And I can't remember. And I'm still forgetting things. (Barbara)

I still occasionally forget what I'm doing but it's getting better. (Maureen)

These women believed that the fatigue and nausea they had experienced were a major factor in their forgetfulness and inability to concentrate. Others had heard or read that 'you're supposed to get vague when you're pregnant'.

Comfort – interactions with family, friends, and work colleagues subcategory

'Feeling comfortable' captures the mood of how all the women experienced their interactions with the people in their environment. Workloads were adjusted, and health professionals reported being given assistance with heavier cases and replaced by other staff when clients were having X-rays or radio-active implants:

When they know you're pregnant – they treat you as fragile. (Sheila)

My family seem to be a lot more concerned about me and make a bit more of a fuss, and though it was strange to start with, it's quite nice. (Margie)

Eleven colleagues at work are pregnant so it's no novelty. We're all complaining of the same things. The only difference that I've noticed is that I've ceased to be known by my name. I am now called 'mom'. And I say 'No, no, I'm Susan, and I have an identity somewhere!' (Susan)

A few women expressed disappointment at their family's reaction to their pregnancy. They felt that some family members were not as interested or supportive as they would have liked them to be:

For years my mother has been saying: 'Get pregnant, get pregnant', you know, because I'm 35 now, and then once I got pregnant, it was just 'well, you've done it now, and that's that' – no more interest. (Maria)

People walk into you when the supermarket is crowded. They don't care. But one day at the petrol station a young man held the door open for me. I wouldn't have got that at any other time at a service station. (Sheila)

Acceptance – interactions with the health-care system

Concurrent with the new found sense of physical and mental well-being, was the acceptance that their pregnancy and delivery may not be straightforward, and that they may not always be in control of events. Some women had additional ultrasounds and four women had genetic screening tests.

There was a marked change in the women's affect when they discussed the ultrasound procedure which they considered the highlight of the pregnancy. They experienced fear and anxiety before, and sometimes during, the ultrasound until the sonographer indicated that all appeared well with the fetus:

The ultrasound was great. The sonographer was very professional and informative. It was lovely to see the baby. (Merryl)

It was just amazing! Before I had the ultrasound I thought: Am I really pregnant? But then I saw the arms and legs and I knew there was something there. It was just so hard to comprehend. (Maria)

Control

During the second interview, only seven women appeared interested in discussing their feelings about control. The focus had changed from wanting to be in control of events to accepting responsibility, being assertive, and making choices based on knowledge:

I've been reading a lot and I've realised I'm not on my own in having anxiety and fear about what's in store for me. I think the authors are encouraging us to take responsibility and make choices. (Susan)

I feel more grounded but that doesn't mean I'm in control. I've relinquished control to a degree. I can't control the changes – I think I've accepted that. (Maureen)

I want to make decisions about my care, and if the doctor says you should do X, I want to be in a position to discuss it with him, but he knows better than I do and will make the ultimate decision. (Diane)

The women wanted information about the progress of labour and delivery and to participate in a meaningful way in decisions about their care.

Portrait of the third trimester – 'Feeling a little better, but when will it end?'

The third trimester extends from about 27 to 40 weeks gestation although a 'term' pregnancy may be from 37 to 41 weeks gestation.

Discomfort – the physical subcategory

The third trimester interviews were conducted at 36 – 38 weeks gestation. The physical symptoms were highly variable. A return of tiredness or fatigue was experienced. Sleeping or lying down was a problem for most of the women. Five women experienced heartburn; they were eating smaller meals and eating their last meal of the day earlier than usual to avoid heartburn. The women reported that their baby had 'dropped' sometime between 32 and 37 weeks gestation:

I've felt extremely well physically, emotionally, and cognitively. I know the baby has a good chance of surviving. I feel more confident about making plans. I seem to be getting through the day a lot better. (Amy)

This trimester has been difficult physically because of my high blood pressure and very swollen legs and ankles. I had to walk more slowly, I got tired so easily, and I couldn't catch my breath. (Barbara)

I don't know exactly when it was but I was feeling really good – I was loving being pregnant and enjoying this growing bulge in front of me. Lately I've started feeling tired again. It's different from the tiredness in the first trimester which was all consuming. This is a bodily tiredness. (Jane)

Every now and then I still get nauseated and vomit. My back aches and my feet get really tired. I have to stop and rest during the day. I feel energetic one day and flat the next. (Merryl)

Stable – the emotional subcategory

Stable is how most of the women felt emotionally during

the third trimester. It appears that the women did not, in general, experience increased mood lability or mood swings during their pregnancy, and in this respect, changes in emotional responses for these women, are not noteworthy:

I feel more stable now. I had an extremely stressful time at work – I was anxious about getting maternity leave and being made redundant. I received very little support from other colleagues. (Merryl)

I had heard a lot about emotional changes and was expecting this 'blast', but it never arrived. I think I've been more relaxed even in this pregnancy. (Jane)

The only time I got upset was when the doctor dismissed my complaints. He knew I was a medical practitioner. If he could intimidate me like that, I'd hate to think of how other women would feel. (Grace)

Normalcy – the cognitive subcategory

Of the six women who experienced cognitive dysfunction during the first trimester, two women felt that they had returned to normal by the second trimester and four women still reported problems into the early weeks of the second trimester. Two women expected their cognitive problems to continue because 'it's hormonal':

I must admit that I've been checking myself a few times because I was scared that I might become vague. My colleagues told me that pregnant women become vague and forgetful during pregnancy. (Jane)

The nurses on the ward told me to expect mood and cognitive changes but I haven't. I have no difficulty remembering my patients or their details. (Margie)

I started to write things down to make sure I didn't forget what I was doing, so I don't know whether I was vague or just expected to be. (Merryl)

Needing assurance – interactions with family, friends, and colleagues subcategory

The desire to keep in touch with family members and assurance that family would be available to them characterises the third trimester. They were socialising much more – 'eating out, having tea parties and making up for the time when I won't be able to do it any more'. There was a feeling of relaxation and excitement preparing the baby's room. They were feeling very heavy and tired, having difficulty getting around easily, experiencing interrupted sleep, and wishing it was all over:

I miss my mother a lot at the moment. I almost feel like saying to her: 'Just ring me every day at the moment mum' – I'm almost wanting that from her. (Beth)

My family has been great. My mother-in-law cleaned the house for me, my mother took three weeks off work to cook for

me, and my parents visit every second day. I feel very spoiled. (Grace)

I'm disappointed that my partner didn't take the classes seriously and he hasn't been much support around the house either. He whinges. My parents have been very helpful and supportive. (Sheila)

Teamwork – interactions with the health care system subcategory

The concept 'teamwork' best characterises the feelings and attitudes of the women at this time. They appeared to recognise the need for teamwork throughout labour and delivery. They had become familiar with their role in the health system and had all attended antenatal education classes. There was an impression that now they were reconciled to placing themselves in the hands of the health professionals in the cause of wanting a good outcome for their pregnancy. At the same time, most of the women did not want to totally relinquish responsibility or control.

Pain relief, epidurals, gas, and pethidine injection were discussed at the classes, and it appeared that most of the women intended asking for epidural analgesia soon after the commencement of labour.

For the women having 'shared care' it appeared that the postnatal hospital stay was limited to three days. For some, this was a source of concern:

We were told at the last antenatal class that the hospital has reduced the stay yet again. They've now cut it down to two nights and three days. It's just ridiculous. The midwife told us: 'It's now 48 hours post delivery, so that's why it's important to make the most of that time with us and learn what you want to learn'. (Merryl)

I won't be able to have my baby in the birthing centre now because it's breech. I'm very sad because I have got to know the midwives there and they have been fantastic, and the obstetrician too. I'm a bit annoyed now just realising how differently you are dealt with in the main part of the hospital compared with the birthing centre. (Beth)

There were also some positive comments about the doctors:

I feel lucky because I've got a doctor who will allow me some choice. Some obstetricians would automatically tell a woman with a breech presentation that she'll have to have a Caesar. But it's not necessarily so. (Diane)

My obstetrician is happy for me to make decisions. I'd like to think that I have some control over what happens to me, but if necessary, I may have to rely on the medical staff, that's what they're trained for. (Amy)

Antenatal education classes

When asked about their experiences in the classes, most

women were satisfied with the information about labour and pain relief, however, they indicated that they expected there to be some information on how to look after their baby and about breast feeding. They were disappointed that these issues were not addressed comprehensively:

There was nothing much on baby care. That's what my husband and I actually commented on – that they focus so much on that day – on labour and delivery, like only in the last half hour, well, OK, now we've got this baby, what do we do with it? (Merryl)

They spoke about baby massage but didn't demonstrate it, also baby's sleeping patterns but not much about infant care as such. They were pretty much saying: 'There's no rule', and if you have any worries, give them a call. (Beth)

I've spoken to other girls and we all thought that they could have put a bit more into the baby side of things. I mean they'll teach us a few of those things in hospital but by that stage we'll all be in such shock we won't know what's going on. (Beth)

We had one session on parenting. A couple came back to the class with their 16 week old baby to talk about the first 6 weeks at home. Everyone was very focussed on parenting. (Diane)

Breast feeding

Most of the women had received some information about the benefits of breast feeding, but generally the let-down reflex, potential difficulties with inverted or flat nipples, various positions for feeding, or how to get the baby to 'latch' on or attach to the breast were not discussed:

I think perhaps one of the most important things I learned in the classes about breast feeding is that if things aren't going right you don't just plod on, you ask for help before the situation gets too bad. I know of so many women who are put off early, and I dearly want to breast feed. (Amy)

They didn't tell you much about breast feeding and the problems. They just said that there was a Nursing Mothers' Association. They could just as well have given us a sheet of paper with instructions on it – it would have been more useful. (Grace)

Discussion

There are many personal intervening variables that may influence a woman's experience of pregnancy and the meanings she attaches to those experiences. While the literature indicates that there are some commonalities among experiences (Stoppard 1996, Adelaide 1997, Eisenberg et al. 1997, Fallows 1997, Llewellyn-Jones 1998), there are clearly many differences too. The factors that influence a woman's pregnancy include her philosophy on life, health status, education, culture, financial status, support network, life experiences, her partner and important others in her life, and not least of all, her own particular needs and expectations.

All the women reported changes in partner and family relationships, and this finding appears to be common (Stoppard 1996, LeBlanc 1999). Support was very important to all 13 women. They felt insecure and sought frequent reassurance that important others really wanted this pregnancy. This extended to health professionals also. There are studies on support during labour (Kennel et al. 1991, Davis-Floyd 1992, Fallows 1997), but little information on the need for, and importance of, support throughout pregnancy. The support a pregnant woman receives may play a major part in how she feels about herself and thus, her life experiences.

Control emerged as an important issue particularly in the first trimester. Control is mentioned in some literature (Stoppard 1996, LeBlanc 1999). One study reports that in a sample of 61 mothers, more than 60% rated their birth performance poorly because they did not feel in control (Mackey 1990). In her in-depth anthropological study Davis-Floyd (1992) identified women who 'seem to judge most situations by the degree of control they feel they can maintain' (p. 195), and Maushart (1997) suggests that perhaps women need to 'sustain an illusion of control' (p. 114) over their bodies.

The classes were probably the major source of information for the women, and while studies (DiMatteo et al. 1993, Everitt et al.1993, McKay & Yager-Smith 1993, Barclay et al. 1997) have repeatedly indicated that women want information about parenting, the programmes do not reflect consumer needs. Childbirth/parenting classes were considered helpful but pregnant women and their partners wanted information on baby care, behaviour, sleeping patterns, and self-care. Conflicting and sometimes unhelpful information was given which resulted in confusion. Other studies show that the classes did not prepare the women for the reality of birth and parenthood (DiMatteo et al. 1993, MacKay & Yager-Smith 1993), and that women wanted more information about infant care, feeding and behaviour (Imle 1990, Hiser 1991,). Regarding programmes, the Review (1990) identifies several areas of need: lack of clarity on principles for childbirth education, absence of accreditation process and standards for childbirth educators, and inadequacies in the educational preparation of health professionals. In a survey of public and private sector agencies in the Australian Capital Territory (ACT), O'Meara (1993) found that goals and objectives were poorly defined, and planning and co-ordination were inadequate. Leach (1994, p. 241) says that childrearing is probably the most onerous life task people undertake, and yet society offers less preparation for it than for any other task.

Breast-feeding advice and experiences have been

discussed at length in the literature (Donnelly et al.1986, Eisenberg et al.1997, Kitzinger 1997, Maushart 1997). The women related the same issues and concerns others have been reporting over the past 15 years. It is likely that the ability, or lack thereof, to breast feed, may have a marked effect on a woman's perceptions of herself as a new mother.

Similarly, information about cognitive changes during pregnancy appears in the popular literature (Stoppard 1996, Eisenberg et al. 1997, Fallows 1997). Llewellyn-Jones (1998) believes a pregnant woman 'no longer has the clarity of mind and precision of thought she had before pregnancy' (p. 205) and she fears she is becoming 'cow-like', and LeBlanc (1999) thinks that as pregnancy progresses a woman's thinking 'may become a little scatty' (p. 41). In their study, Ales and Norton (1989) found no changes in ability to concentrate or in emotional status, that is, ability to cope with stress, and Schneider (1989) found no changes in ability to think or learn during pregnancy. Some women were told to expect changes (forgetfulness, absentmindedness, difficulty concentrating) by the midwife conducting the class. This advice appears contrary when pregnant women are about to attend childbirth/parenting classes for the purpose of learning about important issues and could well affect how she feels about her ability to cope with a new baby.

The women's experiences in this study are neither exhaustive nor conclusive. In the most personal and intimate aspects of feelings and meaning, the experiences remain unique, and for many women the enormity of the experience may remain non-verbal and untold to the researcher.

Implications for health care

Pregnancy is a difficult time for most women and health professionals are in a position to make the experience comfortable and satisfying for women. Since antenatal education classes appear to be a major source of information for pregnant couples, it is of concern that pregnant couples are not given adequate information about baby development and behaviour and how important it is to interact appropriately with the baby from the time she or he is born. The many hours spent discussing the stages and progress of labour, that may or may not eventuate, could be more usefully spent discussing parenting issues. Clearly, antenatal education classes need to be stringently evaluated.

Health professionals should focus on preparing women for the often dramatic changes in the first trimester at their antenatal visits because usually childbirth/parenting classes only begin at 28 weeks gestation. The shock and distress the women experience could thus be circumvented. It would be benefcial to pregnant couples if the person conducting classes could explore with them their understanding of 'natural' childbirth, their need for support, the issue of control, and the couple's coping mechanisms. Such a discussion would be helpful in preventing feelings of disappointment or failure if their ideal of 'natural' childbirth is not achieved.

Current programmes should be examined with a view to establishing national guidelines (e.g. philosophy, teaching/learning strategies, content, evaluation). Educators conducting classes should be appointed on the basis of their teaching qualifications, aptitude, and knowledge.

REFERENCES

Adelaide D 1997 Mother love 2. Random House, Adelaide
Ales RL, Norton ME 1989 Changes in functional status during pregnancy. American Journal of Medical Sciences 297: 355-360
Australian College of Midwives Inc 1999 Reforming midwifery: a discussion paper on the introduction of Bachelor of Midwifery programmes into Victoria. Australian College of Midwives Inc, Melbourne
Barclay L, Everitt L, Rogan F et al. 1997 Becoming a mother - an analysis of women's experience of early motherhood. Journal of Advanced Nursing 25:719-729
Brodie P 1999 The experience of Australian team midwives: implications for practice. Proceedings: Australian College of Midwives Inc. 10th Biennial Conference, Melbourne.
Brown S, Lumley J 1994 Satisfaction with care in labour and birth: a survey of 790 women. Birth 21(1): 4-13
Callaghan H 1993 Health beliefs and children: Is it illness or a normal life event? Journal of Australian College of Midwives 6(1): 7-11
Campbell R, MacFarlane A 1994 Where to be born? The debate and the evidence, 2nd edn National Perinatal Epidemiological Unit, Oxford
Davis A, Evans F 1991 The Newcastle community midwifery care project. In: Robinson S, Thomson A (eds) Midwives,

research and childbirth, Vol 2. Chapman & Hall, London
Davis-Floyd RE 1988 Birth as an American rite of passage. In: Michaelson K (ed) Childbirth in America.
Anthropological perspectives. Bergin and Garvey, Beacon Hill, Mass
Davis-Floyd RE 1992 Birth as an American rite of passage. University of California Press, CA
DiMatteo MR, Kahn KL, Berry SH 1993 Narratives of birth and the postpartum: analysis of the focus group responses of new mothers. Birth 20(4): 204-211
Donnelly C, Giblin R, Oddie U et al. 1986 Feeling our way. Experiences of pregnancy, birth and early parenting. Penguin Books, Maryborough
Duden B 1993 Disembodying women. Perspectives on pregnancy and the unborn. Harvard University Press, London
Eisenberg A, Murkoo HE, Hathaway SE 1997 What to expect when you're expecting. Angus and Robertson, Sydney
Everitt L, Schmied V, Rogan F et al. 1993 The postnatal experience of new mothers. In proceedings of International College of Midwives 23rd International Congress, Vancouver
Fallows C 1997 Having a baby. Tien Wah Press, Milsons Point, NSW
Glaser B, Strauss AL 1967 The discovery of grounded theory: strategies

for qualitative research. Aldine Publishing Co, New York

Glikison A 1991 Antenatal education - whose purpose does it serve? MIDRS Midwifery Digest 1(4): 418-420

Goer H 1995 Obstetric myths versus research realities. BerginGarvey, New York

Gregg R 1995 Pregnancy in a high-tech age. New York University Press, New York

Hancock A 1994 How effective is antenatal education? Modern Midwife 4(5):13-15

Health Department of Victoria 1990 Having a baby in Victoria. Final Report of the Ministerial Review of

Birthing Services in Victoria, Health Department of Victoria, Melbourne

Hiser PL 1991 Maternal concerns during the early postpartum. Journal of Academy of Nurse Practitioners 3(4): 166-173

Imle M 1990 Third trimester concerns of expectant parents in transition to parenthood Holistic Nursing Practice 4(3): 25-36

Johnston J 1998 An investigation into midwifery practice in Victoria. Australian College of Midwives Inc, Melbourne

Kennel C, Klaus M, McGrath S et al. 1991 Continuous emotional support during labour in a US hospital.

Journal of the American Medical Association 265(17): 2197-2201

Kitzinger S 1997 The new pregnancy and childbirth. Doubleday, Sydney

Kvale S 1996 InterViews. An introduction to qualitative research interviewing. Sage, USA

Lazarus ES 1994 What do women want?: issues of choice, control, and class in pregnancy and childbirth. Medical Anthropology Quarterly 8(1): 25-46

Leach P 1994 Baby and Child. Penguin Books, Middlesex

LeBlanc W 1999 Naked Motherhood. Random House, Australia

Llewellyn-Jones D 1998 Everywoman. Faber and Faber, London

Maushart S 1997 The mask of motherhood. Vintage, Sydney

Mackey MC 1990 Women's preparation for the childbirth experience. Maternal–Child Nursing Journal 19(2): 143-173

McKay S, Yager-Smith S 1993 What are they talking about? Is something wrong? Information sharing during the second stage of labour. Birth 20(3):141-147

National Health & Medical Research Council 1996 Options for effective care in childbirth. Australian Government Publishing Service, Canberra

O'Meara L 1993 Childbirth and parenting education – the providers' viewpoint. Midwifery 9:76-84

Redman S, Oak S, Booth P et al. 1991 Evaluation of an antenatal education programme: characteristics of attenders, changes in knowledge and satisfaction of participants. Australian & New Zealand Journal of Obstetrics and Gynaecology 31(4):310-316

Reinharz S 1992 Feminist methods in social research. Oxford University Press, Oxford

Rice PL, Ezzy D 1999 Qualitative research methods: a health focus. Oxford University Press, Melbourne

Rowley M 1995 Evaluation of continuous midwifery care. Final Report to the Commonwealth Department of Human Services and Health, Australian Government Publishing Service, Canberra

Schneider Z 1989 Cognitive performance during pregnancy. Australian Journal of Advanced Nursing 6 (3):40-47

Sarantakis S 1994 Social research. MacMillan, Basingstoke

Spradley JP 1979 The Ethnographic interview. Holt, Rinehart and Winston, New York

Stoppard M 1996 New pregnancy and birth book. Wing King Tong, Hong Kong

Strauss AL 1987 Qualitative analysis for social scientists. Cambridge University Press, Cambridge

Strauss A, Corbin J 1990 Basics of qualitative research. Grounded theory procedures and techniques, Sage Publications, Newbury Park

Summers A 1998 The lost voice of midwifery. Collegian 5(3): 16-22

Victoria Women's Council 1995 Getting to the heart of Victoria. Victorian Government, Melbourne

Women's Health Resource Collective and Centre for Development and Innovation in Health 1993 Mapping the models. Centre for the Development and Innovation in Health, Melbourne

Midwifery 2002; 18: 238-249

Early pregnancy care

Jo Coggins

A review of current literature reveals a wealth of research and information regarding antenatal care issues later in pregnancy such as screening, schedule of antenatal care, preparation for labour and breastfeeding and evaluation of antenatal education classes. In contrast, comparatively little exists regarding care in the first trimester. The Midwives Rules and Code of Practice (UKCC, 1998 pp17-18) states 'midwives are responsible for providing midwifery care to a mother and baby during the antenatal, intranatal and postnatal periods' and 'have a role in prescribing/advising on the examinations necessary for the earliest possible diagnosis of pregnancies at risk'. Why therefore do two of the largest European antenatal care studies (Clement, Sikorski and Wilson, 1996; Sanders, 2000) identify women's dissatisfaction with care received during this time? There is a considerable mass of evidence supporting the positive influence of early pregnancy care upon pregnancy outcomes, including perinatal/maternal mortality rates (Enkin, Kierse, Nielson et al, 2000) and women's choices regarding breastfeeding and homebirth (Pownell, 1994; Ward, 2000). Clearly, it is time for midwives to re-examine their role and responsibilities in the first trimester, and develop their practice accordingly for the sake of the profession itself and for the women and families it serves.

The article contains a concise review of the main anatomical and physical changes occurring in early pregnancy, considering both maternal body systems and that of the developing embryo/fetus. This is followed with discussion of the resulting physical, social, psychological and emotional needs of women during this time. Evidence to support this originates from a wide range of sources including databases such as MIDIRS, Bandolier, The Cochrane Library and Cinahl, a number of professional journals and a selection of midwifery textbooks. Anecdotal evidence, borne from my own clinical experience and discussion with friends and

family is also included. An understanding of the changes experienced by women in early pregnancy, and an insight into the needs that they have expressed, will demonstrate the relevance of the midwife's role at this time, and, importantly, how quality midwifery care in early pregnancy can potentially reduce complications later on, thereby increasing successful pregnancy outcomes and improving women's experiences. Potential benefits to midwives include greater job satisfaction and a reduction in unnecessary costs (Sanders, Somerset and Jewel, 1999), which may result in improved recruitment and retention of staff, thereby easing presently heavy workloads (Pownall, 1994).

Physiological changes occurring in the mother during early pregnancy

Following conception, the mother's body is subjected to a multitude of changes, largely determined by alterations in hormone levels (Bennett and Brown, 1999). Such changes facilitate development of the fetus and prepare the mother for labour and lactation. I have chosen to focus on just some of the main internal hormonal changes known to have a noticeable effect on the mother's feelings of physical and psychological wellbeing (see Table 3.2.1).

Six to ten days following conception, the trophoblast (early embryo) secretes human Chorionic Gonadotrophin (hCG), which in turn stimulates the corpus luteum to increase production of oestrogen and progesterone. This is to maintain pregnancy and prevent menstruation. Levels of hCG are significantly raised until approximately ten weeks of pregnancy, at which time the placenta becomes functional and takes over the role. A rise in hCG is associated with a number of extrinsic effects on the mother. Nausea and vomiting is experienced in over 70% of women (Sweet 1997), as is a heightened sense of smell often leading to a sudden

Table 3.2.1

Hormone	Effect of pregnancy	Internal effect on mother	External effect on mother
Progesterone	Increasingly secreted by corpus luteum from 0-10 weeks until placenta is functional	– Relaxes smooth muscle – Dilatory effect on vessels – Slower peristalsis/gut emptying – Softens ligaments – ↑ Plasma/RBC volume – ↑ Iron metabolism – ↓ Blood pressure	– Constipation – Heartburn – Muscular aches/pains – Anaemia – Tiredness – More prone to fainting
Oestrogen	Increasingly secreted by corpus luteum from 0-10 weeks until placenta is functional	– ↑ Proliferation of breast tissue and ductal systems – ↑ Vascularity of uterus – ↑ Hygroscopic effects on gums	– Breast swelling/tenderness – Gingivitis – Ptyalism
Human Chorionic Gonadotrophin (hCG)	Secreted by trophoblast from 6-10 days after conception	– Heightens olfactory senses – Alters taste – Alters thyroid activity and basal metabolic rate	– Dislike for noxious substances – Nausea – ↑ Appetite – ↑ Fat deposition
Melanocyte Stimulating Hormone (MSH)	Secreted by anterior pituitary gland from conception and throughout pregnancy	– Deeper skin pigmentation	– Body image issues – May lead to chloasma

distaste for odorous substances, i.e. coffee, tea, fried foods. It is also known to raise a mother's basal metabolic rate, leading to an increase in appetite (Bennett and Brown, 1999).

The gradual rise in oestrogen and progesterone accounts for a majority of the 'minor disorders of pregnancy' commonly experienced by women in early pregnancy. Until the introduction of more sensitive pregnancy tests, it was often these changes that first alerted women to their pregnancy. Oestrogen is responsible for proliferation of ductal systems in the breasts and can lead to the characteristic breast tenderness experienced by women within as little as four weeks following conception. James, Steer and Weiner et al (1999) report links between increased oestrogen levels and the disorders 'ptyalism' and 'gingivitis'. The former refers to increased salivation and is a result of oestrogen's hygroscopic effects, and the latter describes inflammation and bleeding of the gums. Although not known to be harmful, such a symptom could understandably be worrying to a pregnant woman unaware of its cause.

Progesterone has many functions in pregnancy including the relaxation of smooth muscle and peripheral vasodilation. The former can result in slower emptying of the gut causing 'heartburn', and more commonly, constipation. Ligaments and joints are also affected and may cause considerable aching, especially around pelvic and back areas. Anecdotal evidence from my community based colleagues suggests this is one of the most frequently reported causes for concern in women requesting advice, usually because the pain is feared to be related to miscarriage. The dilatory effect on a mother's blood vessels can result in a mild reduction in blood pressure and for some women may cause extreme tiredness or lightheadedness. A physiological rise in plasma volume of up to 50% occurs to counteract this.

Simultaneously there is a 20% increase in red blood cell production (erythropoiesis) to meet the demands of the developing feto-placental unit. This is known as a 'physiological haemodilution' although controversy exists regarding the potential for a pathological anaemia to occur as a result of insufficient iron to match the increased demands for haemoglobin synthesis during erythropoiesis. Coggins (2002) highlights the risk of iron deficiency anaemia in pregnancy for those women with insufficient iron stores at the onset. This may necessitate iron supplementation in later pregnancy and is associated with a number of physical and psychological issues for sufferers. Identification of such risks in early pregnancy enables midwives to offer women beneficial dietary advice that may prevent such an occurrence.

For 90% of women one of the earliest outwardly noticeable signs of pregnancy is deepening of skin pigmentation around the areola of the nipple (Sweet, 1997). This is a response to increased activity of Melanocyte Stimulating Hormone (MSH), a role of which is to increase deposition of melanin around the nipple in preparation for lactation. In later pregnancy it is responsible for skin changes such as the appearance of the linea nigra and the darkening of the perineum. In some women its effects can extend to the face and arms creating a 'pregnancy mask' (Enkin, Kierse and Nielson et al, 2000). This is 'Chloasma' and although not known to be harmful to mothers or babies, could potentially raise psychological issues for women regarding their body image and facial appearance.

Social and psychological issues in early pregnancy

Having outlined some of the physical changes experienced by women in early pregnancy, it is equally important to acknowledge the psychological and social issues, as the three areas are inextricably interlinked.

Two of the largest European antenatal studies – the South East London Antenatal Care Project (Clement, Sikorski and Wilson et al, 1997) and the Bristol Antenatal Study (Sanders, 2000) identified women's dissatisfaction with emotional and psychological support in early pregnancy.

This is concerning, considering that 'offering emotional support, advice and reassurance' is frequently documented as a fundamental aspect of antenatal care (Clement, Sikorski and Wilson, 1997; Sweet, 1997; Bennett and Brown, 1999; Dunkley, 2000). There are a number of psychological, emotional, social and cultural issues that may affect women's experiences of early pregnancy (see Table 3.2.2), and it is imperative midwives have an awareness of these issues and address them appropriately. This will encourage women to form partnerships with their midwife, in which, through mutual communication and understanding it is likely they will feel empowered early in their pregnancy, and therefore better prepared for issues and events arising in the second and third trimesters, and the postnatal period.

Development of the embryo/fetus during the first trimester

So far, emphasis has been on women's wellbeing in early pregnancy. However, additional evidence to support the argument for improving midwifery care in the first trimester is also found when considering development of the embryo/fetus during this time. There are some key facts relevant to midwives:

- Major regions in the embryo's brain are formed by the 4th week of pregnancy
- Organogenesis (development of fetal organs) is virtually complete by the 8th week of pregnancy
- Poor maternal diet is associated with cardiac malformations in developing embryos (Moore and Persaud, 1998).

Midwives hold equal responsibility for fetal and maternal wellbeing in the antenatal period (UKCC, 1998), so it seems ironic that a majority of women are first receiving midwifery care at a time when the most significant period of development in their baby's life has already occurred! Sanders (2000) found the average gestational age at booking to be eight weeks, with a significant proportion of women being seen even later, at nine to twelve weeks. Therefore, it would seem midwives are missing the opportunity to offer women vital information that could benefit the health of their unborn baby.

Table 3.2.2 Psychological, emotional, social and cultural issues in the first trimster

Is the pregnancy planned/wanted?
Changing body image (breast swelling, waist thickening)
Feeling unwell yet pregnancy not evident to others
Relationship issues/ lone mothers
Fears of miscarriage
Anxiety regarding transition to parenthood
Anxiety regarding screening and fetal wellbeing
Career/employment issues
Financial issues
Lifestyle changes/altered coping mechanisms
Religious/cultural traditions and expectations

Midwifery care in early pregnancy: what do women want?

Little research exists specifically regarding women's needs in early pregnancy, and many of the studies that are published were performed in America (Ciliska, 1983; Lane, 1997; Maybruck, 1988). However, during the South East London and Bristol studies (Clement, Sikorski and Wilson, 1996; Sanders, 2000) whose focus was primarily on women's satisfaction with the number of antenatal visits they received, it became clear that women want midwifery care earlier in pregnancy. In both studies, women expressed:

- The booking interview is too late to receive important dietary/lifestyle advice
- Given a choice, midwifery care is preferable to GP care in early pregnancy
- Talking with a midwife in the early weeks is reassuring and confidence building
- It isn't necessary to 'book' earlier but it is important to have access to a midwife either in person or via telephone during the early weeks
- Meeting a midwife earlier makes discussing sensitive issues such as screening easier
- Early contact with a midwife is beneficial to both nulliparous and multiparous women.

Midwives interviewed during the Bristol study (Sanders, Somerset and Jewell, 1999) agreed that women need improved access to care and advice when first discovering they're pregnant. 'Over-the-counter' pregnancy tests are now able to confirm pregnancy at three to four weeks (Enkin, Marc and Nielson et al, 2000) and it is crucial that women are able speak to a midwife at this time if they choose to do so. Despite these findings, access to midwives in early pregnancy still isn't routinely offered to women and in my experience women aren't informed adequately of their rights to midwifery care. For many women, the GP's receptionist continues to be the only point of contact prior to booking!

The benefits of early pregnancy midwifery care

The benefits of early pregnancy midwifery care are numerous. Not only do women gain a better service in which their needs are adequately met, it also offers midwives the opportunity to exercise another fundamental aspect of their role in the antenatal period. That is, to identify 'at-risk' pregnancies as early as possible and to address potential complications quickly in the hope of achieving a better outcome, i.e. referral of mothers with known medical conditions such as diabetes or epilepsy. Meeting women earlier in pregnancy also allows for earlier advice and support with lifestyle alterations, such as stopping/reducing smoking. Smoking is a known risk factor for undesirable pregnancy outcomes (RCM, 2001) and yet at present only approximately one quarter of all women who smoke give up in pregnancy (Enkin, Kierse and Nielson et al, 2000). Midwives have an increasingly active role in this and other public health issues, a matter that is now being addressed by government policy (DOH, 2000; RCM, 2001). The involvement of midwives in initiatives such as the 'Sure Start' programme further supports the argument for midwifery care in the early antenatal period, and ideally, preconceptually (Pownall, 1994).

Earlier midwifery care may also reduce the need for medical intervention in later pregnancy, which is associated with increased risk of intervention at delivery, including increased risk of induction of labour and Caesarean section (Villar, 1997). This has multiple effects. It improves women's experiences of pregnancy and childbirth by maintaining normality, and consequently reduces strain on services and costs by, for example, minimising the length of stay in hospital and reducing attendance at consultant clinics. This in turn, ensures the needs of those women requiring joint consultant/midwife care can also be met more effectively, i.e. less waiting time for clinic appointments.

Considering existing staff shortages and consequently heavy workloads, it is likely that midwives will have reservations about finding time to adjust current schedules of early antenatal care or introducing new early pregnancy services. I believe the issue of early pregnancy midwifery care is an example of where only slight change to existing services is necessary to reap a wealth of benefits. For example, there may be no need to introduce 'formal' clinics. Perhaps it is enough to offer a telephone service or to allocate a time of day when a midwife is available in her office if women want to 'drop in'. It would be interesting to hear readers' views and experiences, and to know how other midwives are addressing this issue.

Conclusion

This article has reviewed and highlighted the importance of midwifery care in the first trimester of pregnancy. Having revised the physical, psychological and emotional changes experienced by a majority of women in early pregnancy, I hope to have clarified the role of the midwife at this time, and the potential benefits of offering earlier midwifery care. Midwifery services should be sensitive to the needs of the women and families it serves, and in light of available evidence, the issue of care in early pregnancy would appear to be an area where perhaps we need to revise our practice and further our research, to examine the current services available to women in early pregnancy, such as 'early bird' clinics and 'meet-a-midwife' sessions, and discusses their effectiveness. Using recent government policies and position papers currently relevant to midwives' practice, emphasis needs to be placed on how existing early pregnancy services might be improved.

REFERENCES

Bennett VR, Brown LK (Eds). 1999. Myles Textbook for Midwives. 13th edition. Edinburgh: Churchill Livingstone

Ciliska DK. 1983. Early Pregnancy Classes as a Vehicle for Lifestyle Education and Modification. Canadian Journal of Public Health, 74(3), 215-217

Clement S, Sikorski J, Wilson J et al. 1996. Women's Satisfaction with Traditional and Reduced Antenatal Visit Schedules. Midwifery, 12, 120-128

Clement S, Sikorski J, Wilson J. 1997. Planning Antenatal Services to Meet Women's Psychological Needs. British Journal of Midwifery, 5(5), 298-305

Coggins J. 2001. Iron Deficiency Anaemia: A Midwife's View. MIDIRS Midwifery Digest, 11(4), 469-474

Department of Health. 2000. The NHS Plan: A Plan for Investment, a Plan for Reform. London: HMSO

Dunkley J. 2000. Health Promotion in Midwifery Practice: A Resource for Health Professionals. London: Harcourt Brace & Company

Enkin M, Keirse MJNC, Neilson J et al. 2000. A Guide to Effective Care in Pregnancy and Childbirth. 3rd edition. Oxford: Oxford University Press

James DK, Steer PJ, Weiner CP & Gonik B (Eds). 1999. High Risk Pregnancy: Management Options. London: Harcourt Publications

Lane B. 1997. Promoting a Great Start. International Journal of Childbirth Education, 12(2), 24-26

Maybruck P. 1988. Early Pregnancy Classes. International Journal of Childbirth Education, 3(2), 17

Moore K, Persaud T. 1998. The Developing Human: Clinically Orientated Embryology. 6th edition. USA: Harcourt Brace & Company

Pownall G.1994. Preconception Care: Are Midwives in Danger of

Missing the Boat? Modern Midwife, 4, 34-35

Royal College of Midwives. 2001. The Midwife's Role in Public Health. London: RCM

Sanders J, Somerset M & Jewel D. 1999. To See or Not to See? Midwives' Perceptions of Reduced Antenatal Attendances for 'Low-Risk' Women. Midwifery, 15, 257-263

Sanders J. 2000. Let's Start at the Very Beginning... Women's Comments on Early Pregnancy Care. MIDIRS Midwifery Digest, 10(2), 169-173

Sweet BR (Ed). 1997. Mayes Midwifery: A Textbook for Midwives. London: Bailliere Tindall

United Kingdom Central Council. 1998. Midwives Rules and Code of Practice. London: UKCC

Villar J, Khan-Neelofur D. Patterns of Routine Antenatal Care for Low-Risk Pregnancy. In: Neilson JP, Crowther CA, Hodnett ED, Hofmeyr GJ (eds). Pregnancy and Childbirth Module of the Cochrane Database of Systematic Reviews [updated 2 December 1997]. Available in the Cochrane Library [database on disc and CD-ROM]. The Cochrane Collaboration; Issue 1. Oxford: Update Software; 1998. Updated Quarterly.

Ward A. 2000. Early Pregnancy Sessions: A Formative Evaluation. The Practising Midwife, 11(3), 40-42

The Practising Midwife 2002; 5(9): 14-17

Exercise in pregnancy

Debbie Howells

Exercise is important for everybody to be aware of for healthy living, but also increasingly within special populations. We as midwives are working with one particular special population – pregnant women. If we are looking at the health of our clients and future generations it is important to have some basic knowledge in this area.

Exercise in the prenatal period has many benefits. These are listed in table 3.3.1.

In 1993 an American study found that healthy women who had exercised moderately throughout their pregnancy had perceived their labours to be less painful than those who had not exercised throughout. This is possible due to the increase in endorphin levels (Hanlon, 1995).

As with anybody starting an exercise programme, health screening is vital at the start of the programme and all the way through. Women know their own bodies and although the following article indicates the current guidelines and recommendations it is important to stress that they are guidelines only. Women should be encouraged to be in tune with their own bodies and exercise within their own comfort zones, which vary greatly from top athlete to new exerciser.

Table 3.3.2 indicates some important screening considerations prior to pregnant women starting an exercise programme. There are relative contraindications, which do not mean that a woman cannot exercise, merely that she should take extra caution or seek extra professional help first. Absolute contraindications, however, are when a woman should stop exercising and seek professional advice.

Exercise in pregnancy is about maintaining fitness in preparation for labour and birth, particularly with the more conditioned client. In the conditioned client, during the first trimester, provided there are no problems, they can continue working at their normal exercise level, excluding any highly competitive sports, or sports such as horse riding. Moderate exercise is calculated by heart rate, working at 70–75% MHR (Maximum Heart Rate) for 15 – 20 minutes, 2–3 times a week, which is known as the aerobic training zone. (Maximum heart rate = 220 - age x 70 or 75%)

Women will often find that they will achieve this rate

Table 3.3.1 Benefits of exercise in pregnancy

Improve minor ailments of pregnancy such as constipation and varicose veins (this is because of an improvement in circulation)
Increase endorphin levels
Reduce leg cramps
Help reduce normal pregnancy oedema
Decrease risk of intervention in labour
Better chance of quick postpartum recovery
Increased body awareness
Strengthened abdominal muscles
Enhanced muscular balance
Help with relaxation

Table 3.3.2 Contraindications

Relative contraindications
  Extremely under weight/over weight
  Essential hypertension
  Anaemia
  Thyroid disease
  Diabetes
  Multiple pregnancy
  Palpitations/arrhythmia
  Breech presentation after 28 weeks gestation
  (although more research is needed on this)

Absolute contraindications
  PIH (Pregnancy Induced Hypertension)
  Pre-eclampsia
  Cardiac disease
  IUGR (Intra Uterine Growth Restriction)
  History of three or more miscarriages
  History of premature labour
  Placenta praevia
  Unexplained vaginal bleeding

more quickly in their pregnancy – this is because of an increase in stroke volume and cardiac output, and hence the subsequent rise in RHR (Resting Heart Rate). The cardiovascular system is already working extra during pregnancy, so it is also important to stress to women that they should be aware of how they are feeling, and to keep themselves well hydrated and drink fluids before, during and after exercise. Theory books will often point out that the risks, and teratogenic effects, of overheating are worst in the first trimester, so adequate hydration is important. However, in healthy women, thermo–regulation changes, and pregnancy lowers the set point for sweating, so this improves the ability to keep the internal core cool once the temperature has started to rise (Clapp, 1998). A longer warm up and cool down (recovery period) would accommodate this.

Deconditioned women would also benefit from starting an exercise programme in pregnancy, however the recommendation here is to start at 50-55% MHR and build up, maintaining moderation for as long as they feel comfortable throughout their pregnancy. The old saying, 'a little frequent(ly) is better than a lot seldom' is certainly true, and deconditioned clients can experience beneficial effects just by starting at this level of 5 minutes building up.

Women can also work out their own intensity using Borg's scale of perceived exertion. This is a scale of how hard you think you are working during exercise. Table 3.3.3 shows these exertion levels. It relates to the responses experienced during exercise and is based on the correlation between perceived exertion, heart rate and oxygen consumption. For example, level 17 would indicate an approximate heart rate of 170bpm (very hard) (Premier, 1999). Women should generally not work harder than 13 (somewhat hard).

The main principals of an exercise programme should be FITT (Fitness Professionals, 2001) as described in Table 3.3.4.

Suitable aerobic exercises for the pregnant participant are low impact aerobics, aqua natal/aqua aerobics, gym programmes, brisk walking, swimming, prenatal exercise classes or studio cycling/spinning (however, studio cycling is only appropriate for the first two trimesters). It is important that if a pregnant woman continues in a mainstream class she tells the instructor that she is pregnant so that adaptations can be made for her.

A study in America by Clapp (1998) investigated the effects on the fetus of women who exercised through their pregnancy. The study looked at fetal heart rates during labour and found evidence that the babies of mothers who exercised moderately tolerated the stress of contractions much better, and there was a decreased risk of fetal distress. Clapp carried out umbilical cord sampling of the babies after birth, and found low levels

Table 3.3.3 Borg's rate of perceived exertion

6
7 very very light
8
9 very light
10
11 fairly light
12
13 somewhat hard
14
15 hard
16
17 very hard
18
19 very very hard
20

Table 3.3.4 FITT

F	Frequency (2-3 times per week)
I	Intensity (low to moderate) dependant on comfortable levels for women
T	Time (15-30 minutes is the current recommendation)
T	Type of exercise

of erythropoietin, which indicates that oxygen supply was more than adequate. Erythropoietin is a hormone found in amniotic fluid and is released when oxygen levels are low, stimulating the body to produce more red blood cells. This would show as high levels if oxygen supply were not enough. Also, the instance of meconium being passed in the utero in labour was much lower in the women who had exercised during pregnancy.

Conditions of the neonate in the exercising group were also examined, and although the babies generally had less subcuticular fat, they had no problems maintaining their temperature or blood sugars and generally adapted to extra-uterine life better than the control group, valuing intermittent stress and stimuli as a positive thing. Babies in the groups where mothers exercised appeared more settled.

It is suggested that the sound and vibratory stimuli provided by exercise before birth may also accelerate the development of the baby's brain (Clapp, 1998).

Muscle conditioning is an important component of any exercise programme but specifically in pregnancy it can also relieve common ailments. Posture changes in pregnancy mean that mean that women often have ante-prior pelvic tilt, which increases lumbar lordosis, particularly as pregnancy and the uterus enlarges. Working the transverse abdominis and contracting it with pelvic floor exercise will help decrease the lordosis, and also help with back pain and improve core stability of the trunk. The pelvic floor muscle group is the inferior wall of the trunk. In order to correct posture during pregnancy, tilt the pelvis under, pull the baby towards the spine and pull the shoulders back. As the breasts also enlarge, shoulders can become rounded and increase thoratic kyphosis. Working the upper back muscles, in particular trapezius and rhomboids, will help with this (Baum, 1998).

Ordinary curl-ups should not be done after 12 weeks because of the direct strain on the rectus abdominis muscle, and diastasis recti will occur in approximately 30% of pregnancies, more commonly in multiparous women (Egger et al, 2000).

Important points to consider are that women should avoid exercising in the supine position after 20 weeks because of inferior venal compression and supine hypotensive syndrome. Avoid any wide leg/abduction movements or squats in the last timester because of softening of the pelvic joint.

Many exercise classes specifically for pregnant women will have a flexibility and relaxation session. Stretching in pregnancy does help in prevention of muscle injury, but because of the increase in progesterone, softening muscle tissue, women should not developmentally stretch, and should do maintenance stretches only. The cool down will also prevent blood pooling to the extremities, causing sudden hypotension.

Summary

This article is a brief overview of a vast area of interest, in which we are learning that women can be encouraged to help their bodies cope with the physiological adaptations of pregnancy, and to enjoy what is a usually very special time in their lives.

Although the studies carried out have only been very small, moderate exercise has not shown any harmful effects in healthy pregnant women, and these findings encourage us, as healthcare professionals, to support women in their choice to exercise during pregnancy, with known beneficial outcomes for both mother and baby.

Further Reading

Baddeley S. 1999. *Health Related Fitness During Pregnancy*. Mark Allen Publishing Ltd
Champion N, Hurst G. 2000. *Aerobics Instructor's Handbook*. AC Black
Gallo B. 1999. *Expecting Fitness*. Renaissance Books

REFERENCES

Baum G, 1998, Before and after childbirth. In: Baum G. Aquarobics: the training manual. London: Harcourt, Brace & Co
Clapp J. 1998. Exercising through your pregnancy. USA: Human Kinetics
Egger N, Champion N, Boltan A. 2000. Special populations and exercise instruction. In: Egger et al. The fitness leader's handbook. London: AC Black

Fitness Professionals Tutorial Handbook. 2001. Pre & Postnatal fitness design. London
Hanlon T. 1995. Fit For Two: The Official YMCA Prenatal Exercise Guide. USA: Human Kinetics
Premier Training & Development Ltd. Training Manual: Exercise To Music. Trowbridge: Premier Ltd

The Practising Midwife 2002; 5(4): 12-13

Teenage pregnancy

A sociological and psychological perspective

Hilary Pilcher, Kim Lyon

The sociological exclusion unit's report (HMSO. 1999) on teenage pregnancy not only stresses the need to reduce teenage conceptions, but highlights the need to support those young people who elect to continue with their pregnancies, and consequently aims to reduce the long-term adverse effects associated with early parenting. So what aspects of support are effective in reducing the 'adverse effects' of teenage pregnancy?

The adverse effects of teenage pregnancy have been well documented (Irvine et al. 1997; Olaussen et al, 1999) and include increased incidence of pregnancy-induced hypertension, premature births and low birth weight babies.

However, the evidence to link adverse effects with teenage pregnancy per se remains controversial and some literature indicates that poor outcomes may be an indication of confounding factors such as belonging to a lower socio-economic group (Peckham, 1993; Barrel, 2000; Phoenix, 1989).

This article gives us the opportunity to reflect and share our practice and experience of supporting young parents. Hilary Pilcher is a midwife and has been in post as a Teenage Pregnancy and Parenting Co-ordinator since April 2000. Kim Lyon has a degree in Playwork and has worked for the health service for the last fourteen years. We hope that this article will dispel the myth for the reader that teenage parents are by definition inadequate parents, unable to cope with the complex and diverse roles of parent. They are in fact competent social actors in their own right (Qvortrup et al, 1994) and are able to make positive choices and decisions about their own lives and those of their children, even though they are still children themselves.

Our aim is to raise the parents' self-esteem, in the belief that they are more than able to be 'good enough' parents. This model of supporting parents through pregnancy and the transition to parenthood is in part influenced by the work of the parenting charity PIPPIN (Parents in Partnership – Parent-Infant Network). The model of support empowers parents by exploring issues that affect the individual parent, raising their self-esteem, and stating that:

'...Once this self esteem is gained, once parents feel good about themselves, each parent's secure experience can then help them to perceive their own child as someone worthy of respect, protection and security.' (Parr, 2000)

Training opportunities

PIPPIN was set up in response to a longitudinal study that 'examined the psychological needs of women, men and couples becoming parents' (Parr, 1997). The programme is thoroughly evaluated and has sound evidence-based principals and theories. There are various levels that can be accessed for training, from courses that enable facilitators to integrate PIPPIN's approach into ongoing work, to becoming PIPPIN Practitioners, Project Workers or trainers.

PIPPIN training programmes do not offer 'quick fix' solutions or 'off the shelf packages' but provide an opportunity to learn in a way that mirrors how effective parenting education programmes need to be facilitated. For some time, studies have given rise to concern that traditional parentcraft classes do not meet all the needs of parents, and in many cases are ineffective (Nolan, 1998; Hancock, 1994; Combes & Schonveld, 1992; RCM, 1999). From available evidence Parr (2001) summarises:

'...An overview of selected studies that suggests effective parent-based preventative interventions for the pregnancy and postnatal period need to:
- Begin early (preferably in pregnancy)
- Include a focus on interpersonal/ couple relationships
- Focus on the attachment relationship between parent and child
- Be delivered by suitably trained and supported individuals

- *Be evaluated*
- *The evaluation needs to demonstrate the progress by which the intervention achieved its benefits for effective and safe replication into the wider community.'*

Supporting the whole family

PIPPIN offers midwives an opportunity to experience a special way of 'being with' women. It also positively encourages fathers' involvement and increases awareness of the baby as an individual from the outset. PIPPIN focuses on the emotional and psychological needs of the family as a whole, and sessions are run in a supportive atmosphere not as instructional 'chalk and talk' classes. PIPPIN programmes and practice underpinned with PIPPIN philosophy give parents opportunities to gain confidence in their ability to make their own decisions around parenting, do not give unrealistic expectations of any aspect of the transition to parenthood, and promote the importance of communication.

Hilary completed PIPPIN training in 1999, which led to her PIPPIN Practitioner and Project Worker status. Since then PIPPEN has been integrated into her practice as a midwife. Prior to the training she felt that she practised reflectively, but she is now also able to reflect on how she was parented, how she is a parent and all of this impacts on her interactions with parents.

Kim has also completed a five-day PIPPIN programme, 'Educating For Early Family Life'. The course aimed to enable participants to refocus their approach to prevention rather than crisis intervention and to facilitation and support rather than teaching and directing.

Parent-infant attachment and interactions from birth all stem from the strong relationships that occur within a family and, as the child gets older, the relationships they form in the wider world. But an individual's feelings towards, and attachment to, his mother will last a lifetime. They can affect his sense of security in other relationships, and even during adulthood, at times of stress, this attachment behaviour will be revisited (Bolwby, 1998). This is especially prevalent during pregnancy when a woman seems to need her mother, to support and protect her through this transitional period. Optimal attachment makes it more likely that the parents and the greater community will be able to promote the healthy personality development of the child (Bowlby, 1998; Stern, 1998).

Window of opportunity

The intergenerational links to attachment behaviour must not be ignored or trivialised. Pregnancy is a 'window of opportunity' to explore feelings aroused personally about the pregnancy and the impact on the immediate and extended family.

Young people are often very open to reflective dialogue, and a floodgate of emotions can be opened. The issues raised are phenomenal and they must be explored and resolved before the parents-to-be can begin to discuss the needs of their own baby during pregnancy, labour and the early days of the child's life. Steele (1997) gives us strong evidence to support this, stating that

'...how infant-parent patterns of attachment reflect nurture more than nature comes from careful study of the childhood histories of parents.'

Fraiberg et al (1980) discuss these 'transient invaders', the ghosts from the past, the experiences of being parented. Fraiberg writes that although parents remember their own experiences of being parented, they do not remember the feelings evoked at the time. Even in the most extreme cases of abuse, it hurts too much to remember, so they put it to the back of their minds. Fraiberg explains why the cycle perpetuates and is not broken, clearly demonstrating the need to confront these demons from the past and lay them to rest. Failure to do so, with the support of a sensitive facilitator, during parenthood, may in some cases result in

'...insecurely attached infants, leading to a "mismatch" in maternal response' (Parr, 2000)

We work in a geographical area which has the seventh-highest rate of under-18 pregnancies in the country and the fourth highest rate of pregnancies in those under 16. The reasons that young people become pregnant are as complex as the society in which they live. One of the issues often raised is the link to education. There is a common belief that adolescent girls drop out of education because they are pregnant, but recent research substantiates anecdotal evidence that pregnancy occurs following expulsion from school (Barrel, 2000).

Another observation is that many young people become pregnant, take their GCSEs and leave, and a few (usually those who are supported) continue or return to their studies. However, they are about to become parents and deserve as many opportunities as any other parent, so that the risks of social exclusion are reduced.

Applying new skills

In our area, referrals are made through the midwife to Hilary, who then arranges, with consent, to meet the young women at home. The young women can invite other people to be present, and they often choose to share the meetings with their mothers (Birch, 1997; Rozette et al, 2000). The young women are able to verbalise both negative and positive feelings relating to their pregnancy, sharing these feelings with the other people present. This demonstrates that the professional who is present and listening is not going to be judgmental or prescriptive but supportive.

Wherever appropriate the partner's involvement is positively encouraged: they are also prospective parents who need to be supported. Even in modern society the father's role is often undermined, and in the case of young people, circumstances such as age and domestic arrangements can mitigate against their long-term involvement.

As the relationship is nurtured, so is the young person's confidence. The young people are given the opportunity to develop their own long-term informal and formal support networks, increasing the likelihood of long-term positive outcomes (Wilson, 1995). The intervention of support may involve group work, one-to-one meetings or family groups, but is always facilitative.

Our catchment area is large and groups are facilitated throughout the community and at the Young Parent Education Unit. The groups that are co-facilitated are less demanding as both the skills and the challenges are shared.

The facilitator needs to be constantly aware of the changing needs of the group and the developing group process. Part of that awareness is acknowledging the participants' age: it is important to provide age-appropriate resources. A patronising attitude is never appropriate.

A flexible programme is necessary to address the physical and emotional aspects of the transition to parenthood, whilst acknowledging the needs of the young adult (Parr, 1997; Wilson, 1995). Wide-ranging issues are explored as they emerge during the pregnancy, and these can be revisited postnatally.

Cultural expectations

Childhood is a social phenomenon which is clearly defined by the culture in which a child lives. It brings with it a set of expectations and societal norms: these do not, for many, include becoming pregnant in the adolescent years.

The 'problem' of teenage pregnancy has been constructed by society as an issue about age (James & Prout, 1997; Postman, 1994) but the underpinning belief system goes that much deeper. The ideal of the innocence of childhood – some feel – is lost forever for girls who become pregnant in their teens. They have defied their assigned position in society as dependent, weak and incompetent.

'Pregnancy is a clear indication of sexual activity, and as such, loss of innocence' (Phoenix, 1991) and some will say that these young girls, by entering parenthood at such

an early age, are forfeiting their childhood/adolescent years.

Learning to play

A parent and child play session has evolved which builds upon the foundations developed in the antenatal period, but also includes the child. The group meets at the Child Development Centre, with access to a well-equipped playroom and multi-sensory room

Play and Playwork have a significant role to play in supporting parents and young children, focusing on those parents who are also children themselves. The 'older child', the parent, is able to explore her relationship with the infant through play.

Play can promote and enhance parent-infant attachments. Only through play experiences/environments that offer 'fun, freedom, and flexibility' are the needs of the child and the parent met on equal terms (Brown, 2000). Play empowers children to be able to make choices and decisions about their lives.

The medium of play allows the playworker to provide support that develops the 'self', addressing the needs of the young parent for positive regard, acceptance, respect and warmth, and developing the individual's self-actualising tendencies (Rogers, 1995; Kagan, 1971; Ewen, 1994). Billington (1989) when discussing parent education and young parents states

'A woman who has a sense of self worth is able to meet her child's needs and to provide appropriate childcare'.

A willingness to enter the child's world through shared play experiences can enhance a woman's relationship with her child.

Conclusion

Teenage pregnancy may not always be a problem per se, although it may well raise complex issues within our society. However, it is clear that, given support, young parents can be confident in their abilities to parent.

Becoming a parent may also refocus their lives as their responsibilities for the baby are realised; positive aspirations and directions often emerge.

Some young parents find a new determination to seek success, not only as full time parents but also as individuals who are confident, socially included citizens in our society.

It is also clear that the support offered to these young people must be ongoing, consistent, flexible, based on the needs of the individual, grounded in clear evidence-based principals and continually evaluated.

REFERENCES

Barrel M. 2000. Educational experiences of adolescent mothers. The Practising Midwife, 3(9), 30-2

Billington. 1989. 45 Cope Street: Working in partnership with parents. Health Visitor, 62(5), 156-7

Birch DML. 1997. The adolescent parent: A 15 year longitudinal study of school age mothers and their children. Journal of Adolescent Health and Welfare, 10(1), 17-25

Bolwby J. 1998. A secure base: clinical applications of attachment theory. London: Routledge

Brown F. 2000. Compound flexibility (S.P.I.C.E Revisited). A paper for Play Education's 2nd Theoretical Play Meeting, "New Playwork - New Thinking?" Malting Conference Centre, Ely, Cambridgeshire

Combes G & Schonveld A. 1992. Life will never be the same again. London: Health Education Authority

Ewen RB. 1994. An Introduction to Theories of Personality. New Jersey: Lawrence Erlbaum Associates

Fraiberg S, Adelson E, Shapir V. 1980. Ghosts in the nursery: A psychoanalytic approach to the problems of impaired infant-mother relationships. In: S Fraiberg (ed). Clinical studies in infant mental health. London: Tavistock Publications

Hancock A. 1994. How effective is antenatal education? Modern Midwife, 14(5), 13-15

HMSO. 1999. Social Exclusion Report: Teenage Pregnancy. London

Irvine H, Bradley T, Cupples M and Booham M. 1997. The implications of teenage pregnancy and motherhood for primary health care: Unresolved issues. British Journal of General Practice

James A & Prout A (eds). 1997. Constructing and Reconstructing Childhood. 2nd edition. London: Falmer Press

Kagan J. 1971. Understanding Children: Behaviour, motives and thought. New York: Harcourt Brace Jovanovich

Nolan ML. 1998. Teenage pregnancy: A challenge for the government and nation. RCM Midwives Journal, 1(5), 152-4

Olaussen PO, Cnattingius S, Haglund B. 1999. Teenage pregnancies and risk of late fetal death and infant mortality. British Journal of Obstetrics and Gynaecology, 106(2), 116-21

Parr M. 1997. Description of a study evaluating a new approach to preparation for parenting for women and men in the transition to parenthood. Hertfordshire longitudinal study. Revised draft. Unpublished thesis. University of East London. PIPPIN 1997

Parr M. 2000. Why PIPPIN was developed: Description of a study evaluating a new approach to preparation for parenting for women and men in the transition to parenthood. Hertfordshire: PIPPIN Herts Study (1989-1993) revised 17/01/00. Unpublished PhD thesis

Parr M. 2001. PIPPIN Making Changes Pre-Requisite Study Day Handbook PIPPIN

Peckham S. 1993. Preventing unintended teenage pregnancies. Public Health, 107, 125-33

Phoenix A. 1989. Influences on previous contraceptive use/ non-use in pregnant16-19 year olds. Journal of Reproductive and Infant Psychology, 7, 211-25

Phoenix A. 1991. Young Mothers. Oxford: Polity Press

Postman N. 1994. The Disappearance of Childhood. USA: Vintage Books

Pugh G, De'ath E, Smith C. 1994. Confident parents, confident children: Policy and practice in parent education and support. London: The National Children's Bureau

Qvortrup J, Bardy M, Sgritta G, Wintersberger H (eds). 1994. Childhood Matters. Avebury Press

Rogers C. 1955. Client Centred Therapy. Boston: Houghton-Mifflin

Royal College of Midwives. 1999. The transition to parenting : An open learning resource for midwives. London: The Royal College of Midwives Trust

Rozette C, Houghton-Clemmey R, Sullivan K. 2000. A profile of teenage pregnancy: young women's perceptions of the maternity services. The Practising Midwife, 3 (10)

Steele M. 1997. Intergenerational cycles of attachment: recent advances in research on parenting. The Parenting Forum. Briefing Sheet No: 6

Stern D. 1998. The Motherhood Constellation. London: Karnac Books

Wilson J. 1995. Caroline: A case of a pregnant teenager. Professional Care of Mother and Child. 5(5), 139-40, 142

The Practising Midwife 2002; 5(2): 25-27

Parent education
Preparing for life after birth

Judith Schott

Most expectant parents embark on parenthood with virtually no preparation save their own experience of being parented. Many hold a new baby for the first time when their own is placed in their arms. The most common cry heard in the first few weeks after the birth is, 'Why didn't somebody tell me it would be like this?' It is not only after the birth that parents realise that they need information and skills. Research confirms that expectant parents are interested in preparing for the practical and emotional challenges that a new baby will bring (O'Meara, 1993; Nolan, 1999; Singh and Newburn, 2000). So what part can antenatal classes play in preparing parents for the realities of life after birth?

Class leaders are in an ideal situation to lay the foundations for effective parenting. They see expectant parents on a regular basis over several weeks, and have time to build up trust and rapport. They can raise issues, offer information, teach skills and suggest strategies for managing new demands. They can encourage people to share their hopes and concerns and to build their own support networks.

Some class leaders feel that it is hard to get expectant parents to look beyond birth, and anyway there is so much to say about labour that there is little time for anything else. Labour, crucial though it is, seldom lasts longer than twenty-four hours, so although this view is understandable, it has several negative consequences. It can become a self-fulfilling prophecy and perpetuate the myth that the birth is the goal. It also encourages the idea that people only become parents once their baby is born, even though the mother's body is already nurturing and protecting their baby, and expectant parents have already made dozens of decisions which affect their baby's welfare.

Practical approaches

Class structure and style

The structure of the course and the style and approach of the class leader can have a strong influence on parents' ability to focus on life after birth.

A structured programme that states exactly what will be covered in each session allows those who are preoccupied with labour to limit their attendance to certain sessions and to miss classes that cover life after birth. A less structured programme which outlines the topics and issues to be covered in the course, without stating exactly what will be covered when, is more likely to keep people coming.

Active participants learn better than passive recipients. Class leaders who deliver large amounts of information are less likely to prepare parents for labour than those who actively involve parents in their own learning. Passive recipients are therefore less likely to be able to focus on the transition to parenthood (Wiener, 2002). So, in the first class, it is important to turn the class from an audience with a speaker into an interactive learning group (Schott and Priest, 2002: 29-43) and to use active learning techniques throughout the course

Starting with their priorities

Whatever the structure and style of the course, parents coming to classes are very naturally preoccupied with the prospect of labour and may not appear to be looking further ahead. The key to enabling parents to focus on parenting is to deal with their priorities first. Once labour has been tackled to their satisfaction, they will be more able to consider what comes next.

Putting parenthood on the agenda

This does not mean leaving all mention of parenthood

until later classes. When they are setting their own agenda for the course, parents could be invited to consider including topics about life after birth (Schott and Priest, 2002: 35-37). In addition, the class leader can briefly mention the baby or some aspect of parenthood in every single class. This encourages parents to look beyond the birth and can be done by:

Including the baby's experience. Try bringing the baby's point of view into every topic and issue. In this way parents are reminded that their baby is affected by everything that happens. What might contractions be like for the baby? What might it be like to be born? What sort of welcome would help the baby adjust to the bright, noisy, cold world? What are the effects of various procedures on the baby? What is it like for the baby to be monitored? What are the effects on the baby of opiates? A Caesarean birth? An epidural? Entonox?

Words and actions. These convey subtle but powerful messages about parenthood and babies. Talking about 'life after birth' is likely to be more meaningful to parents than the more clinical phrase 'postnatal period'. No babies are 'it', so it is important to use 'he' or 'she' when talking about them, alternating the sex frequently. Choosing an attractive doll and handling as if it were a real baby provides parents with useful visual images from which they can learn without a word being said.

Drawing analogies between current experiences and parenthood. The unpredictable and inevitable nature of labour is like the erratic and continuous needs of a new baby. The disturbed sleep of late pregnancy mirrors broken nights after the birth. The tiredness of early and late pregnancy is like the exhaustion of early parenting. Babies literally come between a couple who want to hug in pregnancy and are just as intrusive once born. The way nauseated women eat in early pregnancy is similar to the way new babies breastfeed – little and often.

Linking skills for labour to parenting skills. The skills parents are taught for pregnancy and birth can be useful once the baby is born. For example, 'a relaxed parent is more likely to be able to soothe a fretful baby' – 'babies like to be stroked and massaged. Tired parents might enjoy it too!'

Encouraging parents to notice their unborn baby's behaviour. Each baby has his or her own patterns of activity and rest. Some are prone to hiccough. Some seem to quieten when the father puts his hand on the mother's tummy. A few object when a woman sits for too long. Many become active when the mother relaxes. Some startle at loud noises. Starting a class with a round asking, 'How has your baby been this week?' or 'Does your baby seem to have any likes or dislikes?' can help a group of parents focus on their babies and appreciate that each one is an individual.

Allocating time for life after birth

There is no way that class leaders can equip people for parenthood. Parenthood is a process of evolution. The needs of a newborn baby are different from those of a toddler. A five-year-old makes different demands from a ten-year-old, and the parents of teenagers may need a whole new set of skills and strategies. However, effective leaders can help parents to make the transition to parenthood by offering a balance of information, practical skills, strategies, and time for reflection. This can be done in a variety of ways.

Using active learning techniques. In addition to discussion and small group work there is a range of approaches that can help expectant parents to think about life after birth (Schott and Priest, 2002: 97-107). However, these will only work when parents feel relaxed and comfortable with each other and if the course has been interactive from the start.

Exploring expectations. During pregnancy, an expectant parent moves from being a child of their parents to being the parent of their child. For better or worse their expectations and assumptions about parenthood are rooted in their own experience of being parented. Childhood experiences may have been positive or negative, or more usually a combination of the two. When a couple become parents there are two sets of attitudes and assumptions. Some may be similar but others may conflict (Daws, 1997). Most couples will benefit from talking and listening to each other so that they can learn about each other's views, feelings and ideas about parenting. They can find out about their partner's expectations and think about how they will share chores and baby care as well as finding time for each other.

Class leaders can help people to explore and share their ideas and expectations by setting up small groups. Parents could be invited to discuss what will be good and what will be hard about being a parent, or be offered situation cards which describe a scenario and offer suggestions for coping strategies (see Figure 3.5.1, overleaf). The main thing is to get people talking and thinking, and in the process the leader can offer the relevant information and suggest ways in which parents could deal with different situations.

Balancing the joys and the challenges. Discussions about parenthood tend to be polarised. Parents are either presented with idealised images of relaxed parents holding a beautiful, contented baby, or they are bombarded with dire warnings about how chaotic life will be. Class leaders can balance these extremes by giving realistic information coupled with skills and strategies to manage the difficulties, and also by discussing the pleasures – the sense of pride and

Figure 3.5.1 Sample situation card from *Leading Antenatal Classes a practical guide*.

Toby is four weeks old. Recently he has been fretful and hard to pacify from about 5pm onwards. It is two am and he still has not settled. Louise and Tom are both exhausted. What could they do?

- Feed and change Toby once more, then put him down and let him cry for a bit to see if he will settle?
- Take him into bed with them?
- Take him out in the car to see if that will soothe him?
- Decide that one of them should sleep while the other takes Toby into another room?
- Put Toby in a sling and walk around for a bit?
- What else?

What changes could they make to deal with this pattern?

- Make sure that Louise eats lunch and tea and rests during the afternoon so that her milk supply remains good in the afternoon and evening?
- Talk to the midwife or health visitor?
- Ask a supportive friend or relative to come in and dilute the situation?
- Arrange for help with household chores?
- What else?

achievement that parents can feel, the indescribable feel and smell of a newborn baby nestling in one's arms – the joy of the first smile – the satisfaction of watching them grow.

Including what babies can do. A great deal is known about what unborn babies can do. From early in the pregnancy, babies can suck, swallow, yawn and show preferences for certain tastes. They can hear and perceive light. They respond to the mother's activities and moods and show preferences for different types of music (Chamberlain, 1987: 34 and 52. Klaus and Klaus, 1998: 3). In other words, unborn babies are alert and aware individuals.

A baby is born with all senses working. Their facial expressions can convey feelings ranging from pleasure to rage. Contrary to popular belief, babies smile very early, sometimes at birth if the experience has been gentle (Chamberlain, 1987: 54). After some time resting quietly on the mother's chest, a baby is capable of moving towards and finding the mother's nipple unaided. Within hours of birth, babies show a preference for their own mother's odour (Klaus and Klaus 1998:10-18).

Immediately after a straightforward birth during which the mother has received little or no medication, new-born babies are often alert and calm for a considerable period of time. They are often extremely interested in the world about them, show a preference for people rather than other objects. They also respond to human voices, especially those that they have heard before birth. Above all, they are fascinated by faces and will look at them intently. A series of photographs, designed for use in antenatal classes, called *Ethan's first half hour* (The Children's Project, 2001), taken from a

video of a newborn baby's first interactions with his parents, demonstrates quite clearly that, not only is the baby fascinated by his parents' faces, within the first half hour of his life he can interact. The father holds the baby about nine inches from his face. Then he sticks out his tongue while the baby watches intently, and after a few seconds, baby Ethan sticks his tongue out too (Murray and Andrews, 2000).

Armed with this sort of information and visual evidence and, given time, peace and quiet after the birth, parents can begin to learn how to communicate with their son or daughter. If they hold the baby about nine inches from their face, support her or his head and pay gentle and sensitive attention, they will probably be rewarded by discovering that their baby is highly responsive and fascinated by them.

Including how babies communicate. Babies are different, some are more relaxed and cuddly than others, some cry more. Some are outgoing, others are easily over stimulated and need more peace and tranquility. Even very young babies are extremely expressive. They convey their needs and moods not only by crying but also through their level of eye contact, their facial expressions and body movements. Parents who learn to notice subtle changes in their baby's moods can recognise early signs of distress and prevent it escalating. They can also develop ways of minimizing or avoiding situations that upset their baby (see Murray and Andrews, 2000 for practical approaches).

Teaching practical skills. Many parents want to know how to bath, feed and change their baby. Telling parents that they will be shown these skills when the time comes may satisfy some but leaves others feeling let down and unprepared. Early discharge from hospital may also leave little time for teaching these skills and, as a result, parents may go home feeling ill-equipped and anxious. It may also difficult to include partners after the birth, who should ideally be taught alongside their partners.

If practical skills are not included in classes, it is important to explain why and to be sure that parents will be shown what to do at another time. Class leaders who do include these skills in classes need to decide the best way of covering them. This is not always straightforward.

The role of the demonstration baby bath has been questioned. McLoughlin (1996) suggests that watching an expert bath a baby in unfamiliar surroundings and with equipment that may not be available at home may be intimidating rather than empowering. It is quicker and possibly more useful to use a doll to show parents how to wrap and hold a baby in order to wash her face and head, and then how to hold a baby safely while bathing him and lifting him in and out of the water. Then pass dolls and towels around so that each person can practise.

Parents need clear factual and balanced information on the pros and cons of breast and bottle feeding and, depending on the choices they make, they also need to know, for example, how to position a baby at the breast or how to sterilise bottles and make up feeds. However, the UK Baby Friendly Initiative (UNICEF, 2001: 24) states that instructions on how to make up feeds are best given on an individual basis, and that demonstrations in front of a group are unlikely to equip people to make up feeds properly. Contrary to popular belief, the Initiative does not preclude giving factual information about bottle feeding in a class, so in units that have achieved Baby Friendly status, the only thing that should be omitted to a group is a demonstration of how to make up bottle feeds.

Bringing in a mother, father and new baby. This works best if the baby is under six weeks old, as expectant parents are less likely to identify with an older baby. It is important to take care when choosing whom to ask, as the total focus of the class will be on the parents and of course, on the baby. The ideal candidates are neither long-winded nor dogmatic. So who should be invited? Someone who had a easy birth or someone who did not? A mother who is breastfeeding and happy to do so in front of the group? Or one who prefers privacy for feeds or is bottle feeding? A couple, or a mother by herself?

It is important to plan how to structure the session. It can be run it as an informal discussion, or guided by the leader asking the parents questions that will encourage them to talk about certain issues. The latter enables the leader to invite the visiting parents to talk about feelings, reactions and coping strategies as well as factual events.

REFERENCES

Chamberlain D. 1987. The Cognitive Newborn, a Scientific Update. British Journal of Psychotherapy, 4(1), 30-71

Daws D. 1997. Family Foundations. New Generation, September issue. London: The National Childbirth Trust

Klaus MH and Klaus PH. 1980. Your Amazing Newborn. Cambridge Massachusetts: Perseus Books

McLoughlin A. 1996. Trial By Water. British Journal of Midwifery, 4(4), 204-8

Murray L and Andrews L. 2000. The Social Baby: Understanding babies' communication from birth. The Children's Project, CP Publishing, Freepost SEA 10364, Richmond, Surrey TW10 7BR. www.childrensproject.co.uk

Nolan M. 1999. Antenatal education – where next? Journal of Advanced Nursing, 2(11), 534-8

O'Meara C. 1993. An evaluation of consumer perspectives of childbirth and parenting education. Midwifery, 9(4), 210-19

Schott J and Priest J. 2002. Leading Antenatal Classes – a practical guide. 2nd edition. Oxford: Books for Midwives

Singh D and Newburn M. 2000. Becoming a father: men's access to information and support about pregnancy, birth and life with a new baby. London: The National Childbirth Trust

The Children's Project 2001. Ethan's first half hour – a series of ten A4 photographs for use in classes, available from The Children's Project Ltd. (see address above)

UNICEF, 2001. Implementing the Baby Friendly Best Practice Standards. UK Baby Friendly Initiative

Wiener AJ. 2002. The brick wall of labour. The Practising Midwife, 5(2), 38-9

The Practising Midwife 2002; 5(6): 37-39

The brick wall of labour

Andrew Julian Weiner

I am a child psychiatrist working in a Child and Adolescent Mental Health Service in Hertfordshire. In my line of work there is a big focus on promoting the emotional wellbeing of children. Antenatal parenthood education classes are one area of routine professional practice that can be used to promote the emotional wellbeing of children. If mothers and fathers can emotionally prepare for parenthood there is evidence that they will be in better shape to care for their babies (Parr, 1996). This in turn means that babies will get a better start in life, and may then go on to cope better with the emotional challenges of childhood.

Last year I was invited, along with a midwife tutor and two psychologists, to take part in a project to see if midwifery-led antenatal classes could focus more on the issues around parenthood. However, many midwives at the local hospital told me that the project would fail. They said it was a well known fact that pregnant women cannot think about parenthood until after the baby is born. On further investigation I found that this view had been expressed in a press release by the Royal College of Midwives (RCM, 1997), and that there was some research to support it (Bliss-Holtz, 1998; Handfield & Bell, 1995). In the report on midwifery services by Coombes and Schonveld (1992) it was reportedly noted by professionals that women found it very difficult to think beyond the birth. They named this phenomenon 'The Brick Wall of Labour'.

Because of the concern that our project would fail, it was agreed that the first step was to look for evidence of the 'Brick Wall of Labour' in local antenatal classes. I sat in on some hospital antenatal classes and found that despite the midwives' attempts to raise the topic, little or no discussion was taking place about parenthood issues.

Hitting the wall

In one class a midwife gave information about the importance of cuddling babies and how difficult life could be with a new baby. The group sat silent and impassive. In another class, after discussing the details of Caesarean sections and forceps delivery, a midwife showed a video about the first year in a baby's life. After the video, the midwife asked if there were any questions but there was silence. One woman finally said that she could not prepare for life with her baby because until it was born she didn't know what kind of baby it was. So here it was: the 'Brick Wall of Labour'.

Then during the coffee break, the midwife left the room to organise something and one expectant mother came up to me and started chatting. She confided in me (quietly) that she talked to her unborn baby every night before she went to sleep. She said she was a bit worried that this was not normal. She thought she might be going a bit mad. Where was the Brick Wall now?

Lecturing

These silent groups had one thing in common: the midwives were giving a great deal of information in a lecture type format. The lecture style is the most common teaching style in antenatal classes. One study found that 9 out of 10 classes used a lecture format (Underdown, 1998). However, two of the classes I observed had very different format, they were run in a facilitative way. As I will describe, the facilitative approach had a major impact on the Brick Wall phenomenon.

In the facilitative classes ample opportunity was given for the group members to get to know each other, and contributions from the group were listened to actively, valued and expanded on. Ideas from the group were sought first then discussed. Information was given in short bursts and videos were hardly used. The midwives leading these groups were sensitive to the feelings of the group and would make humorous remarks or stop for tea break when the group seemed tired, bored or anxious. During tea breaks the midwife would be available for informal conversation. The women in these groups talked a lot about the impending arrival of the baby and their feelings about this. Feelings of intimacy and mutual support developed and the whole experience felt warm, emotional and safe.

So, in the lecture style groups women were unwilling or unable to think with midwives about issues to do with babies, where as in the facilitative groups they were keen to do so. It is not easy to talk openly with strangers about one's hopes and fears for parenthood; it is far easier to ask about practical matters such as labour and childbirth. It became clear to me that it was the lecture style that created the Brick Wall.

Facilitation

After my observations of classes, the midwife tutor and I decided to take a set of classes ourselves, in the facilitative style. This brought to light further insights into the Brick Wall of Labour. Early on in the classes, two women spontaneously said that they were finding it difficult to think beyond the birth. Our approach was to take opportunities to find out more about these thoughts. One woman said that she had been fine with her pregnancy until her husband was driving her to her first class. It then dawned on her that the pregnancy was getting near the end and the labour that she dreaded was getting close. This made her anxious. She was terrified of the pain and the thought of blood. She thought labour involved 48 hours of constant pain, and that the 'waters breaking' would be catastrophic. Over the course of the classes, with the opportunity to discuss these fears in a safe setting, she visibly grew in confidence and was much more relaxed. In her evaluation of the classes she was full of praise for the groups, said she felt prepared for enough labour and had valued the discussion of postnatal topics. The other woman was in the process of moving house, but did not know if they would be able to move before the baby arrived. She said she found it difficult to settle down to thinking about the baby when she did not know where she was going to be living. Giving her the opportunity to talk about this seemed to help. In the evaluation form she said the postnatal topics were useful.

Towards the end of our set of classes, during a discussion on the topic of life with a baby, a third woman seemed unwilling or unable to focus on this and was asking the midwife lots of questions about labour. I commented that it seemed hard for people to think about babies at the moment. The woman responded that she had gone to visit a friend who had just had a baby. She said she couldn't her eyes off the little baby in the cot. She said she couldn't believe she was going to have a baby too; that a real baby was going to come out of her

body and that it was going to be hers! This woman's experience of being 'unable to focus on the baby' was provoked by a very powerful exposure to the reality of motherhood. These feelings temporarily overwhelmed her. Behind her difficulty in focussing on parenthood lay a very touching and pertinent point that was of great value to the whole group, including myself and my midwife colleague.

In the lecture style classes that I observed, midwives were giving as much information as they could. Every detail of the childbirth process, and of possible complications of labour, was given. Forceps were regularly brought along for women to see. A review of the history of antenatal classes shows that this approach is a backlash to the patronising way antenatal classes were taken in the 1960s and 1970s (Oakley, 1980). Then, classes were focused on relaxation, and encouraging women to be passive and unquestioning recipients of (male) medical care. In the 1980s and 1990s there was a shift towards openness and transparency. Women were given as much information as possible to be equal participants in their care. The phrase 'Knowledge is Power' has been used to describe this ideal (Hancock, 1994). Recently this approach has been criticised (Nolan, 1999). In the process of imparting knowledge a midwife demonstrates to her clients beyond any doubt where the expertise really lies. This is actually disempowering for women.

Disempowerment

In the lecture style antenatal classes I observed some chilling examples of disempowerment. For example in one class a particularly graphic video was shown of a woman during childbirth. The woman had hoped for a labour without pain relief but she was in a lot of pain, and everyone watching was very relieved when she accepted that the doctor should administer an epidural. After the video had finished one vocal man told the group he was glad he wasn't the one having the baby. The women in the group became prickly and annoyed. The men muttered to each other about going to the pub after the session. This annoyed the women even more. At the end of the session the couples left in silence looking unhappy and dejected. The women were left feeling alone and unsupported by their partners. The video had proved just how traumatic childbirth could be and just how much a midwife is needed. In this anxious and isolated state of mind it is understandable that all one's attention is focused on surviving the labour. So, while some women have difficulty thinking beyond the birth, this does not amount to a 'brick wall'. The 'Brick Wall of Labour' that is seen by many midwives is a by-product of the didactic, disempowering, lecture style approach to antenatal education, and the insensitive use of anxiety-provoking teaching materials. If, on the other hand, a sensitive, facilitative approach is taken, where women have access to a safe and secure setting where fears can be accepted, listened to and worked through, women are able and willing to discuss intimate issues around babies and parenthood.

Training

Training is required to run a group in a facilitative style, and one needs to enter the training with a certain humility and sensitivity. With the current staffing crisis in midwifery it is easy to see that the status quo will prevail for the some time ahead, but step by step, if more midwives can see the benefits of a facilitative approach a gradual shift in practice should be possible. The results would be very rewarding for all concerned, midwives, parents and babies.

REFERENCES

Bliss-Holtz J. 1988. Primiparas' prenatal concern for learning infant care. Nursing Research, 37, 20-4

Coombes G, Schonveld A. 1992. Life will never be the same again. London: Health Education Authority

Hancock A. 1994. How effective is antenatal education? Modern Midwife, May13-15

Handfield B, Bell R. 1995. Do childbirth classes influence decision making about labour and postpartum issues? Birth 22, 153-60

Nolan ML. 1999. Antenatal Education: Past and future agendas. The Practising Midwife, 2 (3), 24-7

Oakley A. 1980. Women confined: Towards a sociology of childbirth. Oxford: Martin Robertson & Co

Parr MA. 1996. Support for couples in the transition to parenthood. University of East London Department of Psychology: Unpublished PhD thesis.

Royal College of Midwives. 1997. Press Release: Midwives Criticise Labour's Antenatal Plans. London: RCM Press Office

Underdown A. 1998. Investigating techniques used in parenting classes. Health Visitor, 71, 65-8

The Practising Midwife 2002; 5(2): 38-39

Parent education
Should it include relaxation and breathing?

Judith Schott

Relaxation and breathing were once a standard part of most antenatal education courses, but in some areas this is no longer the case. The exact reasons for this omission are unclear, however there are several contributing factors. One is lack of class time and the pressure to cover increasing amounts of technical information. Another is that most midwives have had little or no training to teach relaxation and breathing and so, understandably, lack the confidence to teach them. Some midwives do not see the point of teaching relaxation and breathing because they have never seen women use them effectively in labour.

So why teach relaxation and breathing awareness?

The ability to release unwanted tension is a life skill which can be used in everyday situations and can benefit everyone. The overwhelming majority of women experience pain in labour and research into pain management has highlighted a number of relevant factors.

- Pain and the anticipation of pain provoke anxiety which results in muscle tension and leads to the release of pain-inducing substances. The result is an escalating cycle of pain–anxiety–tension (Craig, 1989, Read, 1950).
- Pain is a powerful respiratory stimulus (McDonald, 1999) and breathing inevitably alters during labour. Some women are able to 'just let go and go with the flow'. However, others become tense and panic. Teaching breathing awareness can enhance women's ability to release unwanted tension, and to help them to respond flexibility to the demands of their body and to feel in control of their behaviour. It can also be used as a distraction technique and can help people to maintain their equilibrium in many other stressful situations.

- Pain and emotional distress increase cortisol and cateholamine levels which can affect the length and intensity of the labour (McDonald, 1999).
- Relaxation has been shown to increase people's ability to tolerate pain. Relaxation and controlled breathing can also increase their ability to deal with anxiety, and can improve feelings of control over stressful and painful experiences (Turk and Okifuji, 1999; Weisenberg, 1999; Crothers, 1994). Slade et al (1993) observed that personal satisfaction is strongly associated with the ability to control pain.
- Expectations of pain and stress tend to be fulfilled. People who have developed coping strategies and who believe that they can manage their pain, cope better than those who feel helpless. Confidence in coping strategies can influence the body's own pain relieving and immune responses (Weisenberg, 1999).

Many parents expect to learn relaxation and some come to antenatal classes especially for 'the breathing'. If they are not taught, women may feel let down. If the scope of relaxation and breathing as a method of pain management is not discussed, women may have unrealistic expectations and be shocked in labour when they do not experience the pain relief they anticipated.

So as well as offering a range of approaches (see below), it is essential to be realistic about what these skills can achieve. Relaxation and breathing cannot eliminate pain – they are coping strategies that can help people to manage pain and stress and to conserve energy. They can be a focus of attention, a distraction from the pain, they can help reduce pain perception and enable people to tolerate it better (Crothers, 1994; Spibey et al, 1993).

Who teaches these skills?

Some health professionals believe that relaxation and

breathing should only be taught by specially trained 'experts'. In reality, the ability to teach them effectively can be learned by anyone who takes the time to think through the issues and to gather ideas and information and to develop and practise these skills. The ability to teach them enables class leaders to vary the pace and focus of the class and to link the information with coping strategies.

Being able to teach relaxation and breathing can also enhance clinical practice, for example, when supporting a woman through a long labour, helping a new mother to establish breastfeeding or to cope with a crying baby or a rebellious toddler. These skills are especially important for intra-partum care. It is unrealistic to expect a woman who has been taught the relaxation skills, to apply them in the turmoil of labour without continuous encouragement and support, especially in a high-tech environment (Nolan, 2000; Spiby et al, 1999). So there is an argument for all midwives, whether or not they lead classes, to be able to teach women how to relax. After all, most if not all midwives have at some time or other during their clinical practice said to a woman 'Now just relax!' Telling a woman what to do has limited value. Showing her how to do it is likely to be much more effective!

Incorporating relaxation and breathing awareness into the antenatal course

Relaxation and breathing are often talked about as separate skills, but in reality they are closely intertwined. It is very hard to let your breathing flow without being relaxed, and hard to relax if your breathing is tense and controlled. Linking the two enables people to enhance their awareness and their ability to use both to help themselves in labour and with the day-to-day stresses of life.

Frequency

In order to acquire and develop these skills, people need plenty of practice. They also need to believe that they can use them effectively (Spiby et al, 1999; Weisenberg, 1999). It is tempting to hope that everyone goes home and practises assiduously between each class. In reality, many people don't. They are more likely to benefit and develop confidence if they are offered frequent opportunities to practise during classes. This need not take up too much time. Short sessions within each class are often more effective than one or two long ones and people who are reluctant are more likely to participate. If relaxation and breathing skills are taught in separate sessions, people who don't fancy the idea can opt out and will therefore miss out, and the ability to link them to the topics under discussion is lost.

Timing

If relaxation is included in several classes, try varying the timing. It can be used to change the pace and atmosphere and can also be linked directly to the topics under discussion.

Variety

If parents are only taught one approach, the leader will please some of the people all the time and the rest not at all. There is a wide variety of approaches to teaching relaxation and breathing awareness, and offering different methods keeps people interested and helps to ensure that everyone finds an approach that suits them. It is important to choose the least threatening and most practical approaches for early classes, leaving the more reflective and personal approaches until the people are feeling more confident and at home in the group.

Choices include (starting with the least threatening, most practical approaches)

- Contrasting tension with relaxation
- Linking relaxation to breathing – letting go on the outward breath.
- Linking relaxation to posture and positions
- Quick relaxation techniques
- Relaxation, breathing awareness and managing pain
- Visualisation
- Touch relaxation (see Schott and Priest 2002 for practical descriptions).

Establishing the relevance of relaxation and breathing

People seldom take the trouble to learn anything new unless they can see how it will benefit them. Acting on the assumption that teaching relaxation is 'a good thing for parents to learn, so let's just get on with it', or announcing 'now we are going to do relaxation' may mean that some class members switch off. A more inviting approach is to start by helping people to consider how releasing tension can help them in everyday situations. There are several ways of doing this.

You could ask:

'What changes do you notice in your body when you are in a stressful situation? Imagine for example that you are late for an important meeting... You are on a bus or in a car, stuck in a traffic jam and time is ticking by.' Group members may volunteer responses or you may actually see people tense their shoulders and fists.

You could elicit further responses by asking:

'Where else do you tense up? What happens to your jaw muscles? To your breathing and your heart rate? Anyone get a

dry mouth? Feel hot and bothered? How do you feel when you have all these physical reactions to stress? Can you think clearly? Do you arrive calm and in good shape? What difference would it make to reduce these responses to stress?'

You could also establish the relevance of releasing tension to manage pain, or you could invite the class to imagine being in pain. For example:

'Have you noticed what happens when you stub your toe? What's the first thing you do? Hold your toe? Tense up? Hold your breath? What else? Have you noticed that a second before you actually feel pain you've already tensed up in anticipation? Does the tension help? Next time try breathing out and letting go.'

You could follow this with a short, simple introduction to relaxation which offers people an opportunity to find out what it feels like to let go. Afterwards you could suggest that, during the following week, they pay attention to their physical reactions when they get tense or when they hurt themselves. Ask them to notice where they tend to tense up first, and where the tension spreads to. Then suggest they try letting go and notice how that feels.

With this approach you are already linking the topics of relaxation, stress, breathing and pain. You can build on this when talking about labour and parenting in subsequent classes.

Some women may think that relaxation is irrelevant because they are planning to have an epidural or an elective Caesarean. You could invite them to think about how it could help them in early labour, or whilst having an epidural inserted. Women anticipating a Caesarean section could practise relaxation lying down, using a sheet or pillow to simulate the screen the screen that will be across their upper chest during the operation.

Relaxation is equally useful for labour partners. It is hard to remain relaxed when you are tired and worried. Labour companions also need to conserve their energy and keep as calm as possible, both for themselves, and for the woman in labour. Tension and stress are highly infectious and easily transmitted from one person to another.

In later classes participants could think about the relevance of relaxation to parenting. For example:

'Imagine that your baby is four weeks old. He or she has been waking several times each night and you are getting more and more tired as the days pass. She or he has been restless and crying on and off all evening. It is 2am, you have fed and changed your baby and he or she is still crying and won't settle. How might you feel? Physically? Emotionally? How might releasing your tension help you/your partner? Help your baby to settle?'

Or you could lead relaxation with a visualisation about life after birth.

Relaxation can also be the central peg to which the skills and attitudes specific to labour can be attached (see fig 3.7.1).

The following points can help to make the sessions go well.

- Model a relaxed and unhurried approach. A brisk business like manner is unlikely to put people at their ease.
- Expect everyone, including partners, to join in and 'give it a try'.
- Keep sessions short, especially if you sense reluctance. It helps if you say at the beginning how long the session will last.
- In the first session, tension can be reduced by acknowledging that it is strange and perhaps difficult to come into an unfamiliar place, to be surrounded by strangers and then asked to let down one's guard and relax.
- Make sure that the room offers sufficient privacy. Feeling overlooked is inhibiting.

Figure 3.7.1

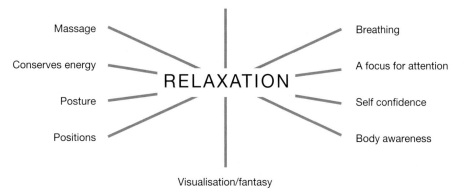

From *Leading Antenatal Classes. A Practical Guide*, Schott and Pries. Books for Midwives 2002

- Try to keep noise and interruptions to a minimum. However, if these do occur it is worth pointing out that being able to relax with activity around will be useful for everyday situations, for busy labour wards, and for parenting.
- Think about the positions you suggest that people adopt. Getting expectant parents to lie down is time consuming and people may find it embarrassing. It can be a great position for imagining that you are walking through a forest at dawn to meet your inner self. But it fails to prepare people for the rigours of labour, which is more like being at sea, in a force ten gale, with thirty-foot waves rolling in at regular intervals. Nor does it prepare people for the stresses of everyday life and parenting, most of which have to be dealt with on the hoof, not lying down in a darkened room! Invite people to practise whilst sitting on a chair, standing, leaning on something or someone.
- Encourage people to get comfortable and to change position if they want to. Many feel they have to keep quite still and are embarrassed to move despite being uncomfortable. They won't learn much about relaxation in these circumstances.
- Make sure that your voice sounds relaxed. Speak clearly and ensure that everyone can hear you. Remember that you are much more likely to go too fast than too slowly. Unless you are leading a standing relaxation which should not last longer than a few minutes, you cannot talk too slowly! Leave pauses between phrases. Though they may be familiar to you, they are new to the parents, who need time to think and act on what you are saying.
- Do the relaxation yourself (without losing the ability to lead the session!). This will help you get the pace right.
- Choose your words carefully. Instructing people to 'relax' can be counterproductive. It may not mean anything to people who have never thought about relaxation before. Most of us have been told to 'just relax' in a tone that makes tension and irritation far

more likely responses. Instead, choose everyday language and use words and phrases which actually describe the range of sensations that people can experience when they relax. For example: 'loose...floppy...heavy...warm...soft...let yourself sink into your chair...smooth your forehead...feel the weight of your legs against the seat of the chair, allow the chair back to support you'.
- Giggling and laughter are ways in which people release embarrassment. If you allow them, things will work better in the long run than they would if you try to avoid or suppress them.
- Encourage people to yawn if they feel like it. It does not mean they are bored! It is an excellent way of releasing tension.
- Mention that some women may feel their babies becoming more active as they relax. By suggesting that the babies enjoy it when their mothers relax, you begin to encourage parents to see their baby as a responsive and sensitive individual.
- End the session gradually. Encourage people to start by becoming aware of their surroundings, then move slowly and maybe stretch and yawn.
- Afterwards, invite people to review in pairs (fours in a couples class) by asking some open questions: *'What was that like?...What did you enjoy...find helpful?...What was hard?...What did you notice about yourself?'* This will help people to think back on what they experienced and, at the same time, give you some useful feedback.

Relaxation and breathing awareness are useful skills for managing unwanted tension and anxiety, and can improve people's feelings of confidence and control. Being able to release unwanted tension can enhance people's ability to deal with the stresses of traffic jams, job interviews, physical examinations, dental treatment, a crying baby or rebellious toddler. It is a good way of encouraging expectant and new parents to take a little time for themselves. It is a strategy for managing pain. It is also an extremely useful skill for stressed health professionals and nervous class leaders!

REFERENCES

Craig KD. 1989. Emotional aspects of pain. In: PD Wall and R Melzack (eds). Textbook of pain. 3rd edn. Edinburgh: Churchill Livingstone

Crothers J. 1994. Labour pains: A study of pain control mechanisms during labour, Journal of the Association of Chartered Physiotherapists in Obstetrics and Gynaecology, 74, 4-8

McDonald JS. 1999. Obstetric pain. In: PD Wall and R. Melzack (eds). Textbook of Pain. 4rh edn. Edinburgh: Churchill Livingstone

Nolan M. 2000. The influence of antenatal classes on pain relief in labour 2: The research. The Practising Midwife, 3(6), 26-31

Read GU. 1950. Childbirth without fear. London: Heinemann

Schott J and Priest J. 2002. Leading Antenatal Classes: A practical guide. 2nd edn. Oxford: Books for Midwives Press

Slade P, MacPherson SA, Hume A and Maresh M. 1993. Expectations, experiences and satisfaction with labour. British Journal of Clinical Psychology, 4 (Nov), 469-83

Spiby H, Henderson B, Slade P, Escott D and Fraser R. 1999. Strategies for coping with labour: Does antenatal education translate into practice? Journal of Advanced Nursing, 29(4), 388-94

Turk D and Okifuji A. 1999. A cognitive-behavioural approach to pain management. In: PD Wall and R. Melzack (eds). Textbook of Pain. 4th edn. Edinburgh: Churchill Livingstone

Weisenberg M. 1999. Cognitive aspects of pain. In: PD Wall and R. Melzack (eds). Textbook of Pain. 4th edn. Edinburgh: Churchill Livingstone

The antenatal cardiotocograph (CTG)

Shirley Andrews

The view of the fetus as a patient began with the discovery that the fetal heart could be auscultated, and fetal heart tones have been used to evaluate the fetal condition for more than 150 years (Sureau, 1996). Variation in the fetal heart rate (FHR) can be predictive, and can be correlated with the health or sickness of the mother or fetus. It is part of the midwife's role to identify whether or not a fetus is at risk by utilising her clinical knowledge and experience, supported by technology to aid diagnosis.

CTG's historical context

CTG is one of a battery of tests that is part of fetal assessment (Cutlan, 2001). It was introduced in the 1960s with claims that it was a tool for reducing perinatal mortality and morbidity – an effective diagnostic aid for detecting fetal asphyxia in labour, which would help prevent fetal deaths and ultimately improve newborn health (Schifrin, 1995). Electronic fetal monitoring (EFM) did not, however, 'catch on' simply on the basis of its objective advantages, but was very much a product of its time. It was a technique that was introduced in the pro-technology, medicalised and hospital-oriented environment of maternity care in the 1970s, where it flourished under the widely held belief that through technological, interventionist medicine mothers would give birth to healthier babies (Anthony & Levine, 1990).

This paradigm shift took place under the influence of the 'Peel Report' (Ministry of Health, 1970). The resulting decrease in the home birth rate led to the technique of intermittent auscultation of the fetal heart (the favoured home birth option) giving way to electronic detection and recording of fetal heart action (Neilson, 1994). Thus, the traditional, but effective Pinard stethoscope was perceived as being obsolete compared to the modern method of EFM (Neilson, 1994). Concurrent with these changes was a fall in the perinatal mortality rate (Erkkola

et al, 1984) and the 'obvious' correlation between the introduction of EFM in the 1970s and the falling perinatal mortality rate was made. 'Success' bred confidence and EFM was introduced for most women, regardless of risk-status (Albers, 1994).

However, debate does surround the relative merits and efficacy of this method (Thacker & Stroup, 2000). While the evidence to support EFM was encouraging, an examination of the evidence surrounding its safety and efficiency was inconclusive, lacked rigorous controls and failed to take into account variables such as improved antenatal and neonatal care, social status, the parity of child-bearing women and the overall improved health of the nation (Edinger et al, 1975). For example, a particularly important change in maternity care was the rise in the availability of screening and diagnostic tests for congenital abnormalities. This increased knowledge about potential adverse intrapartum events for the fetus and led to a subsequent increase in the number of terminations for congenital abnormality. This had a direct effect on perinatal mortality and morbidity rates, since unviable/borderline fetuses that would have appeared in these statistics tended to be shifted into the abortion category (Brook et al, 1974). Also, women's expectations and control of their own fertility were revolutionised with the introduction of the oral contraceptive pill as the favoured method of family planning (Snowden, 1991). Thus, the new technological era that embraced EFM was also a time of great social change, improved reproductive health, choice for women and the transfer of childbirth to a hospital culture. In retrospect, this fast changing environment was not a good one in which to draw rock solid conclusions about the effects of introducing a specific piece of technology.

Looking at the particular conclusions drawn, the studies of the time reasoned that patterns of fetal heart rate traces could be used to indicate signs of fetal hypoxia, pH levels and Apgar scores. Later, randomised controlled trails do demonstrate a lower (and largely consistent) number of neonatal seizures with EFM in prolonged, induced or augmented labours – that is, in women with additional risk factors in labour (Grant et al, 1989). Therefore, we are now in the situation where arguably, in high-risk labouring women, there is demonstrable evidence that EFM is beneficial. Its general application, however, remains questionable from a clinical perspective. That is not to say there that there are not definite advantages to EFM. With a normal CTG trace a practitioner can be reassured of fetal wellbeing because of the low-false negative rate (FIGO, 1987). 92% of consultant-led units consider the CTG, alone or in combination with other tests, to be the most reliable method of detecting fetal distress prior to labour (Wheble et al, 1989). Secondly, many women enjoy non-interventionist tests that directly show them evidence of a healthy fetus. The ultrasound scan is the best example of this (Baillie, 2000), but the sound of a heartbeat can also be a thrilling moment.

CTG interpretation

An important fetal heart rate parameter is its variation, which naturally changes abruptly with the baby's sleep state (Dawes et al, 1990). The healthy baby has frequent episodes of high variation (active sleep associated with fetal movements). Episodes of low variation correspond to quiet sleep and can last for up to 50 minutes. Hypoxaemia is revealed by an unusually low FHR variation (Dawes et al, 1992). Hence, an episode of high variation indicates normality, but as the fetus deteriorates overall variation progressively falls, which can be used to detect the onset of acidaemia (Diogo et al, 2000).

The central problem with EFM lies in interpretation. Indeed, the absence of a uniform policy and the failure to recognise the relationship between fetal hypoxia and the risks of neurological damage have led to the situation of dramatic variation in the interpretation of fetal heart rate patterns among practitioners, and even by the same person at different times (Simkin, 1987). The failure to demonstrate the superiority of EFM over auscultation and the inability to improve birth outcomes may be attributed to the lack of uniformity in naming and interpreting fetal heart patterns. There is usually a consensus of agreement about the baseline, which, while an important prerequisite for analysis (Dawes et al, 1982) does not address the problems arising from analysis of reactivity and variability. So much so, that visual analysis of FHR variation has consistently proved to be unreliable (Albers, 1994; Dawes et al, 1992).

Computerised analysis systems represent modern methods for overcoming the difficulties with variation interpretation. Dawes-Redman is a computer-based system designed for use during the antenatal period only, which analyses the non-stress test. The main test criteria are used to detect placental dysfunction (Pattison & McCowan, 2000) by comparing the subject's signals with data derived from more than 43,000 records. The maximum duration of a record is 60 minutes. In fact, more than 50% of records are stopped after 10 minutes; the average duration of a record is only about 15 minutes. If there is no episode of high variation by 60 minutes, the fetus is considered to be abnormal, and should be reported as such. If there are doubts about fetal health then it may be necessary to use other methods of assessment to supplement the FHR analysis, for example ultrasound scanning (Vintzileos & Hanley, 2000).

It is important at this point to remember that EFM is not a diagnostic device but rather it alerts the practitioner to the possibility of fetal compromise. The information obtained by computer analysis should be taken in an advisory capacity; it should be not used as a short cut for interpretation. Also, techniques of intermittent auscultation do not directly provide information about fetal heart rate variability. Reduced fetal movements can be an ominous sign and may indicate fetal compromise (Albers, 1994), but epidemiological evidence indicates that asphyxia is far more likely to be due to a prenatal event rather than an intrapartum one (Rosen & Dickinson, 1993). Thus, EFM in the antenatal period may provide clues to fetal compromise, however it is unlikely to predict it and prevent it (Neilson, 1994).

The computer can provide objective data, but not a judgement. What it can do is contribute to the high intraobserver and interobserver variation on fetal analysis (Dawes et al, 1990). This is important since even when computerised analysis of the FHR is used, care-providers do not always agree with the results (Bracero et al, 2000). Hence it is important that a midwife does not allow the process of decision-making to shift from the professional to the machine. If that happens then she becomes dependent on a computerised trace analysis and runs the risk of losing the vital midwifery skills of interpretation and understanding (Gibb & Arulkumaran, 1997). Used properly computer analysis may save time, by avoiding the necessity for a second opinion when an ambiguous trace has been obtained and thus has the advantage of supporting midwifery led-care (Dawes et al, 1992). This is time that could be spent with the parents, reassuring them and/or answering their questions.

One of the most common causes of referrals to the antenatal day unit is reduced fetal movements (Gibb & Arulkumaran, 1997). Pregnant women and their care-providers have long recognised the importance of fetal movements as a measure of fetal health (Pattison & McCowan, 2000). Thus, a perceived lack of fetal movement can be worrying for a pregnant woman – her only direct sensory confirmation of the life of her fetus is suspended and she becomes understandably concerned. In most cases the reason is benign, and the lack of movement temporary. However, it can also indicate fetal distress due to, for example, oxygen compromise, or even death.

Women are encouraged to be aware of their babies' movements because fetal activity such as movement perceived by the mother is a reliable indicator of fetal health. Consequently, a lack and/or reduction of movements may be an important alarm signal during pregnancy and is a reason for fetal assessment (Gibb & Arulkumaran, 1997). Unless an ultrasound scan is performed, direct observation of the fetus is not possible, therefore indirect information relating to fetal condition is required. A normal reactive trace is associated with survival of the fetus for one week or more in more than 99% of cases (Parer, 1999). Thus the key decision-making task is differentiating between the normal and abnormal, requiring integration of knowledge from available clinical evidence, from previous experience and the use of clinical judgement (Bates, 2001).

When a woman reports reduced fetal movements in a normal healthy pregnancy, testing for fetal wellbeing is primarily for maternal reassurance (Druzin, 2000). A severely compromised fetus would be expected to demonstrate other symptoms and only then may a selection of tests appropriate to conditions be made (Gibb & Arulkumaran, 1997).

In modern life technology plays a prominent role; we are surrounded by machines with push button facilities, electronic beeps and glowing visual displays. The overwhelming cultural effect of this is to make us believe four things. First, we are in control, second we have choices, third our lives are directly improved by technology and fourth technology is good (conversely, an absence of technology is bad). This is not the place to debate these issues in general, but the point is made to highlight the cultural background in which clients and practitioners inhabit. Midwifery has not been immune to these trends and midwives are now expected to use technology as part of their work (Crozier, 2001). Technology, coupled with the fall in perinatal mortality and morbidity means that our expectations have been raised to the point where we demand to know why anything goes wrong – pregnancy included. It is even argued that women seek out technologies in pregnancy and childbirth in an attempt to feel in control and feel safer (Sinclair, 2000).

Women do worry about a lack of fetal movement and sense something is wrong (Moulder, 1997). Thus, it is understandable that women find fetal monitoring reassuring rather than worrying (Jackson et al, 1983).

However, many believe that EFM can guarantee the safety of their baby (Burnham & Gillmer, 1996). Tests provide probabilities, not certainties and the language used to explain this is regularly cited to be difficult to use and often poorly handled. This may be because midwives often have a strong inclination to reassure women to make them feel better (Moulder, 1997), pandering to their increasing expectations of a perfect outcome for their infant (Burnham & Gillmer, 1996). The fact that women are reassured, rather than apprehensive about the test shows that they are at ease and familiar with technology in general and results are taken unquestioningly. This is understandable in a client, but less acceptable in a midwife, who should understand the questions and qualifications, which surround computerised diagnosis. Communication is the key here.

The computerised CTG is perceived by the health professionals using it as simple and routine particularly in cases of reduced fetal movements. Information giving to women particularly in the antenatal period has been said to be inconsistent and often standard and not adapted to take into account women's understanding of the situation (Kirkham & Perkins, 1997).

Skilling and de-skilling of midwives

Most women prior to labour now have a CTG trace and it is considered a basic competency for midwives to keep up to date with the use of this technology (UKCC, 1996; UKCC, 1998), but also to be aware of its limitations and to ensure they give accurate information to women. It is also a component of being able to offer women choice and it can only be informed choice if the midwife fully understands what she is offering. As technology advances the midwives role will continue to change (Cario, 1985). Technical skills, scientific knowledge, practical abilities and good clinical judgement are all necessary for effective care, but they must be employed in the context of individual situations (Page, 1995). Some would argue that increasing dependence on machinery turns a midwife from a skilled practitioner into a technician (Tew, 1990). Again the question is not should a tool be used, but how should it be used. Is the CTG program making the final diagnosis or the midwife?

A midwife who learns to use a CTG machine and knows how to blend it with her traditional skills has advanced her practice. A midwife who simply presses buttons and relies on a computer-generated number to make her decisions for her is reducing her skill. To be 'with woman' means understanding that women need to be treated as equals in their understanding of their pregnancy. If a test is limited in its meaning then this should be explained. The failure is often not in clinical judgement, but in communication. The women are often discharged reassured, but under the misapprehension that they are guaranteed a perfect baby because the machine said so – which clearly could never be the case.

Conclusion

At present the methods of information gathering about fetal health are limited and EFM is the prevalent aid to the midwife in screening for fetal compromise. In most cases in modern maternity care, EFM represents the routine supervision of the fetal heart, but does not necessarily improve outcomes and certainly does not replace clinically observed evidence. For any test to be effective, safe, and efficient with the provision of consistent reliable information it must be reproducible and not open to misinterpretation. EFM has often been criticised for the overall lack of consistent interpretation by many practitioners. However, used appropriately in conjunction with computerised analysis it is a useful way of confirming normality. It is not, though, a predictive tool for unexpected fetal death. EFM can only provide a snapshot of fetal health at a particular moment and as such is a good way to provide reassurance for that moment in time.

REFERENCES

Albers L. 1994. Clinical issues in electronic fetal monitoring. Birth, 21(2). 108-110

Anthony M, Levine M. 1990. An assessment of the benefits of intrapartum fetal monitoring. Developmental Medicine & Child Neurology, 32, 547-533

Baillie C. 2000. Psychological benefits of routine obstetric ultrasound: are there any? BMUS Bulletin, May, 36-37

Bates C. 2001. Assessing and managing risk in midwifery practice. Clinical risk management series. London: The Royal College of Midwives

Bracero L, Roshanfekr D, Byrne D. 2000. Analysis of antepartum fetal heart rate tracing by physician and computer. The Journal of Maternal-Fetal Medicine, 9(3), 181-185

Brook D, Bolton A, Scrimegeour J. 1974. Prenatal diagnosis of spina bifida and anencephaly through maternal plasma-alpha fetoprotein measurement. The Lancet, 1, 767

Burnham D, Gillmer M. 1996. CTG revisited: how valuable is it? Obstetrics & Gynaecology, November/December, 227-229

Cario G. 1985. Fetal monitoring. Senior Nurse, 2(3), 11-13

Crozier K. 2000. Technology: is it killing the art of midwifery? RCM Midwives Journal, 4(12), 410-11

Cutlan C. 2001. Cardiotocography in Labour. Clinical Risk Management Series. London: The Royal College of Midwives

Dawes G, Houghton C, Redman C. 1982. Baseline in human heart-rate records. British Journal of Obstetrics & Gynaecology, 89, 270-275

Dawes G, Moulden M, Redman C. 1990. Limitations of antenatal fetal heart rate monitors. American Journal of Obstetrics & Gynaecology, 170-173

Dawes G, Lobb M, Moulden M et al. 1992. Antenatal cardiotocogram quality and interpretation using computers. British Journal of Obstetrics & Gynaecology, 99, 791-797

Diogo A, Bernardes J, Garrido A et al. 2000. Sisporto 2.0: A program for automated analysis of cardiotocograms. The Journal of Maternal-Fetal Medicine, 9(5), 311-318

Druzin M. 2000. Antepartum fetal heart rate monitoring. In: Winn H, Hobbins J (Eds). Clinical Maternal-fetal Medicine. London: The Parthenon Publishing Group

Edinger P, Sabinda J, Beard R. 1975. Influence on clinical practice of routine intrapartum fetal monitoring. British Medical Journal, 168, 341

Erkkola R, Gronroos M, Punnonen R et al. 1984. Analysis of intrapartum fetal deaths: their decline with increasing electronic fetal monitoring. Acta Obstetrics & Gynaecology of Scandinavia, 63, 459-462

FIGO. 1987. Guidelines for the use of fetal monitoring. International Journal of Gynaecology & Obstetrics, 25, 159-167

Gibb D, Arulkumaran S. 1997. Fetal Monitoring in Practice. 2nd Edition. Oxford: Butterworth-Heinemann

Grant A, O'Brien N, Hennessy E. 1989. Cerebral palsy among children born during the Dublin randomised trail of intrapartum monitoring. The Lancet, 25th November, 1233-1235

Kirkham M, Perkins E. 1997. Reflections on Midwifery. London: Bailliere Tindall.

Jackson J, Vaughan M, Black P et al. 1983. Psychological aspects of fetal monitoring: maternal reaction to the position of the monitor and staff behaviour. Journal of Psychosomatic Obstetrics & Gynaecology, 2, 97-102

Ministry of Health. 1970. Domiciliary Midwifery and Maternity Bed Needs: the report of the Standing Maternity and Midwifery Advisory Sub-committee Chairman: J. Peel. London: HMSO

Moulder C. 1997. Understanding pregnancy loss: perspectives and issues in care. London: Macmillan

Neilson J. 1994. Electronic fetal heart monitoring during labour: information from randomised trails. Birth, 21(2), 101-104

Page L. 1995. Putting principles into practice. In: Page L (Ed). Effective Group Practice in Midwifery: Working with women. Oxford: Blackwell Science

Parer J. 1999. Fetal heart rate. In: Creasy R, Resnik R (Eds). Maternal-Fetal Medicine. 4th Edition. London: WB Saunders & Co

Pattison N, McCowan L. 2000. Cardiotocography for antepartum fetal assessment (Cochrane Review). In: The Cochrane Library Issue 3. Oxford: Update Software

Rosen M, Dickinson J. 1993. The paradox of electronic fetal monitoring: more data may not enable us to predict or prevent infant neurologic morbidity. American Journal of Obstetrics & Gynaecology, 168, 745-751

Schifrin B. 1995. Mediolegal ramifications of electronic fetal monitoring during labour. Clinics in Perinatology, 22(4), 837-854

Simkin P. 1987. Is anyone listening? The lack of clinical impact of randomised controlled trails of electronic fetal monitoring. Birth, 13(4), 219-220

Sinclair M. 2000. Birth technology: observations of high usage in the labour ward. All Ireland Journal of Nurse-Midwifery, 1(3), 83-88

Snowden R. 1991. Social factors affecting contraceptive use. In: Louden N (Ed). Handbook of Family Planning. Edinburgh: Churchill Livingstone

Sureau C. 1996. Historical perspectives: forgotten past, unpredictable future. Bailliere's Clinical Obstetrics & Gynaecology, 10(2), 167-184

Tew M. 1990. Safer Childbirth: a critical history of maternity care. London: Chapman & Hall

Thacker S, Stroup D. 2000. Continuous electronic heart rate monitoring for fetal assessment during labour (Cochrane Review). In: The Cochrane Library Issue 3. Oxford: Update Software

UKCC. 1996. Guidelines for professional practice. London: UKCC

UKCC. 1998. Midwife's Rules and Code of Practice. London: UKCC

Vintzileos A, Hanley M. 2000. Antepartum fetal assessment by ultrasonography. In: Callen P (Ed). Ultrasonography in Obstetrics & Gynaecology. 4th Edition. Philadelphia: WB Saunders & Co

Wheble A, Gillmere M, Spencer J et al. 1989. Changes in fetal monitoring practice in the UK: 1977-1984. British Journal of Obstetrics & Gynaecology, 96, 1140-1147

Reflecting on Pregnancy

• Which of the issues raised in Zevia Schneider's article do you feel most strongly about? (For instance, some midwives feel most strongly that we should support women in labour, while others feel that informed choice is paramount.) Why do you feel this is the case? Do you feel that this affects the way you practise? If you have had children of your own, have your own experiences of pregnancy impacted on the way you midwife other women?

• What are your views on whether there is a "brick wall" that parents find it hard to see beyond during pregnancy? Although there is evidence that being prepared for parenting has a positive effect on children (as discussed in Andrew Julian Wiener's article), I sometimes wonder if our professional preoccupation with this issue is also partly a reflection of our societal tendency to live in the future rather than the present? What do you think about this?

• How frequently are CTGs being used on pregnant women where you work? How can we make sure that these are used appropriately, and that women are given the kind of information that they need?

If you feel like writing…

• If you agree that relaxation is a useful thing for midwives to teach, would you consider writing your own relaxation exercise to read to women during pregnancy or birth? You can find examples of these in books and on tapes, and you could incorporate the phrases and affirmations you think are important. If you don't like the idea of writing, or of a relaxation exercise, how about a finding or writing a poem that you could read to women while they close their eyes and relax during a break?

If you feel like taking action…

• Has there been any kind of work done with the women in your area to find out what they want and how they feel about the service offered? This doesn't have to be a mammoth piece of research; all you would need is a box, a pack of index cards and a notice inviting women to write their suggestions and comments on a card and post it in the box. It may be that the results of such a survey could be fed into local committees and decision-making processes in order to make services more responsive to women's needs.

Focus on:
Spirituality

SECTION CONTENTS

Antenatal classes and spirituality

An oxymoron or opportunity for transcendancy?

Lorna Davies

We talk about 'holistic care' a great deal in midwifery practice and education. Yet, in reality, how much of what we offer is truly holistic; that is, geared to optimise the emotional, psychological, social, and spiritual experience of the childbearing period for women and their families? Most midwifery practitioners would consider themselves to be skilled at identifying the physical requirements of women. Some of us may even be fortunate to work in a team or group practice, where we get to know each woman reasonably well and have some insight into who she really is, and what factors are affecting her during this pregnancy, enabling us to help her to identify her social and psychological needs. The really thorny issue in the model of holistic care seems to be this matter of spirituality.

As a culture, we are not very comfortable with the whole notion of spirituality. It is an abstract and complex entity that is easier to slot into the box of 'religion', in neat little denominational boxes. That way, it doesn't interfere too much with the main thrust of provision in care within our reductionist pseudo-scientific system.

Jenny Hall, in her book *Midwifery, Mind and Spirit* (2001), rightly points out that any discussion of spirituality is usually confined to the question of 'what religion are you?' at booking interview. This suggests that one's spirituality is restricted to a strict code of religious conformity, and ignores the manifold ways in which human beings utilise a spiritual plain as a form of self-expression.

The spiritual dimension of our humanity is not necessarily defined by holiness or mysticism, though it may be. It may be encountered in acts of collective worship, but it may equally be a profoundly personal and private affair. It may focus on articles of faith, or be a statement of self, which may culminate in a transcendental experience.

I do not intend to undermine the significance of religious faith or practice, or the importance of acknowledging the individual denominational needs of our client group. But I feel that we must recognise that a tick box describing religious conviction or association may do little to inform us of the spiritual needs of women in their pregnancies, birth and postnatal period, and that we must be aware of this fact.

Pregnancy places a woman in a very special place, on a journey from one state of being (woman) to a new state of being (mother). Does this journey have the potential to be transcendental? Is this a concept that we embrace within our current provision of care? Are fathers also on a spiritual journey, that will lead to the development of new elements of the self?

How can we, as midwives, best help new parents on this journey? I firmly believe that we have the capacity to provide such opportunities during the antenatal period, both in an informal capacity on a one-to-one basis with the woman and on a slightly more formal level in parent education sessions in the antenatal and postnatal period.

It would appear that the dominant consideration in antenatal classes in the NHS continues to be the preparation for the physical event, although progress is slowly being made and the psychological and emotional needs of women are being more widely addressed, thanks to the work of antenatal educators such as Andrea Robertson, Judith Schott and Mary Nolan. The recognition that a woman's emotional state may affect her physical state is now broadly recognised. However, the spiritual element continues to be shadowed, and if the model of holistic care is right then the harmony required for total wellbeing may be held in disequilibrium.

We may argue that we facilitate client-led sessions, where the group determine the agenda. Therefore if they request information on the menu of pain relief, then we are duty bound to provide that for them. I would argue that we frequently end up providing them with information that they do not necessarily require, information that they either already have, or have easy access to. I would equally argue that there is no reason why a spiritual dimension could not be included within a discussion on pain and its purpose in labour, instrumental delivery or any other subject considered essential in parent education. In her book, *Birthing from Within*, Pam England (1991) emphasises that regardless of the mode of birth, the most significant factor is that the woman has experienced 'birthing in awareness'.

Pregnancy itself may be considered by the woman to be an intensely spiritual experience. On a physical, psychosocial and spiritual level, it is a rite of passage. A correspondent on a midwifery Internet list recently described birth as the nearest a woman gets to reaching out and touching the face of God. It is not uncommon for a woman who has experienced labour to talk about an out-of-body or other psychic experience.

We know that encouraging a woman to communicate with her unborn child may have some physical and psychological benefits; we may add to this a spiritual advantage.

Fergal Keane, the BBC overseas correspondent, has published a series of letters that he wrote to his unborn son during spells away from his partner during her pregnancy. This simple act has left his son with a legacy that few people would fail to be touched by. Couples attending classes could be introduced to this idea. This may be something that they will eventually share with their child in years to come, or it may remain a private entity, but one that may help them to grow and develop as parents.

I actively encourage parents to keep a log of their experience of pregnancy in pretty much the same way that they would keep a 'baby book' once the baby has been born. This may include reflections on being pregnant or being with someone in their journey through pregnancy; photographs of the mother and father during this period; interesting news items and stories; entries from the grandparents. Women frequently become more aware of their creativity during this, the greatest act of creation, and it may prompt them to write poetry or paint or draw, and these could also be included.

Pam England introduced me to the idea of preparing a 'birthing bundle' for the baby. Couples are encouraged to bring along a number of items for their baby which they have wrapped in a bundle and, if they are comfortable, to 'show and tell' with the group. The items must include something that symbolises the life of one of the grandparents, something from the parents that represents who they (singly or jointly) are, and something that represents the baby itself. I have never ceased to be moved at the offerings that group members have made when I have used this activity in my sessions. Items such as poetry, pressed flowers, family bibles and

patchwork quilts have been offered. The birthing bundle makes the group members consider connections with the past and the future and in doing so gives them a sense of their own place in the world. It also highlights the changing relationship with their own parents at this significant time and lastly it makes them consider the relationship that they want to have with their new baby, often beyond a material level.

Using a spiritual approach in sessions may mean developing an intuitive response in a woman and her partner. We believe that women are particularly intuitive during pregnancy and by helping to strengthen a woman's belief in her intuitive responses we may enable her to achieve an enhanced belief in her ability as a mother. Intuitive responses are almost impossible to quantify and do not therefore sit comfortably within a medical model of care. Women may therefore be wary of sharing what they believe to be irrational responses which may sometimes supersede decisions based on medical information. Encouraging women to talk about their dreams, which are known to be 'different' during pregnancy, may help to strengthen their trust in their own intuitive responses, and encourage them to disclose what they may perceive as unfounded knowledge.

Relaxation and visualisation may offer another means of establishing an intuitive bond between parents-to-be and their future offspring. A basic relaxation exercise can be used initially and when in a relaxed state, the group should be asked to imagine a special place where they would like to be. Get them to think about the surroundings, the sounds, the colours, the temperature. Ask them to consider why this place is so special to them, why is it significant. Then ask them to imagine taking their child to this place and sharing with them. When the group have come out of the relaxation, you can ask them how they feel, where they were, and how it felt to share where they had been.

A further visualisation involves getting the group into a state of deep relaxation before getting them to visualise their unborn baby. A guided imagery can then be used to get them to see the watery world of the baby; to hear the muffled sounds and the growing familiarity of its parents' voices; to imagine its ten tiny fingers and toes and the little toe and finger nails. I have found over the years that this particular relaxation exercise is extremely effective at getting parents to connect with their babies. If couples are doing it together, it is useful if the father sits behind the mother with his hands gently touching her 'bump'. This enables him to make a connection with the baby too and may help both parents to visualise their little one more clearly.

Birth is a rite of passage: as we have already acknowledged, it embraces the transitional acts of woman to mother and man to father. This is a profound event and one that surely deserves due recognition. In other cultures, rituals and celebrations of birth abound. Sheila Kitzinger and Jacqueline Vincent-Priya highlight numerous accounts of such acts of ceremony in their work. However, in western industrialised society, we seem to have lost sight of the sacred value of birth and with it we have lost the sense of initiation that ritual brings to this rite of passage. Ironically we still recognise the importance of ritual in marriage and death, if not the sanctity, but in birth the nearest we get to a ritual is the commercialisation of the American baby shower or the father's pub celebration in the early postnatal period.

I recently met a woman from California, who told me about a tribe of Native American Indians who take the pregnant women from their tribe when they are about 36 weeks pregnant, and involve them in an interesting ritual where they receive a 'make-over'. Someone will massage them; someone else will brush and style their hair. They are adorned with new clothes and jewellery and emerge as a new person, which serves as a metaphor for their new persona as mother. Most women that I know would welcome the thought of being pampered and luxuriated at a stage of pregnancy when one is often tired and weary. Most importantly, this simple rewarding act actively acknowledges the woman's changing status.

The newly revived trend of belly casting could provide a vehicle for exalting the passage to motherhood. This act, which involves creating a plaster cast of the woman's pregnant abdomen followed by decoration of the impression, provides the opportunity for the woman to metaphorically step outside her pregnancy and create something beautiful and eternal from this special period in her life.

Pam England encourages the men who attend her classes to bring in a gift for their partner, without the knowledge of the women. They are then invited to perform a footbath (complete with floating rose petals and essential oils) on their partner, followed by a foot massage. At the end of the ceremony, the man dries the feet of the woman and then presents her with his gift. This is an act of love that is guaranteed to make any woman feel as though she is the most special person in the world, and serves as a wonderful act of initiation into motherhood.

Many of these activities may sound arcane and may leave the reader wondering how they could have any place in the antenatal classes that we are currently able (or willing) to provide. They may consider their clientele to be more interested in the facts, 'spiritually bereft' or simply unready for such an initiation. From personal experience I would suggest that they serve to fulfil those who are involved in a way that defies scepticism.

We know that from the work of many in this field that our current approach to parent education is not meeting the needs of parents-to-be. It may well be that holistic needs are not being met. The idea of trying something so different may fill you with trepidation, but by feeling the fear and doing it anyway, you may be opening a window to the soul that has been denied within a strictly medical frame of reference. The benefits may be as great for the midwife/facilitator as they are for the women and their partners, and may offer a new and strengthened belief in the less concrete elements of becoming a parent.

REFERENCES

England P, Horowitz R. 1991. Birthing From Within. Pantheon Publishing
Hall J. 2001. Midwifery Mind and Spirit. Books for Midwives Press
Keane F. 1996. Letter to Daniel: Despatches from the heart. Penguin
Robertson A. 1994. Empowering Women. ACE Graphics
Schott J, Priest J. 2001. Leading Antenatal Classes 2nd edn. Books for Midwives Press

Nolan M. 1998. Antenatal Education. Baillière Tindall
Kitzinger S. 2000. Rediscovering Birth. Little, Brown
Vincent-Priya J, Odent M. 1994. Birth Traditions and Modern Pregnancy Care. Element Books

The Practising Midwife 2002; 5(11): 19-21

The pregnant Pagan

Amber House

If a woman informed you, during her first antenatal visit, that she was a Pagan, would you know what she meant? Would you know how, and if, her spiritual beliefs would affect her wishes during pregnancy? Your answer may well be 'no', yet at most booking visits, midwives ask women a question about their religion. The aim of this is to gain an understanding of the special requirements and rituals that may be performed during pregnancy and birth, relevant to that religion or belief system (Sweet, 1999). However, such information is often merely recorded, and an opportunity for further exploration is lost (Schott and Henly, 1996).

Spiritual belief has relevance to clinical practice and needs to be incorporated into healthcare. As midwives, the care we give to clients should be appropriate to the individual and promote and protect their interests (NMC, 2002). Spirituality is an individual, personal and basic element of us all; our beliefs and values are woven into the very fabric of our being (Schott and Henly, 1996). If spirituality is important to health and wellbeing, how can Pagan beliefs and spirituality be better recognised and incorporated into midwifery care?

Whilst it is not appropriate to give in-depth detail about Pagan belief and practice, a brief outline and definition follows. The word 'Pagan' derives from the Latin 'Paganius' meaning a country dweller, or one who had their own rustic or regional way of doing things (Pagan Hospice and Funeral Trust [PHFT], 1992). Today, Paganism is seen as meaning ancestral religion (Pagan Federation [PF], 1996) and Pagans regard themselves as those who have retained the wisdom and values of their ancestors (PHFT, 1992). As such Paganism is probably one of the oldest surviving religions and although exact numbers are difficult to obtain, a conservative estimate made a few years ago was that there were 25,000 practising Pagans in Britain, compared at the time with 20,000 Quakers, showing the extent of the belief in the UK (PHFT, 1992). Paganism as a term covers many

traditions, including Wicca, Druidism and The Northern traditions, yet according to the Pagan Federation (1996) all have three fundamental elements in common. These are the veneration of nature (for example, in celebrating the cycle of the year, or respect for the earth as sacred), polytheism (a belief in many different gods or goddesses), and recognition of the feminine face of divinity (or a belief that the divine being can be or is female). Although the meaning of these may differ according to the tradition, this gives a brief overview of the fundamental elements.

There is a small amount of literature available examining the relationship purely between spirituality and pregnancy. Of these pieces, all assume that there is a connection between the two, but for differing reasons. Campanelli (1998) and Wickham (2001) both perceive pregnancy and childbirth as a rite of passage, laden with spiritual meaning and therefore transcending from the physical to the spiritual. Other authors view the connection in terms of the pregnant woman being a symbol of ultimate creativity (Hall, 2001) or a reflection of the Goddess herself (PHFT, 1992). Jennifer Hall also suggests that the experience of being pregnant may stimulate a woman to evaluate her beliefs or may awaken spiritual resources previously buried (Hall, 2001).

If the evidence does conclude that spirituality is important for women during pregnancy, is it already being considered during antenatal care? In order to ascertain whether Pagan beliefs are already being catered for, ten informal interviews with Pagan couples that had experienced midwifery care were undertaken. These were initially instigated by placing requests for views and input on the Internet. Email correspondence was used by the majority who replied, with some couples also agreeing to talk over the telephone. The interviews consisted of requests for a history of their experience of antenatal care, whether their 'carers' were aware of their beliefs, how those beliefs affected their requirements during pregnancy and childbirth, and whether those requirements were met appropriately. Extracts and information from those interviews are below.

Firstly, all respondents stated that their Pagan beliefs made them want a more natural experience of pregnancy, because, as one woman stated, she had a 'bone-deep knowledge that this is what my body is evolved for'. However, all the respondents expressed the view that they would be happy to have whatever intervention was appropriate, as long as it was deemed necessary and with prior discussion. When questioned about any ceremonies or rituals used during the antenatal period, one couple who practice Heathenism held a blot (a ritual involving the gifting of food and drink) to the goddesses, asking for their protection and help, and gave a gift of bread, milk and honey. Another couple that are practising Wiccans had rituals of protection during pregnancy, held at certain times in the lunar cycle. Others didn't hold rituals or ceremonies but used alternative therapies, like herbalism, osteopathy or homeopathy, or meditation, to help them during their pregnancy. When asked whether their midwives knew of their beliefs, most replied that they were reluctant to 'advertise' their beliefs due to fears about lack of understanding. Several women interviewed only told their midwives that they were Pagans at the booking visit, because they were asked their religion. Those who informed their midwives received a variety of responses. One woman said ' the midwife looked at me blankly and told me that she would put me down as an atheist'. Another couple had the response 'A Pagan birth? Oh well, I suppose it'll be all right.' Several respondents used the phrase 'we had to make do', feeling that they were unable to express their spiritual beliefs adequately, when receiving midwifery care. None of the couples stated that they had had their views disrespected, just misunderstood and not considered adequately.

This may be the case for people who practise other faiths, too, but there is a distinct difference. As a midwife, if one wishes to understand more about the religious needs of a couple practising one of the 'mainstream' faiths, there are books and literature available, so that health professionals can give care suited to their needs. There are also strict rituals and rules that these religions abide by, that health professionals can be aware of, and which affect the majority of practising believers of that faith.

Paganism does not have set books, strict rules, or universal ritual. Is this a bad thing? Whilst it does not allow health professionals to learn more about Paganism on a global scale, it gives the opportunity for individual Pagans and couples to explain their faith in their own terms. It also prevents people making assumptions about a person's needs or feelings on a particular matter involving their health or pregnancy.

So, how can Pagan beliefs be better catered for and better understood in midwifery care? Firstly, there is a need for spiritual beliefs to be seen as more than a demographic (Hume, 1999). Asking about a person's belief should be seen as a starting point in identifying potential needs and personal preferences (Schott and Henly, 1996). As much as knowledge of a person's spirituality is not about demographics, it may also not be about spiritual observance or outward practice (Goldberg, 1998). If a woman informs you that she is a Pagan, take the opportunity to learn about her faith and beliefs. Being seen as non-judgemental, sensitive and respectful of another's beliefs, and giving recognition of their faith (Yawar, 2001) allows for further discussion and may be all that is required. This can improve the relationship between midwife and client and therefore improve a woman's satisfaction with her care. As is suggested by the PHFT (1992), write 'Pagan' in the antenatal notes, with a capital 'P', under the place assigned to 'religion' and anywhere else the woman wishes. If a situation arises where the services of a chaplain would normally be offered, this is unlikely to be appropriate. However, do offer to contact someone suitable to their needs, rather than offer nothing at all.

More broadly, the particular requirements of Pagans will not be adequately acknowledged in midwifery practice until the general importance of spirituality is recognised. Health professionals understand the importance of spirituality at the point of death. Midwives need to see and appreciate its relevance at the start of life.

REFERENCES

Campanelli P. 1998. Pagan Rites of Passage. Minnesota: Llewellyn Publications
Goldberg B. 1998. Connection: An Exploration of Spirituality in Nursing Care. Journal of Advanced Nursing 27, 836-842
Hall J. 2001. Midwifery, Mind & Spirit. Oxford: Books For Midwives
Hume C. 1999. Spirituality: A Part of Total Care? British Journal of Occupational Therapy 62 (8), 367-369
McLean C. 1999. Birth Brings More Than a Baby. Alberta Report, 26 (15), 29
Nursing and Midwifery Council. 2002. Code of Professional Conduct. London: NMC
The Pagan Hospice and Funeral Trust. 1992. Caring for the Pagan Patient. London: PHFT
Pagan Federation. 1996. Information Pack. London: Pagan Federation.
Schott J, Henly A. 1996. Culture, Religion and Childbearing in a Multiracial Society: A Handbook for Health Professionals. Oxford: Butterworth Heinemann
Sweet B. 1999. Mayes Midwifery. 12th ed. London: Harcourt

Wickham S. 2001. Reclaiming Spirituality in Birth [online]. http://www.withwoman.co.uk/contents/info/ spiritualbirth.html [Accessed 27th May 2002]

Wright S. 2000. Life, the Universe and You. Nursing Standard, 14 (52), 23

Wright S. 2001. Looking at the Stars. Nursing Standard, 15 (52), 26-27

Yawar A. 2001. Spirituality in Medicine: What is to be done? Journal of the Royal Society of Medicine, 94, 529-533

The Practising Midwife 2002; 5(11): 14-15

Labour and spirituality

Meg Taylor

Some weeks after I gave birth to my second baby I found myself assailed by sadness because I was unlikely ever to give birth again. What I was grieving for was not more babies, but labour itself. I love my children and I am sure that the savage physicality of my feelings for them as babies was coloured by my experience of giving birth. But it is the darkness, pain and otherworldliness of labour that I was lusting for. In considering what it is about labour that drew me, what emerges is something very like a description of certain spiritual practices or the stages on a journey of self-healing.

Labour involves a withdrawal from the world, a regression inwards. Janet Balaskas (1991) writes:

'in the hours of labour you will want to withdraw from the normal day-to-day level of things and your attention will naturally turn inwards, as if the whole world contracts to what is happening in your body. In your mind, time takes on a fresh dimension. Hours can pass in what seems like minutes. It is like being in another world... This great opening of the womb happens only a few times in your life. It is a very deep emotional experience which involves a regression to your most basic and primitive feelings.'

This withdrawal is occasioned by the overwhelming power of the event in simple muscular terms. Concentration on the contractions of this most powerful muscle in established labour precludes preoccupation with anything else – in fact, this self-absorption is one of the signs that labour is established and working. This focus on oneself does not mean that the outside world is shut out. I found myself aware of the passing of time and what my partner and the midwives were doing and thinking. It was as if by focusing inwards I had broadened my awareness. What I could not do was comment on or communicate my experience. There was not time or energy or language to describe this complex working on simultaneous levels. This strange simultaneous narrowing and broadening of awareness is one aspect of the altered state of consciousness which women in labour experience. This

alteration is caused partly by the secretion of endorphins. I believe the secretion of endorphins is facilitated by the rhythmic intensity of the contractions and a rhythmic response to them which involves altered breathing and sometimes chanting.

The time of labour is a special time, time out, a time of transition like twilight. It is a time of heightened awareness. Time moves but the focus is on the instant. And once started there is no going back. An irrevocable threshold must be crossed – the baby emerges under the pubic arch and the woman becomes mother to a new life. Often in labour there is a time of despair, called in the textbooks transition. This occurs just before or around the time that the cervix becomes fully open and the baby can start to move down and be born. This moment of despair must be confronted and worked through, just as the baby must go through the cervix and the pelvis. There is no going back.

The parallels between this experience and various practices designed to enhance spiritual growth are clear. I am thinking particularly of the use of rhythm and chanting both in shamanic ritual and more orthodox forms of worship. Shamanic ritual requires the participant to seek to alter states of consciousness to effect healing or for initiation. The boundaries of the ritual set the event apart from ordinary day-to-day life, as does the altered awareness. There is a withdrawing, often into literal darkness.

Tibetan Buddhism is the result of the mutual influence of Buddhism and shamanistic Bon thought and practice. Walt Adamson (1989) writes of Tibetan Buddhism:

'The Buddhist technology of growth includes many forms of regression... Meditation, the most common feature of Buddhist practice is itself a retreat... It can be a restful nourishing withdrawal into passivity, or it can be a daring descent into the darkest depths of the psyche. The elaborate visualisation practices of the Vajrayana are disciplined regression.'

Labour, ritual, worship, can enable us to be aware of

and enter a Bardo state. Chogyam Trungpa (1992) describes the Bardo as:

'[a] gap; it is not only the interval of suspension after we die but also suspension in the living situation...There are all kinds of Bardo experiences happening all the time... it is like not being sure of our ground, not knowing quite what we have asked for or what we are getting.'

Ornstein (1992) describes a state of consciousness which resembles the altered consciousness of labour:

'a state of darkness, a shift in the receptive characteristics of consciousness, so that sensitivity is increased to a new segment of the internal, personal and geophysical environment.'

To bring this shift about there must be a withdrawal from the day-to-day, a concentration on a single focus – the breath, a candle flame, labour contractions – and the shift in consciousness can be measured using an EEG. One effect of this shift in consciousness is that automatic, habitual responses to stimuli are made conscious. One becomes dehabituated and the world appears fresh. The familiar is seen as if for the first time. (One could perhaps employ the term *jamais vu*. Labour also brings forth something which is seen for the first time: the baby is literally *jamais vu*.) Ornstein also describes a type of perception with a profound sense of unity. He claims that we all have the capacity for mystic experience and that it need not be the result of meditation but can also be produced by fasting, ritual dance, psychoactive drugs, or by a life crisis. Labour and birth form a life crisis. Within our current midwifery practice, is it cruel to deny women this opportunity to confront and work through this crisis?

Marion Woodman (1985) quoting Bruce Lincoln, states that for women initiation should be described in terms of 'enclosure, metamorphosis (or magnification) and emergence' – from where did these images come if not from pregnancy and birth? Birth may also be described in terms of a spiritual emergency (Grof & Grof, 1989; Watson, 1994). It has the potential for women to grow or to face devastation.

A parable which describes an initiation, provides a parallel with labour and which moves me deeply is found in Sara Matiland's novel *Three Times Table* (1991).

Margaret of Antioch was an independent woman; this independence was marked by her Christianity in a secular society and her stubborn refusal to marry. She was a virgin, both in the literal sense and metaphorically, in that her life was not defined by the laws or the wishes of men. As a virgin, she was desired by and consumed by a dragon. Her unusual independence of mind allowed her to find this experience initially amusing, and she laughed at the panic the dragon's arrival had caused her fellow humans. Her laughter so shocked the dragon that he swallowed her alive and whole. In the belly of the dragon she became afraid and her fear communicated itself to the dragon, whose gastric juices started to flow in anticipation. But at the climax of her fear she realised that what she was frightened of was death, and that the process of dying might in itself offer excitement and beauty. So her fear evaporated and turned into a joyful acceptance. And the dragon, feeling the change, opened his mouth and let her out. Margaret of Antioch became Saint Margaret and the patron saint of women in childbirth. She had been reborn of the dragon's belly and during that experience she had faced the darkness that women must face in the depths of their labour.

Margaret has since been demoted by the Vatican, who seem to think this story cannot be true. This is a patriarchal attempt to demote symbol and metaphor. This links in with the power of obstetrics and other male-dominated institutions. The power of the institution is paramount when it comes to making choices – not just the institutions of medicine and doctors, but social assumptions. In recent years attitudes to vaginal birth and Caesarean section have changed, with the former being viewed in parts of the media with distaste and the latter seen as a safe and preferable option.

The myth related above shares similarities with that of Inanna, goddess of the Sumerians, whose power consists of her willingness to divest herself of the worldly and confront death, and with the more familiar story of Persephone.

These stories are stories of initiation, symbolic birth, rebirth. They are stories of survival and transformation. One aim of spiritual practice is to enable us to find the discipline and courage to regard the mundane as offering the opportunity for both survival and transformation. And the mundane includes both birth and death. Chogyam Trungpa (1992) writes of The Tibetan Book of the Dead that it 'is not only a message for those who are going to die and those who are already dead, but it is also a message for those who are already born; birth and death apply constantly, at this very moment'.

Another aim of spiritual practice is to develop an awareness of unity in multiplicity, an integration of the disparate, an acceptance of ambivalence. Labour offers an integration of the physical and the psychic. Endorphins alter consciousness. Consciousness allows the woman to make choices which will enhance the secretion of endorphins – however, the most powerful determinant of the choices most women believe they make is the institution. The hugeness of the experience demands a focus of awareness, a concentration of the physical and the psychic on a single aim. Labour also integrates the spiritual and the sexual. Childbirth is the culmination of a sexual act. It involves the hormones which induce and express excitement and orgasm, but to a huge degree. Beside childbirth, orgasm is puny. But orgasm's relation even to death is explicit in the term la petite mort: orgasm is also a bardo state. In the Bardo, profound change can occur. The work of the contractions of labour, I was told in my Active Birth classes, happens in the moment between the in-breath and the out-breath. And the opening of labour links subtle and gross anatomy. I was especially aware of an open throat, an open diaphragm and an opening cervix, and a channel of energy between these points of anatomy which also correspond to chakas.

The experience of labour is the bridge between pregnancy and afterwards. For me, there was a continuity between the increasing waves of excitement as my pregnancy got bigger, then the tumultuous waves of labour and the rushes of milk and love afterwards. I felt no hiatus. The whole event was charged with a sexual energy and I was sexually active again within a week. Sometimes (mostly?) this continuity is broken by unwarranted medical interventions which make labour a physical and psychic trauma: no longer a bridge but a gap.

There is a concept of a doula – an experienced woman who guides and supports the mother-to-be through labour, just as the initiate is guided by the teacher. Both women in labour and initiates need what Alida Gerslie (1994) calls 'quiet mothering' at this time. Ideally a midwife (whose title means with-woman in Old English) should be able to provide this quiet mothering. This issue of doula and midwife has changed in recent years. A division of labour, with an overemphasis on the medical in what is expected of midwifery care, has become hardened in the economic context of a midwife shortage. In normal cases most prescribed schedules for observations are unnecessary. It is totally unnecessary, for example, to take a woman's pulse every quarter of an hour. To some extent I believe midwives have welcomed this overmedicalisation because it can be seen to enhance prestige and enable the midwife to flee from the emotional heat of caring for a woman in labour.

To give birth one needs to go through the pain of labour, to survive the darkness and the fear, which is the fear of death. To go through this easiest requires acceptance, an opening to the experience, which is also an opening of the cervix. Balaskas (1991) states:

'in a way you need to lose control, to surrender and trust in the birth process which takes place involuntarily without your conscious control. You need to let go of your mind, of everything you know and just let it happen. This is a time to turn inwards, to abandon oneself to the unknown, not to think ahead to what is to come, just to take it moment by moment and let the natural involuntary rhythms of your body take over.'

This is a passive acceptance of a huge activity. Sexuality and regression, eros and thanatos are aspects of the same energy, are mutually dependent.

The opportunities which labour offers for survival and transformation and for integration also allow for profound healing. Labour is healing because any rite of passage which involves confronting and surviving fear, pain and darkness is healing. It is also healing because it both requires and gives strength. It gives what it demands. There is a reflexivity about this which leads me to see labour (and mothering) as a clear and undistorting mirror. There is no distortion because the experience is immense to the point where there is no disguise. Contemplation of this undistorted image is healing because it offers the chance to accept what might otherwise be rejected as negative, parts of oneself that we might prefer to be kept hidden, social and personal shame, physical shame. Women often defaecate in the second stage of labour. This act, which in this culture is usually private and associated with shame, is here public. Ironically (or not) babies exposed to their mothers' faeces get fewer infections because they are able to produce appropriate antibodies. In the Buddhist tradition, meditation provides an undistorting mirror in which to view our own minds and encourages the development of an equanimity such that faeces and roses evoke the same response.

Women, according to Susie Orbach and Luise Eichenbaum (1987), subtly learn that they are intrinsically wrong. The social yardstick is male. And the female genitalia are particularly shameworthy. Labour exposes these shameful areas. Cultural institutions of childbirth enhance the shameful evaluation of women's bodies. While women are no longer shaved in labour (an act which was shown in the 1920s to increase rather than decrease infection and which took over fifty years to eradicate) women are far too often mutilated by episiotomy and operative delivery. This is probably the crudest response to the shameworthiness of the female, but there are many others more subtle.

To some extent the learnt shame is a result of the fear of the powerful. Women's genitalia are both despised and desired. A common graffito is that of a woman with her legs apart. Women seeing this might feel shame at the exposure of the private and fear at the implied violence of that exposure. As they are intended to. But they might also feel pride that what is exposed is the gateway through which we are born, and they may be able to recognise that the fear they feel in meeting this is no greater that the fear that lies behind its expression. There is a powerful ambivalence here.

The greater the negative contained within the ambivalent, the greater the power when this is recognised and acknowledged. Accepting ambivalence can be said to put us in touch with the source of our power if it is accepted that psychic energy is unnecessarily bound up in keeping ourselves cut off from the negative. If the female is greatly despised it is a testament to her power. Accepting ambivalence is healing because it integrates the negative and the positive and reduces the tendency to project what is negative onto others. It is also healing because it puts us in touch with the source of our power. And in childbirth the greatest negative of all is hovering. Margaret of Antioch confronted the fear of DEATH. Modern childbirth practices have as their rationale the obviation of death. They must fail because there is no escaping death. Lama Anagarika Govinda (1992) writes that physical continuity, immortality, does not allow for physical or material difference and neither therefore the capacity for spiritual integration. This is expressed more poetically in the myth cited by Gerslie (1994):

'In the earliest days the first human couple lived in heaven. One day God spoke to them and said: "What kind of death do you want, the kind of death the moon has, or the death of the banana?" The couple did not have a clue and were somewhat panic-stricken at having to make a decision. God therefore explained to them what the difference between the two different kinds of death was. The banana puts forth shoots which eventually take its place, while the moon renews herself. The couple pondered their choice for a long time, then they made up their minds. They thought that if they had chosen to remain childless, then they would have avoided death, but they would also have been rather lonely. There would not be anybody to work with or to care for. They therefore asked God for the death of the banana. Their wish was granted and since that time people do not live on this earth for a very long time.'

The moon does not change its substance. If there is to be growth there must also be differentiation and dissolution.

Giving birth is an involuntary act of great physical and psychic power. I don't mean telepathy – for me the word implies a sense of deeper, unneurotic self. As Caroline Flint says, it is never forgotten (1986). A testament to its power is the lengths to which the culture, expressed as medicine, goes in its attempt to attenuate and control that power. The circumstances in which I gave birth, at home, with loved and trusted attendants, are profoundly different from the norm. I am not seduced by nostalgia for an imagined ideal past or present simpler society.

Many such societies see birth as filthy. Milarepa (1983) described pregnancy as hell:

Driven by lust and hatred / It enters the mother's womb
Therein it feels like a fish / In a rock's crevice caught.
Sleeping in blood and yellow fluid,
It is pillowed in discharges,
Crammed in filth, it suffers pain.

This is truly hellish, though the hell consists not of blood and amniotic fluid, but the values put upon them.

But for years I have listened to the pain of women as they have told me their unexceptional experiences of giving birth, and I should like to see changes for the future in the institutions of childbirth so that labour is not a medical event but more a rite of initiation.

Marion Woodman (1985) states that in genuine ritual both body and psyche are involved. Current practice attends only to the body; I should like to see attention also to the psyche. According to Woodman, such ritual extends body and psyche to the limits. Certainly women in labour feel their bodies to be stretched to the limit and I believe that if more attention were paid to the psychic aspects of birth women would find the physical extremes they encounter more tolerable, they would use less analgesia and anaesthesia and they would find within themselves the resources to survive and transform the experience. But such intensity requires a socially acceptable form to contain within a facilitating environment the ritual.

The containers of the ritual of birth could be the midwives. Midwifery can, as Flint (1986) has shown, be organised in such a way that small groups of midwives practise autonomously and no woman need give birth in the presence of strangers. But to do this, midwives need more financial, institutional, political and psychological support than they get at present.

Redgrove and Shuttle (1999) acknowledge that women who can integrate their sexuality and experience of menstruation are less likely to find labour traumatic. This would require confronting huge cultural and political barriers which render female physiology taboo, even now, even in a culture which has soft porn on mainstream terrestrial TV channels. Also, there are issues of individual trauma such as sexual abuse.

I recognise too that women are afraid and that this fear has deep physical, psychic and cultural roots. Many women may need some prior healing if they are to integrate their experience of birth. For some the event may be, as it is now, the precipitant into psychotic chaos. But for others it may be, as it was for me, the beginning of a process of profound healing and growth.

REFERENCES

Adamson W, Aldridge A. 1989. Open Secrets: A Western guide to Tibbetan Buddhism for Western spiritual seekers. Jeremy P Tarcher Inc

Balaskas J. 1991. New Active Birth. Harper Collins

Flint C. 1986. Sensitive Midwifery. Butterworth-Heinemann

Gerslie A. 1994. Storytelling in Bereavement. Jessica Kingsley Publications

Govinda A. 1992. The Way of the White Clouds. Rider Books

Grof S, Grof C. 1989. Spiritual Emergency: Understanding Evolutionary Crisis. Jeremy P Tarcher Inc

Matiland S. 1991. The Three Times Table. Henry Holt & Co

Milarepa. 1983. In: Meltzer D (ed). Birth. North Point Publishers

Orbach S, Eichenbaum L. 1987. In: Ernst and Maguire (eds). Living with the Sphinx. The Women's Press

Ornstein R. 1992. The Evolution of Consciousness: The origins of the way we think. Touchstone Books

Shuttle P, Redgrove P. 1999. The Wise Wound. Marion Boyars

Trungpa C, Rinpoche S, Fremantle F (translators). 1992. The Tibetan Book of the Dead. Shambala Publications

Woodman M. 1985. The Pregnant Virgin: A process of psychological transformation. Inner City Books

The Practising Midwife 2002; 5(11): 10-13

Finding the spiritual side of birth

Jennifer Hall

There is something about December that always turns my thoughts to birth. I suppose it has a lot to do with the images of birth on Christmas cards and the visions of infant school children popping out baby dolls from underneath oversized blue gowns in Nativity plays! However, when I reflect on what that birth is all about, it is the rawness and earthiness of the whole event that strikes me most. That birth was not in the glossy, pretty-pretty atmosphere of the greetings cards or pantomimes. Neither was it in the cold, clinical whiteness of a labour ward, or even the soft furnishings and candles of a home birth. We are talking real basics here!

Some time ago I recall a BBC programme that attempted to depict, through computer-aided graphics, the Palestine of Jesus' day. The scene of the place of birth showed a round stone building with a platform where the family lived, with an area below which was the home of the animals. The suggestion was that this could have been the 'stable' of the Bible – a dark, dusty place with the profound smells of animal fodder and excrement. There may have been a fire for the family, but little light. Were there midwives there? They may have been too busy with the influx of people in the town for the census. Perhaps Mary and Joseph could not pay them. Perhaps even Joseph distanced himself from the birth itself, if he obeyed the Orthodox Jewish law that said he should not touch a woman when she was ritually 'unclean'. Perhaps he was pushed outside by the midwives as this was 'women's work'. And I have often wondered what happened to the afterbirth. Did the animals get to eat it? Did Mary have to deal with it if Joseph wasn't allowed to touch anything so 'unclean'? It certainly wouldn't have been buried under a rose bush!!

A few years ago I made a visit to the supposed site in Bethlehem. I wasn't too struck by the Church of the Nativity, but more by a chapel nearby celebrating Jesus' first breastfeed. Of course the reality of infant feeding was no bottles or formula then. In the enclosure shared with the animals perhaps the instincts so close to those of animals may have been more enhanced; there would have been no question of not breastfeeding. The symbolism of the time has been further enhanced for me by the birth of one of my daughters two days before Christmas and the debut acting appearance of another as Jesus in a Church nativity at the age of 3 months! (Sighs all round the building...). For me, there is such a basic normality in all this, the simple, symbolic birth – a celebration of new life. Even if you have no belief in the religious aspects of this event it is worth valuing the story as a celebration of the normality of birth.

But I have to believe there is more to life than just the physical and emotional experience of it all. Even Lord Winston at the end of the recent excellent BBC series on human instincts (*Natural Born Heroes*, 13th November 2002) revealed that his own experience as a doctor had led him to recognise there is more – what he called the human spirit. In the past couple of years since my discussion on these issues (Hall, 2000) there has been a glut of books related to healthcare, challenging different dimensions of the issues relating to spirituality (Burkhardt and Nagai-Jacobson, 2002; Chamberlain and Hall, 2000; Koenig, 2002; McSherry, 2000; Orchard, 2001; Swinton, 2001). In midwifery terms, a study has investigated the issues surrounding religious belief and home birth in America (Klassen, 2001) and in the UK a couple of papers have seriously tried to address the issues (Hall, 2000; Walsh, 2002) but midwives have generally been strangely quiet. I say strangely because a) it remains written into our current rules of practice that we should be carrying out spiritual care, and b) the birth of the child has the potential for a profound effect on a woman's spiritual experience and her personal wholeness. Still we recognise the necessity for the meeting of spiritual needs at the end of life, but there is little discussion for what is going on at the beginning.

Although the beginning of this article mentioned in

passing an element of a religious belief, spirituality and the human spirit is not limited to those who focus on religion as a source of spiritual expression. There is potential for spirituality in all humans and the expression of this may come in many forms. The fact that there is a raw earthiness in the act of childbirth leads women to the very roots and bareness of their being. They are bordering the very edges between life and death. A recent challenging paper describes women experiencing out-of-body experiences during labour (Kennedy, 2002). The closeness of women to the spiritual realms during childbirth is something that we should not ignore. Are we being so blind as midwives as to ignore these experiences and to classify women as odd if they voice them to us? Do we just back off and suggest the chaplain or the psychiatrist come for a visit? Perhaps in reality women don't feel comfortable in making explanations to us about the reality of their actual experiences. Perhaps it is just too raw and painful for women to address initially; it may take months or years to relate the depth of such profound changes.

I recognise, too, that many women are just too fearful to get anywhere near the experiences I am talking about. It is a risky business to 'let ourselves go' to this extent, and sadly many women do not feel safe enough with us as health carers or within our clinical birth environments to reach such an intensity of experience. It is no doubt the option of sitting in a birth pool away from the edge and the probing hands of fussy midwives is an alternative some women choose to make. I recognise too that there are many midwives out there who are scared to watch women experiencing the true intensity of normal birth as it is too close to the sexual and too far away from their own experiences – they would rather intervene before it exposes their own vulnerability as women. Birth opens us all wide and for some midwives the pain may be too hard to bear.

There is much work to be done to be able to understand more of the processes relating to providing a place where women can experience birth spiritually as well as physically. We need to know how to give spiritual care and who should give it. But I don't think we should be ignoring it. Meanwhile, I am off to the Nativity play, to be reminded about the real normality of birth and place Christmas in context again.

REFERENCES

Burkhardt MA, Nagai-Jacobson MG. 2002. Spirituality: Living our connectedness. Delmar

Chamberlain TJ, Hall CA. 2000. Realized religion: Research on the relationship between religion and health. Templeton Foundation Press

Hall J. 2000. Midwifery, mind and spirit: Emerging issues of care. Oxford: Books for Midwives

Hall J. 2000. Spiritual midwifery care: Old practice for a new millenium. British Journal of Midwifery 8(2): 82

Kennedy HP. 2002. Altered consciousness during childbirth: Potential clues to post traumatic stress disorder? Journal of Midwifery and Women's Health 47(5): 380-382

Klassen PE. 2001. Blessed events: Religion and home birth in America. Princeton University Press

Koenig HG. 2002. Spirituality in patient care: Why, how, when and what. Templeton Foundation Press

McSherry W. 2000. Making sense of spirituality in nursing practice: An interactive approach. Edinburgh: Churchill Livingstone

Orchard H (ed). 2001. Spirituality in health care contexts. London: Jessica Kingsley Publishers

Swinton J. 2001. Spirituality and mental health care: Rediscovering a forgotten dimension. London: Jessica Kingsley Publishers

Walsh D. 2002. How's your spiritual life going? British Journal of Midwifery 10(8): 484

The Practising Midwife 2002; 5(11): 4

Let us pray

Shirley Webber

I work with Vonnie, Jane and Lesley, my inspirational colleagues of many years, sharing a tremendous professional relationship which is complemented by aspects of our social and domestic existence.

We share a common goal: amongst our case load of approximately 380 ladies a year we encourage home birth when clinically appropriate, with about 25 a year to our credit.

Recognising and owning our midwifery expertise is just as essential as recognising our limitations and there is a fragile element of the notion we call 'informed choice' – we prefer to adopt a policy of 'keep your options open'. The professional paradigm may prefer 'knowledge' over experience, but you can't beat experience. Childbearing may be a biological event but it is also psychosocial and it is lived in the community. We have all culturally acquired 'ways of being' and 'ways of knowing'.

When my pager bleeped at me at 11.45 on a cold winter morning, it was that feeling of 'knowing' that instinctively told me it was a home birth. We had five home births due within the next three weeks, two expected on the same day. Today it was Liz calling. She was not due for another week, but as she shared the same EDD with another, I was quietly thankful. I knew Liz would not linger and I also knew we had an eager student midwife working with us who would be especially delighted as Liz had given permission for students to attend.

Liz, Mike and their son Luke, were a special family to us. Mike was the local curate and Liz a primary school teacher, and sadly and unexplainably they had lost their previous baby who died in the last trimester of a much wanted and longed for pregnancy. There is no greater grief than the grief following the death of a child. When they came back to us in late spring to book their new pregnancy we were delighted and were not surprised that they asked for a home birth, as attending the hospital would only bring back previous heartache. We were also reassured by the knowledge that Liz had given birth to Luke quickly and without intervention.

I drove through the rounded Devonshire hills which offered little resistance to a wind heavy with the promise of snow. Arriving at their home I found Liz, smiling and blowing reassuringly.

Fetal heart was 'happy', membranes intact, a nice 'show' evident and a few distinctive fetal movements confirmed that it was happening and all was well. After a coffee and a chat I suggested I pop back to the health centre, just five minutes away, to inform my colleagues and collect Pam, our student. Liz and Mike were happy to phone me as soon as they wanted me to return, so off I went.

I had no sooner sat down with some of my colleagues when the phone rang. It was Mike. 'I think you had better come back!' he said. Vonnie agreed to be second midwife and Pam, our student, although still at the 'watching' stage was thrilled to come along.

Liz progressed rapidly and without any analgesia or prompting from us she ruptured her membranes and spontaneously gave birth to a beautiful 8 lb baby girl within an hour of our arrival. Mike cut the cord with our supervision and baby Elly went straight to her mum. Perinium intact, estimated blood loss minimal, but as every midwife knows, it's not over until that placenta puts in an appearance. Syntometrine had been given, in accordance with Liz's wishes, and after what looked like a respectable time I noticed what looked like a separation bleed and dissent of the cord. I released the clamp and let the cord bleed, then applied gentle controlled cord traction but was met with adamant resistance. I thought, there is no rush, we will tidy up our mess, put the kettle on and wait. Baby was by this time on the breast nuzzling and sucking like she had done it all before while Mike looked on adoringly, unaware of our quietly growing concern.

I suggested Liz might like to try and empty her

bladder. She happily agreed and we hobbled out to the bathroom in comic fashion clutching inco pads, kidney bowls and clamps between her legs. Nothing happened. We tried applying traction whilst standing, hoping gravity would help, but it did not. Then I suggested an intermittent catheter. By now Liz had realized that we had a problem and she agreed immediately.

We had success there, but still no placenta. Time was ticking by, and still the expected bleed did not come. Then Pam, our student, qualified in several alternative disciplines, suggested a shiatsu foot massage. Knowing the use of reflexology in this area we agreed; however, the placenta had not read the research and refused to budge. We watched, we waited, we felt for encouraging signs but there were none. Elly continued to feed contentedly, but we began to feel demoralised. Tenderly, I explained to Liz and Mike that it had now been an hour since Elly's birth and the placenta was causing some concern. I felt it was in their best interest to transfer to the hospital for removal of the placenta. Their anguish was palpable, one of total disbelief. It was then that Mike requested the most unusual and unresearched proposition, 'Can we try prayer?'

A fleeting glance round the room at my colleagues, reassured me that yes, anything was worth a try. So we put down our bags and towels and stood silent and humbled by another person's faith. Mike placed his hands on the offending fundus and prayed. When he had finished he asked that I try again.

Unconvinced and rather dubious I once again applied some tentative pressure to the cord, and out it came, a Matthews Duncan and almost complete except for one missing cotyledon (which put in an appearance the next day) and still minimal blood loss.

Amongst much rejoicing we midwives said a silent prayer of our own. We were glad we had 'kept our options open', recognised our limitations and most of all there was a way of 'knowing' that we had all underestimated the power of prayer.

The Practising Midwife 2002; 5(4): 16

The placenta

Symbolic organ or waste product?

Rosamund Davies

Throughout recorded history, the placenta has been an object of interest. Two thousand years ago Aristotle recognised the importance of complete delivery of the placenta, and since that time the placenta has been examined and studied.

In the West today, the delivery of the placenta seems of little significance to women. The midwife knows the woman is not safely delivered until the third stage is complete but the placenta itself has no significance in western culture. The woman may think of it as something repellent, ugly, even 'monstrous', which is disposed of by professionals. Occasionally women ask to see the placenta. It is usually only for a minute, and most are surprised by its size, colour or appearance. The fact that it is part of a woman's body, and has been nurturing her baby for the whole gestation, is miraculous. Should it be dismissed so lightly?

Visualisation techniques

Today, we can view the placenta before delivery, by 'non-invasive techniques; radionuclide scintigraphy, ultrasonography and magnetic resonance imaging' (Panigiel, 1993). Ultrasound has been used since its inception to visualise the placenta, its size and thickness. It has proved difficult to relate this to the growth of the fetus, partly because of difficulties in differentiating between the uterine wall and the placenta, and because of the abundant blood supply in the area. However, modern visualisation techniques have undoubtedly had beneficial effects in diagnosing placental problems, especially in women who may have experienced problems before. Simply being able to locate the placenta can provide early warning of conditions such as placenta previa, which could prove fatal. Ultrasound imaging is also essential for chorionic villus sampling and cordocentesis; one scientific process relies upon another.

Real time scanning is now so sensitive that the internal structures of the placenta can be identified. The villus-free regions of the placenta lobules, sometimes called placental 'lakes', have been identified. 'These echo-free structures should in future be referred to as "the central region of the placental lobe"' (Muller, 1993). This command would seem to have more association with landmarks on the moon than with the delicate and intricate structure that maintains the life of the fetus until birth.

A diagnostic tool

Despite extensive research, 'our knowledge of the early phases of human embryogenesis and the establishment of extra embryonic tissue is limited' (Ohisson et al, 1993).

Advances in medical science now make it possible to detect some genetic disorders, chromosomal abnormalities and metabolic defects by examining the placenta. Women carrying a genetic disorder, such as Huntington's Chorea, can now be offered prenatal diagnosis, and subsequent termination if desired. However, Godsen (1993) suggests that 70% of women carrying a chromosomally abnormal fetus are not identified in any of the known risk groups.

As more invasive procedures are initiated in the name of science and progress, have we lost sight of the aesthetic properties of this magnificent organ?

Function of the placenta

The placenta is the link between mother and fetal life. The placenta produces a number of hormones that maintain the pregnancy, notably oestrogen, which reaches astronomic daily levels by term, equivalent to that of a thousand premenopausal women's daily production (Casey & MacDonald, 1993). Progesterone is responsible for maintaining the pregnancy until term, with the assistance of relaxin.

The placenta also helps with the maintainance of haemostatic balance, and acts as a partial barrier to fetal infection. Fox (1991) argues that the placenta delays rather than prevents infection reaching the fetus. The risk of ascending infection is lessened by the barrier of intact membranes and the antibacterial properties of amniotic fluid. The placenta has contact with the maternal blood and immune system (Fox, 1993).

Monitoring the placenta

When the placenta appears to fail, the broad term 'placental insufficiency' is meted out. The amount of investigation, diagnosis and research available on this 'condition' is phenomenal. Wallenberg (1990) suggests that the term placental insufficiency has been used indiscriminately to explain inexplicable cases of fetal distress, intrauterine growth retardation and perinatal mortality. He adds that there is evidence, both clinical and experimental, that the fetus may have some control over maternal cardiovascular adaptations to pregnancy.

Fetal surveillance is ongoing, with new techniques for doing so being employed continuously. Magnetic resonance spectroscopy is another method of viewing the placenta and gaining information about fetal wellbeing. It is a non-invasive technique; however, a single examination could take up to one and a half hours (Weanling et al, 1991).

The caul

The 'caul' once had great significance. Roman midwives used to steal cauls – they brought large sums from those who considered them to be good luck charms. This left the child at a disadvantage, as it should never be parted from its caul. In European tradition, the caul was 'the seat of the external soul; it symbolised the passage between the world of lost souls – of stillborn children, murdered adults and soldiers slain in battle – and the land of the living' (Gelds, 1991). In England it is thought to be lucky if a baby is born within the membranes. Legend has it that the child will be protected from death by drowning, and cauls were in great demand among sailors at one time.

Cutting the cord

'In many parts of South America it is thought that if the cord is cut there is nothing to pull the placenta downwards and it will rise up in the mother's body and choke her' (Priya, 1992).

In France, the cord was taped to the woman's thigh until the placenta appeared. Louise Bourgeois, a French midwife, always employed this method and having performed over two thousand deliveries, 'had not had her hand in the womb more than twice' (Gelds, 1991).

In different parts of the world, there is considerable significance attached to cutting the cord. The length of cord cut is also important. The Malayan midwife cuts the cord to the length of the baby's finger, the Yeo measures to the baby's knee, in Mexico as wide as the hand and the Cherokee Indian measures up to the baby's shoulder (Priya, 1992).

Different implements for cutting the cord are used the world over, from bamboo sticks to scissors and leatherworkers' knives. After this it may be cauterised or have herbs applied to it.

The Japanese have historically kept the whole cord and give it to their daughters on their wedding day.

The lotus placenta

Perhaps there are spiritual benefits of a far-reaching nature even beyond our perception that are conferred by the placenta. Scholes (1989) says, 'It seems, *in utero* the placenta has a physical function, but once out of the womb, while still attached, its function is purely metaphysical.'

The 'lotus' placenta describes the act of leaving the placenta attached to the baby until the cord separates. In this way the baby has time to adapt to its new world and the parents remain cocooned, slow down and recover from the birth as a family. There is no rush to clothe the baby, or pass it round to relatives and friends. Scholes (1989) suggests cord cutting to be a violent act and that the fetus and placenta share the same etheric field aura. She says, 'While the placenta remains attached after birth, the etheric field around the baby is sealing off properly and when complete, the cord drops away. The complete field results in a stronger immune system because it is stronger field energy... Family members' etheric auras can be healed by being in contact with the Lotus baby.'

Gelds (1991) also suggested that the placenta's nourishing capacity could continue after birth until the cord was cut.

Caring for the lotus placenta should not cause a problem. Scholes (1989) suggests patting the placenta dry, salting it liberally on both sides and taping it to a disposable nappy for drainage. It should be changed and salted daily, kept dry and put near the baby. Some people fashion a special bag for the purpose. Once the cord has dropped off, it can be buried in a place designated for the purpose.

Retained placenta

Evil spirits and magical powers were thought to influence the speed with which the placenta was delivered. Different methods employed to expel a delayed placenta included sniffing red pepper to induce sneezing or stuffing the woman's hair into her mouth to induce vomiting.

'In medieval Germany a retained placenta was treated by first cutting a cross into the mother's back with a knife. This was then plunged into the earth with a suitable Christian charm which exorcised the worms in the womb that were withholding the placenta' (Priya, 1992).

Hippocrates used to deliver babies onto goatskin bags filled with water, while the mother sat on a birthing chair. After this, he let the water out of the bags, which helped the placenta to deliver by gravity.

Post-partum haemorrhage was treated with massage (rubbing up a contraction) and a variety of herbs, and sometimes prophylactically with tea before birth. These methods are remarkably similar to the 'modern' methods used today.

Disposal of the placenta

Despite acknowledgement of the placenta's incredible qualities, it is still considered a waste product to be disposed of after birth. In other cultures, disposal of the placenta is an important task, and often one which is the solemn duty of the father.

The Yoruba tribe believe the child is supernaturally attached to its placenta and it is buried with great care (Priya, 1992). Priya says, 'The Malays call the placenta "little brother" which develops during the second month within the womb. As the baby grows, it grows away from its "sibling", and hence develops the umbilical cord. When the baby is born this "little brother" is buried somewhere near the house' (Priya, 1992).

The Guatemalans put the umbilical cord of a baby girl under the hearthstone to ensure that she remains at home to help in the house, while that of the son is hung up in the granary to help him work in the field.

The Cherokee bury their placentas over the amount of mountain ridges they wish to space their family by – one ridge for one year and two ridges for two years. The father buries it with chanting and great ceremony (Priya, 1992).

Gelds (1991) reminds us that the placenta 'simply could not be neglected: the child's future career depended on it because the child inevitably suffered from the repercussions of any misadventure on the part of its double.'

It would seem a disastrous course of action to treat the placenta casually – it must be protected from harm and buried or disposed of with reverence.

Placental opotherapy

Since the time of Hippocrates the afterbirth was used as a medicament; as a folk remedy for a retained placenta (powdered placenta in a glass of water) or for the treatment of freckles, tumours or warts (Gelds, 1991). It was thought that the afterbirth from a boy was more efficacious than that of a girl, despite the fact that the organ had been housed by a woman.

The healing properties of the placenta have been used in France to prevent cracked nipples. This was achieved by placing the placenta on the mother's breasts (Gelds, 1991). Other 'drug' like properties of the placenta included use in assisting fertility and acting as an aphrodisiac.

Until recently, placentas from hospitals were used in make-up and creams, for their reputed skin-regenerating properties, and for blood products. The advent of HIV has halted this practice and the afterbirth is now incinerated. For all of these practices women's consent has never been sought. This raises ethical issues. Most women may prefer their placenta to be destroyed by the hospital, but in these days of particular awareness of informed consent, it might be as well to ask.

Placentophagy

In today's world, something as base and incongruous as eating the placenta seems socially and morally unacceptable – tantamount to cannibalism! However, Gelds (1991) suggests that revulsion for the placenta is a relatively recent phenomenon. He says, 'Every observation shows that all female animals eat the residue after the birth; sometimes even the males participate in this feast.'

Field (1998) practised placentophagy (the mother eating the placenta) after the birth of her second child. She believed it might alleviate postnatal depression and suggests it is instinctive behaviour in mammals.

Following her home delivery, Jackson (1998) reports she ate four cubes of placenta raw, some later with cucumber and biscuits and finally some fried with bacon. She had expected to find the texture and taste unpleasantly like liver, but instead found it an amazing delicacy.

Both these women reported relief from postnatal depression, which may have been coincidental, but suggests that further research may have benefits.

Conclusion

Studies and investigations of the placenta have been helpful in the scientific study of disease. We can locate its position by ultrasound, avoiding disasters in labour such as undiagnosed placenta previa. However, amidst all this, in the West the spiritual and aesthetic qualities of the placenta have largely been forgotten. With the discernible swing during the past few years toward alternative and natural therapies, perhaps there is an opportunity to bring the placenta back into circulation.

REFERENCES

Casey ML, MacDonald PC. 1993. Placental endocrinolology. In: Redman CWG, Sargent JL, Starkey PM (eds). The Human Placenta. London: Blackwell Scientific Publications

Field M. 1986. An unusual solution. New Generation 5(1): 44

Fox H. 1991. A contemporary view of the human placenta. Midwifery, 7

Fox H.1993. The placenta and infection. In: Redman CWG, Sargent JL, Starkey PM (eds). The Human Placenta. London: Blackwell Scientific Publications

Gelds J. 1992. History of Childbirth. Cambridge: Polity Press (English Translation)

Godsen C. 1993. Genetic diagnosis, chorionic villous biopsy and placental mosaicism. In: Redman CWG, Sargent JL, Starkey PM (eds). The Human Placenta. London: Blackwell Scientific Publications

Jackson W. 1988. Placenta on a plate. New Generation 7 (1): 20-21

Multer LMM. 1993. Ultrasound assessment of the placenta, and clinical assessment of placental growth. In: Redman CWG, Sargent JL, Starkey PM (eds). The Human Placenta. London: Blackwell Scientific Publicationns.

Ohisson R et al. 1993. The molecular biology of placental development. In: Redman CWG, Sargent JL, Starkey PM (eds). The Human Placenta. London: Blackwell Scientific Publications

Priya J. 1992. Birth Traditions & Modern Pregnancy Care. Element Books Limited

Panagiel M. 1993. The origin and stricture of the extraembryonic tissues. In: Redman CWG, Sargent JL, Starkey PM (eds). The Human Placenta. London: Blackwell Scientific Publications

Scholes A. 1989. The Lotus Placenta. Homebirth Australia 21: 8

Wallenberg HCS. 1990. Placental insufficiency: pathophysiology and therapeutic approaches. Triangle, 29 April, 171-179

The Practising Midwife 2002; 5(11): 19-21

Labour and birth

I have noted several times in this series that there is a conflict between needing to organise articles into different sections for ease of reading and the realisation that pregnancy is an ongoing journey rather than a succession of clearly demarcated or fragmented experiences. The birthing woman, for instance, will not see the difference between 'first stage' and 'second stage' anywhere near as clearly as her midwife does. Rosemary Mander's article, which questions what we mean by 'transition' and how women experience this, concurrently opens up discussion about the importance of midwifery observation and the flow of labour. This article also considers some questions around pain and how midwives can be with women, a debate that is continued in the qualitative research carried out by Ingela Lundgren and Karen Dahlberg, who interviewed Swedish midwives about what it was like to be with women in pain. One of their key concepts is of the midwife as an 'anchored companion', and they explore aspects of midwifery practice that are similar for midwives everywhere.

One of the key debates in recent years has been around what we actually mean by 'normal birth'; whether, for instance, we take normal to mean 'natural', 'average', 'uncomplicated', 'vaginal' or something else entirely, and whether normal birth really matters. Following on from the issues raised about this in section 1, Belinda Phipps' article, based on women's responses to a questionnaire sent out by the NCT, shows just how much birth does matter to women, and proposes the introduction of another term, 'straightforward vaginal birth'. A complementary midwifery perspective to this debate is offered by Gill Skinner, who looks at the promotion of normal birth and suggests a number of areas for possible action.

Chit Ying Lai and Valerie Levy interviewed Hong Kong Chinese women about their experiences of vaginal examination and their results are a reminder of the kinds of things that are important to the women who experience this intervention. Meanwhile midwives are still exploring other signs of progress in labour, which may reduce or eliminate the need for routine vaginal examination. I really enjoyed interviewing Jean Sutton for the article we wrote together on the rhombus of Michaelis, not only because I am passionate about reclaiming midwifery knowledge, but because Jean herself is so infectiously excitable about this area. She outlines the anatomy of this area well enough that any midwife who has not yet discovered the way a woman's back 'opens' during labour will be able to do so after reading this article.

Finally, Jennifer Wrightson adds another perspective to the debate on CTG monitoring with a review of the history and evidence in this area which will help midwives (and especially those of us who have begun to practise midwifery since the 1970s, when CTGs became widely used) better understand the context of this technology.

The transitional stage
Pain and control

Rosemary Mander

After an initial search of the literature, one might be forgiven for thinking that the transitional stage of labour is a uniquely North American phenomenon. This impression is confirmed after consulting databases such as CINAHL, MEDline, Web of Science and MIDIRS. While this stage of labour features in texts and other literature originating in the US (Volger, 1993; Bobak & Starn, 1993), it barely rates a mention in the major UK midwifery textbooks (Bennet & Brown, 1999; Stables, 1999). The reason for this US interest in this stage of labour will eventually become apparent. Perhaps disconcertingly, 'the transition' is also emphasised by a number of websites which are clearly intended for parents.

The transitional stage at the end of the first stage of labour can be difficult, as you may be quite uncomfortable and yet not be allowed to push (handbag.com:family, 2001)

[aromatherapy] can be used to lift mood and allay fatigue, especially in the transitional stage of labour, when it's common to feel tired and discouraged (Active Birth Centre, 2001)

The nature of the transitional stage

The definition which has been suggested for the transitional stage of labour (or simply 'transition') is:
'when the cervix dilates from about seven centimetres to ten centimetres' (Smith et al, 1973).

Such a narrow definition may be appropriate in a highly medicalised birthing environment, but in a setting where midwifery skills are utilised, the diagnosis of the transitional stage is likely to be easily made on the basis of changes in the woman's behaviour. Robertson's diagnostic criteria include a sudden change in behaviour, as well as restlessness (1994). The other typical features of the transitional stage include loss of perspective, shaking and uncharacteristic irritability (Tucker, 1996). Both Robertson and Smith and colleagues report the woman's limited tolerance of her birth companion,

partner or attendant. These authors also refer to her frank and honest articulation of her likes and dislikes at this time, which may be unfettered by the usual politeness and can be interpreted as rudeness. These articulations are likely to include non-verbal sounds, such as groaning or shouting.

One of the reasons for these challenging manifestations may be the overwhelming urge to push, which the woman is likely to first experience during the transitional stage. If the woman is for some reason being discouraged from following the dictates of her body, she is likely to vent her feelings on those nearest to her. The woman's feelings of distress following such a veto on pushing are clearly demonstrated in the observational research by Bergstrom and colleagues (1997). Smith and colleagues, like Tucker, emphasise the threat which the transition carries to the woman's coping mechanisms may no longer function and she is at risk of 'losing it'. It is at this point that both Robertson and Tucker report that the woman who is in labour in the maternity unit may declare her intention to go home. Similarly, many midwives will have attended the woman who, following an uncomplicated first stage, in the transitional stage requests a Caesarean. According to Leap (2000), such intentions and requests are voiced only in 'a panic moment'.

Smith and colleagues draw attention to 'drowsiness' as one of the signs of the transition, but this interpretation may not be correct. Although eye closing is a well-recognised feature of even the unmedicated transitional stage, this is unlikely to be due to any involuntary change to consciousness. Leap (2000) explains how the woman experiencing the transitional stage needs to draw on all of her reserves of energy and strength. In order to access these reserves she is required to become supremely focused. Such a high level of level of concentration is achieved by the woman effectively distancing herself and withdrawing from the activities and the people round about her. Part of the effort to concentrate in this way involves her closing her eyes. Leap's interpretation is endorsed by Vogler, who reflects on the woman's 'decreased ability to listen or concentrate on anything but giving birth' and links it to 'extreme pain' of the transition (1993).

For the midwife who has come to know the woman and her behaviour, the transitional stage may be easily diagnosed using signs such as these without having to resort to the intrusion of a vaginal examination.

Pain in the transitional stage

The problem which Leap (2000) identifies in relation to the diagnosis of the transitional stage relates to the woman's pain behaviour. Leap recognises the possibility that the midwife may confuse the woman's behaviour in the transitional stage with the signs that the woman is experiencing the more severe and pathological pain of abnormal labour. Following her definition of the transitional stage as 'the very end of the first stage of labour', Kitzinger (1987) goes on to state that 'It is often the most difficult part of labour, but may last for only a few contractions'. It is my personal observation that, as mentioned already, the woman begins to despair of her ability to give birth to her baby successfully without medical intervention. This despair erupts at the time when her contractions are becoming more intense in preparation for the birth and when she feels there is little she can do to help herself. This psychological low point, when combined with seemingly unproductive and increasingly severe pain, correlates with the mental and physical pain which has been labelled 'total pain' by Saunders (Baines, 1990).

Total pain

The concept of 'total pain', which was introduced by Cicely Saunders in 1964 in a very different context of caring for people with cancer, Saunders recognised the multidimensional nature of the pain that such people are likely to encounter. She identified a form of pain which was not just physical pain, but which featured additionally psychological, social, emotional and spiritual elements. The real significance of this form of pain is that it is not amenable to being ameliorated by the relatively simple pharmacological techniques on which healthcare personnel ordinarily rely. Thus, this form of pain requires different approaches which may offer a disconcerting challenge to those in attendance. The complexity of total pain requires a range of interventions if the person experiencing is to be assisted, and these interventions extend beyond the usual drugs, into the areas of humanity which are threatened by total pain.

Saunders described total pain in terms of presenting a problem of finding meaning; this is because such pain is seemingly without time, without ending, without meaning and brings with it an aggravated sense of isolation and despair (Clark, 1999). In this way, this concept of total pain during the transitional stage may be contrasted with the more 'purposeful' pain of the earlier first stage and the more active pain of the second stage (Langford, 1997).

It is clear that the experience of total pain is entirely appropriate to the woman in the transitional stage of labour. At this time her pain is likely to have assumed psychological, social, emotional and spiritual characteristics in addition to its physical reality. These additional characteristics relate to the despair which the woman encounters after labouring through the first stage and feeling that the birth may be no nearer than when her labour began.

There is a further aspect of total pain, which may be relevant in the context of the care of the woman in the transitional stage of labour. This is the concept which Saunders introduced to demonstrate the reaction of staff who may have depleted their psychological and emotional reserves by their over-exposure to pain. These personnel may experience a form of 'burn out', which means that they have no further reserves on which to draw and find themselves falling back to 'retreat behind a technique' (Saunders, 1981). In labour this retreat is likely to take the form of an obstetrical intervention – a quick fix.

Pain intervention

As shown by Leap, it is essential for the person in attendance to be able to recognise the onset of the transitional stage if appropriate intervention is to be used. It may be more likely, though, that such recognition will avoid the use of inappropriate and potentially iatrogenic intervention.

Such inappropriate intervention would involve some degree of acquiescence to the woman's requests during momentary panic, as mentioned previously. In a midwifery-based maternity system such as still exists in the UK, it may be that agreement to a request for a Caesarean late in labour may not be successful. A panicky request for epidural analgesia at this time, however, is not only likely to be successful and is likely to be iatrogenic through causing delay in the completion of the first stage and the lengthening of the second stage (Howell, 2001).

Although the midwife herself is not usually categorised as a pain intervention, in this situation this label may be justified. The actively supportive presence of the midwife may be all that is required to assist the woman in working through the transitional stage to reach the second stage. During these 'few contractions' mentioned by Kitzinger (1987) the midwife is in position to provide the woman with informational support (Langford et al, 1997). Such an explanation of the phenomena giving rise to the woman's overpowering feelings, may be sufficient to empower her to deal with them.

Additionally, at this time the woman may be encouraged to employ the pain control techniques which she has previously found to be successful. During the transitional stage finding a suitable position may, once more, assist with controlling pain, as well as facilitating the progress of labour. The use of articulation, already mentioned as a sign of the transitional stage, has been found by some women to be an effective coping mechanism (McCrea, 1996), although some midwives and other labour ward personnel regard this strategy as problematic (Leap, 2000).

The significance of the transitional stage

The main reason the significance of the transitional stage is given limited attention in the UK literature and practice, but given considerable exposure in North American literature may be due to the highly medicalised birthing environment there. This is simply because the transition does little more than provide an early warning of the imminent birth and the need to inform the medical practitioner so that he is able to 'catch' the baby.

The work of Bergstrom and colleagues (1997, mentioned above) is significant in this context because it focuses on the second stage. While clearly demonstrating the distress which a woman experiencing medicalised labour may endure at this time and, particularly, how this distress may be aggravated by unthinking adherence to a medical protocol, these authors never actually mention the transitional stage of labour *per se*. At the same time as they emphasise the aggravation of the woman's distress in the transitional stage, these authors indicate a likelihood that such aggravation may be due to errors in clinical observation. The result being that one woman may be inappropriately prohibited from pushing, while another may be required to push on an incompletely dilated cervix. In their conclusion, these researchers quote Varney:

'Failing to listen to the woman is one of the biggest mistakes a practitioner can make' (1997)

The transitional stage is also significant in a more purely midwifery oriented sense. What this means is that this stage of labour is crucial in defining the difference between midwifery practice and obstetric practice. This is because, as Bergstrom and colleagues indicate, vaginal examination to ascertain cervical dilation is not the totally objective observation which it is supposed to be. The diagnosis of the transitional stage moves observation on to a higher level, as it is a far more woman-centred and subjective skill. The diagnosis of the transitional stage is essentially a midwifery observation and as such is dependant on knowing the woman, her behaviour and recognising any changes in her behaviour. It is not possible to enter a room where a woman is in labour and observe that she is in the transitional stage in the way that Bergstrom and colleagues observed medical practitioners attempting to diagnose the second stage.

A valid diagnosis of the transitional stage, if it is to be accurate in order to facilitate appropriate care, depends on considerable background knowledge of the woman and her labour. Providing appropriate care requires that the midwife should work with the woman through being an actively supportive presence. Thus, this midwifery diagnosis and care provision are uniquely midwifery skills which are dependent on the nature of the relationship between the woman and the midwife. I suggest that these are skills which may be used to provide a benchmark of quality midwifery practice.

Conclusion

The transitional stage may serve as a shibboleth, that is a test of the quality of midwifery care. No other healthcare provider has either the opportunity or the skills to establish the supportive relationship on which effective care in the transitional stage must be founded. It may be argued that midwives have to decide whether they are prepared to accept the challenge which the transitional stage offers to their professional skills.

REFERENCES

Active Birth Centre. 2001. Aromatherapy during Labour. www.activebirthcentre.com/pb/pbusefultiparomainlabour.html
Baines M. 1990. Living with Dying: The management of terminal disease. Oxford: OUP
Bennet VR, Brown LK. 1999. Myles Textbook for Midwives. Thirteenth Edition. Edinburgh: Churchill Livingstone
Bergstrom L, Seidel J, Skillman-Hull L, Roberts J. 1997. "I gotta push.

Please let me push!" Social interactions during the change from first to second stage labour. Birth, 24(3), 173-80
Bobak IM, Starm JR. 1993. Third Trimester. In IM Bobak & MD Jensen (eds). Maternity and Gynecologic Care: The nurse and the family. 5th Edition. St Louis: Mosby.
Clark D. 1999. Total pain, disciplinary power and the body in the work of Cecily Saunders 1958-67. Social Science & Medicine, 49 (6), 727-36

Handbag.com:family. 2001. Labour. www.handbag.com/family/b4baby_labour2/

Howell CJ. Epidural versus non-epidural analgesia for pain relief in labour (Cochrane Review). In: the Cochrane Library, Issue 3, 2001. Oxford: Update Software.

Kitzinger S. 1987. Giving Birth: How it really feels. London: Gollancz

Langford CPH, Bowsher J, Maloney JP, Lillis PP. 1997. Social support: a conceptual analysis. Journal of Advanced Nursing, 25(1), 95-100

Langford J. 1997. The legendary pain of labour. New Generation, 16(1)6-7

Leap N. 2000. Pain in Labour: Towards a midwifery perspective. MIDIRS Midwifery Digest 10(1), 49-53

McCrea BH. 1996. An investigation of rule-governed behaviours in the control of pain management during the first stage of labour. Unpublished DPhil thesis. University of Ulster

Robertson A. 1994. Empowering women: Teaching active birth in the '90s. Camperdown, Australia: ACE Graphics

Saunders C. 1981. Current views on pain relief and terminal care. In: Swerdlow M (ed). The Therapy of Pain. Lancaster: MTP Press Ltd

Smith BA, Priore RM, Stern MK. 1973. The transition phase of labour. American Journal of Nursing, 73(3), 448-50

Stables D. 1999. Physiology in childbearing. London: Bailliere Tindall

Tucker G. 1996. National Childbirth Trust Book of Pregnancy, Birth and Parenthood. Oxford: OUP

Varney H. 1997. Varney's Midwifery. 3rd Edition. Boston: Jones & Bartlett

Volger JH. 1993. The First Stage of Labour, in: IM Bobak & MD Jensen (eds). Maternity and Gynecologic Care: The nurse and the family. 5th Edition. St Louis: Mosby

The Practising Midwife 2002; 5(1): 10-12

Midwives' experience of the encounter with women and their pain during childbirth

Ingela Lundgren, Karin Dahlberg

Objective: to describe midwives' experience of the encounter with women and their pain during childbirth.

Design: qualitative study using a phenomenological approach. Data were collected via tape-recorded interviews.

Setting: Sahlgrenska University Hospital, Göteborg, and Karolinska Hospital, Stockholm, Sweden in 2000.

Participants: nine experienced midwives with between 12 and 28 years of midwifery practice.

Key findings: the essential structure was described as a striving to become an *anchored companion. To be a companion* is to be available to the woman, to listen to and see her situation mirrored in her body, and to share the responsibility of childbirth. To be *anchored* is to show respect for the limits of the woman's ability as well as one's own professional limits. Five constituents can further describe the essential structure: listening to the woman; giving the woman an opportunity to participate and to be responsible; a trusting relationship; the body expresses the woman's situation; and to follow the woman through the process of childbirth.

Implications for practice: the basis for maternity care should give an opportunity for midwives to be anchored companions. This could be done by emphasising listening to the woman, participation, responsibility, a trusting relationship and a clear understanding of the professional limits and the limits of the woman's ability.

Introduction

The experience of childbirth is a major life event that can influence the woman for many years (Simkin, 1992). One of the most important aspects of the total birth experience is the support received from the midwife (Hodnett, 1999; Lavender et al,1999; Waldenström,1999). Support increases the breast-feeding rate, has a positive impact on mother-baby 'bonding' and leads to fewer interventions (Hemmiki et al, 1990; Hofmeyr et al,1991; Zhang et al, 1996). Support during childbirth also reduces the length of labour (Klaus et al, 1986; Zhang et al, 1996). The support should include 'continuous presence, the provision of hands-on comfort, and encouragement' (Hodnett 1999, p.1). The quality of the relationship between the woman and the midwife is a key factor for good support during childbirth. Several studies have described women's experiences of the relationship with the midwife. The midwife can be described as caring/empowering versus uncaring/discouraging, as a 'cold professional' versus 'warm professional', and as a friend (Halldorsdottir & Karsldottir, 1996, McCrea et al, 1998, Walsh, 1999). Women express a need for the midwife's presence and trust during childbirth (Berg et al,1996; Fraser, 1999, Hodnett, 1999; Seibold et al,1999).

The relationship between the woman and the midwife also has an impact on the woman's experience of pain. A good relationship between the midwife and the woman will tend to alleviate pain (Niven 1994; Bergum 1997). Waldenström et al. (1996) have shown that support by caregivers has a positive effect on women's total birth experience, while pain relief does not explain any of the variations in women's responses. By being 'a warm professional' and by being present, the midwife can have a positive influence on the women's experience of pain during childbirth (McCrea et al, 1998; Lundgren & Dahlberg, 1998). To summarise, there are in-depth studies that describe women's experiences of the relationship with the midwife. However, knowledge about midwives' experiences of the encounter with the woman and her pain during childbirth is limited. The aim of the study reported here was to describe midwives' experience of the encounter with the woman and pain during childbirth.

Methods

To be able to describe the encounter between the midwife and the woman and her pain during childbirth it is necessary to enter deeply into the experience. This is possible using a phenomenological method, based on a lifeworld approach (Dahlberg et al, 2001). The emphasis is on the phenomenal field (Merleau-Ponty, 1976). The purpose of phenomenological research is to describe phenomena as they are lived and experienced by individuals. The phenomenological analysis seeks to uncover the meaning of humanly experienced phenomena, based upon the subjects' descriptions (Dahlberg et al, 2001). The phenomenological method involves some basic elements. According to Giorgi (1997), the phenomenological method means description. Firstly, the analysis is based on the subjects' concrete and experiential descriptions of the phenomenon. Secondly, this method also means a descriptive analysis of the data, in other words, no interpretation is made. On the contrary, Giorgi emphasises that the aim is to stay with the phenomenon precisely as it is given. Giorgi (1997) further advises researchers within phenomenology to acknowledge what he calls the phenomenological reduction. This means that the researcher holds in abeyance such theoretical and experiential knowledge, preconceived notions or expectations that otherwise would interfere with an open-minded description of the phenomenon. During analysis, the researcher moves from understanding the interview text as a whole, through understanding the single meaning units of the text, to a new whole where the essential meaning of the phenomenon is illuminated (Dahlberg et al, 2001).

Inclusion and exclusion criteria

The head midwife at Sahlgrenska University Hospital, Göteborg and Karolinska Hospital, Stockholm selected midwives and was asked to choose 'experienced' midwives working in the unit. In Sweden there are about 1500 registered midwives; 65 at Karolinska Hospital and 100 at Sahlgrenska University Hospital, who provide care during childbirth. All the experienced midwives in the units were informed, and they were asked to tell the head midwife if they were willing to participate. The head midwife at Karolinska Hospital selected three of the 65

midwives and none declined to participate. The head midwife at Sahlgrenska University Hospital selected six of the 100 midwives and none declined to participate. By letting the head midwife at the unit select the midwives attending this study, bias concerning their knowledge of the researchers' identity was minimised.

Conduct of the study

Permission to conduct and tape-record the interviews was obtained from each midwife and they were assured that all information would be treated in confidence. The midwives were interviewed on one occasion by one interviewer (IL). The interviews were conducted in a private setting, a room normally used for conversation, in the hospital and lasted between 60 and 90 minutes. The initial question was 'Can you tell me about the experience of the encounter with the woman and pain during childbirth?' The midwives were encouraged to describe all their feelings and experiences.

Data analysis

The data were analysed following the descriptions of Dahlberg et al (2001) and Giorgi (1997). The interviews were transcribed and primarily analysed by the interviewer (IL). Each interview was first read to bring out a sense of the whole, and after that meaning units were marked. The meaning of the text was organised into different clusters by 'unpicking' the meaning of the text and relating the meaning units to each other. In the final stage, the essence of the investigated phenomenon, a description of what has been revealed was formulated. Through a transformation from the subjects' naïve description to a language meaningful for midwifery, a new understanding of the phenomenon was developed. Ethical approval to undertake the study was obtained from the Ethics Committee at the hospitals. Access to undertake the study was obtained from the physician in charge at the hospitals.

Findings

Sample

The sample consisted of nine midwives from Sahlgrenska University Hospital, Göteborg and Karolinska Hospital, Stockholm, Sweden. The midwives were 38–52 years old and had 12–28 years of midwifery practice. Midwives in Sweden have full responsibility for providing care in normal pregnancy and childbirth. Midwives in the community provide all antenatal care if the woman is healthy and has a normal pregnancy. Antenatal care is provided as part of the community health care system.

The midwives interviewed in this study were providing care for women during childbirth at the two university hospitals. To verify the findings from the analysis, quotations from the midwives are reported and the midwives are given numbers to maintain anonymity.

The essential meaning of midwives' experience of the encounter with the woman and her pain during childbirth

The midwives' approach to the woman and her pain during childbirth was described as a striving to become an *anchored companion*. *To be a companion* was to be available for the woman, to listen to and see her situation mirrored in her body, and to share the responsibility of her childbirth. To be available was to be open, to establish a trustful meeting, and to follow the woman through the process of childbirth. To listen to the woman was being sensitive to the wishes and the needs of the woman. If verbal communication was hindered, the midwives could see the condition of the woman through the expression of the woman's body. The expression of the eyes, the face, and the whole body were important signals to the midwife. The non-verbal communication through the woman's body increased as the process of childbirth proceeded. If this process was disturbed and the limit of the woman's ability was exceeded, the midwife could notice this through the expression of the woman's body. To share the responsibility for the childbirth meant that the focus should be towards the woman's needs and desires. It also meant that the woman had a responsibility to express herself to the midwife, and a willingness to go through the childbirth and meet the pain during childbirth. According to the midwives, there was a risk of being burnt out if the midwife took all the responsibility for the childbirth. To be *anchored* was to show respect for the limits of the woman's ability as well as the midwife's professional limits. To show respect for the limits of the woman meant that the midwife had a responsibility to ensure that the woman did not exceed the limit of her ability and that the pain did not become too much for the woman. When the woman was in this state, the midwife could try to interrupt this development by, for example, a more distinct communication and by establishing eye contact. To respect the professional limits meant to support the woman's capacity to see the normal process of childbirth, but also to see the boundaries of complicated childbirth.

The essential structure can be further described by its five constituents: listening to the woman; giving the woman an opportunity to participate and to be responsible; a trusting relationship; the body expresses the woman's situation; and to follow the woman through the process of childbirth.

Listening to the Woman

By being open and listening to the woman, the midwives tried to understand her unique situation and her desires. One of the approaches described was to begin by asking the woman open-ended questions, instead of using a standard protocol. When they first met it was important that, by creating a feeling that she was there solely for the woman and had all the time needed, the woman felt that the midwife was on hand. The midwives tried to make the woman feel that she could be herself and express her thoughts and feelings, because the woman's innermost needs are likely to emerge during childbirth. This was described as meeting the woman as a unique individual in an open-minded way. One midwife illustrated this by saying:

The way, in which you ask is important, often you have a standard question, when did it start, what is the pain level etc. But instead, ask her open questions; how has the last day been, do you feel ready to give birth, what do you think and feel about the childbirth and so on. And sometimes I think you can meet the woman there and find out things that would not have been expressed otherwise. (Midwife 6)

Listening to the woman included a shift of focus in childbirth, from the midwives themselves to the woman. The woman's needs and desires should be the focus and not those of the midwives. The midwives' task was to support the woman in her decision. The midwives also tried to encourage the woman to express her own needs concerning childbirth and to use the woman's knowledge. Sometimes this was a problem because the woman could not express any explicit desires:

It is not the midwife's obligation to bear the woman's pain and feel that she is pleased afterwards because the woman could stand the pain. That is not my obligation; it is to support the woman according to her wishes. If she knows what she wants then OK, but sometimes she doesn't know that, then you have to make that decision together. (Midwife 2)

If the midwife and the woman first met in a phase of childbirth where conversation could take place, the midwives wanted to take the opportunity to investigate the woman's view of pain. According to the midwives, many women have not reflected on this matter. The woman may know a lot about different pain relief methods, but has not had the opportunity to express what she feels about pain. The midwives' question to the woman was about desired pain relief methods. But the midwives also tried to widen the question to investigate the woman's reflections about pain during childbirth. According to the midwives, these reflections could help the woman to deal with the pain:

Sometimes I ask the woman about her general view of pain, what her opinion about pain during childbirth is. Well, that is, if they are in a latent phase of birth, with cervix dilatation of 3-4 cm. It also helps the woman to reflect about pain. And I also think that just reflecting will help her to deal with it. (Midwife 5)

According to the midwives, listening to the woman was also a confirmation of the woman's experience of pain. This confirmation meant conveying to the woman that the midwife did not ignore her experience of pain. According to the midwives, the confirmation of pain should be combined with an attitude of not increasing the problem:

I think it is very important that her experience of pain is confirmed. That you don't ignore it. If she says that it hurts a lot, I tell her that I can see that and that I know that it can hurt a lot to give birth. Thus confirming her feelings. And you can say that this contraction was very painful. But it is important that you don't make the pain into a big problem. (Midwife 4)

According to the midwives the opportunity to be able to listen to the woman could, however, be limited due to organisational factors of maternity care provision. According to the midwives a major problem was the lack of economic resources for the hospitals. All changes in maternity care in recent years were described in negative terms. The midwives had to care for more and more women at the same time and they often thought that time for the individual person was lacking:

All midwives are very stressed in this situation. And this has been the situation for several years. Every change that happens is always for the worse. This is experienced as very unfortunate in the midwifery profession and I think this is very stressful for me. Not being able to do the job the way you want. I think we lack resources for a genuine encounter with the individuals. (Midwife 4)

The woman's partner could be a resource but also an obstacle to a good relationship between the woman and the midwife. For instance, aggressiveness from the men was described as a problem:

Sometimes I think establishing contact with the father is very difficult. He can be suspicious, worried, and obstruct my contact with the woman. Because he can have a negative attitude, is blunt, and asks a lot of difficult questions. I think this is a bigger problem for me than the relationship with the woman. (Midwife 2)

The midwives' strategies for overcoming these problems were listening to and seeing the future father. The midwives also described how an active participation by the father influenced the childbirth in a positive way:

And then I asked him, 'How are things for you?' It was like pressing a button. And then I had to listen to him for 15 minutes. And I just listened and honestly thought that he was quite silly. Finally, he asked me my opinion. And I said that I understood his situation and his anxiety, but couldn't say too much about feelings. And I said that the best thing for you is to give your attention to your woman. And help her to give birth to your baby. And you do this best by sitting beside her, supporting her and daring to believe that she can give birth. And this conversation ended in a good experience for both the woman and the father. (Midwife 4)

Giving the woman an opportunity to participate and to be responsible

It was described as important to invite the woman to participate and be responsible for her childbirth. The midwife could support and guide the woman through the phases of childbirth, but the woman must also take responsibility. According to the midwives, the woman's responsibility was to tell the midwife about her feelings, thoughts and desires. The woman must also have a will of her own to give birth:

And I think there is a risk of being burnt out if I am made responsible for things that are not my responsibility. And there is a sharing of responsibility. Then you have to be clear right from the beginning. I can go this far as a midwife but then you have to take over, no matter how painful it is. Perhaps getting burnt out is from trying to be more midwife than is possible, bearing all deliveries on one's own shoulders. (Midwife 5)

According to the midwives, the woman's participation in and responsibility for her childbirth could strengthen her. The intention was to use the woman's own resources and strengthen her self-confidence. The midwives exemplified this by describing how they supported the woman in releasing her need for control and encouraging her to let herself go in the process of childbirth. This was an opportunity for the woman to see her own ability, and be aware of her own body. According to the midwives, the woman's experience of her own strength and her own body's ability could be positive for her:

To use the woman's capacity. What they think about. It takes different time for different women, but I think most women can do this if you give them enough support. And afterwards they can say: 'I can do this. Good Lord, what I can do. My body is capable.' You get so aware of your body's capability. I think this is good for the women. (Midwife 1)

The woman may not, however, be willing to take responsibility. For various reasons the woman may be unprepared for responsibility for her childbirth. Sometimes the woman had not discussed participation and responsibility during pregnancy. There is also an attitude in society that says that you should leave all responsibility to the professionals:

I am surprised that so few women have demands and desires about childbirth. I think they are very compliant. I think this is a pity but there are so many different attitudes in society. 'You know best' they often say. 'I don't know so much.' Actually, I am a little surprised about that. The women very easily put themselves into the hands of the midwives. A lot more women are like that than I would wish. But some midwives may think this is good, the attitudes vary among the midwives. Some midwives may think it's comfortable with women without demands. (Midwife 6)

As examples of women that are not used to taking responsibility over situations in their own lives, the midwives referred to women from other cultures or socially vulnerable women:

Actually, there are some cultural systems where the woman isn't used to expressing her wishes. And maybe this is not allowed in that culture. Once I tried to ask a woman about her wishes concerning pain relief. And she looked at her husband and asked him to decide. And then I felt that I couldn't do anything about that. (Midwife 4)

A trusting relationship

To be an *anchored companion* also meant offering a trusting relationship in order to give the woman trust and security during childbirth. According to the midwives a trusting relationship meant that the woman should feel that the midwife cared about her as a unique person, and that she was not just one in the crowd:

I think it is important that you make it plain that you care about the woman. It is important for me that you have a good childbirth. That I am available for you and that I give you security and care about you. You are not only a patient for me, you are the only one for me right now. (Midwife 2)

A relationship built on security and trust could strengthen the woman's self-esteem, especially if she sensed that the midwife was confident in the woman's capacity to give birth. This support included helping the woman to dare to meet the unknown during childbirth without being afraid. The midwives encouraged the woman to sense what was happening in her body, to be attentive to that and the process of childbirth. The midwives also wanted to support the woman in dealing with the pain by conveying a belief that her body is capable. A big problem though, according to the midwives, was fear. If the woman was afraid, the experience of pain could lead to panic. But an emerging feeling of panic could disappear if the woman had a trusting relationship with the midwife:

I work with them and try to give them trust in their own capacity. And that they dare to cooperate with their body's signals and feel what is happening now. And if they can do so, this panic pain will disappear. And to encourage them to not be afraid of childbirth. (Midwife 1)

Some women with no trust in their own capacity, or in the midwife's support, could have problems in letting go, and could not develop a trusting relationship with the midwife:

And they are always a bit on their guard. They dare not believe. Maybe it is about trust. Trust in several meanings,

trust in her own body, and trust in the process of childbirth and giving birth. And the midwife's trust in believing in the woman's ability to give birth. (Midwife 4)

The body expresses the woman's situation

The midwives could be in contact with the woman even if they could not communicate verbally. Non-verbal communication could occur in some phases of childbirth when the woman did not want to talk:

Many women are very introverted in some phases of childbirth. They are in their own world and will not communicate verbally. But even if they are in their own world I can notice if everything is OK by their body language. (Midwife 9)

The non-verbal communication was bodily communication. The midwives described how they tried to understand the woman's situation by the expression of her body. The most important signals came from the eyes. An important question for the midwives was to interpret whether the woman's eyes were expressing calm, or worry and anxiety. But also the face, the breathing, and expressions of the whole body were important signals to the midwife. The woman told the midwife about her situation by the posture of the body, by tensions, and by perspiration:

If you take her hand you can feel if she is sweaty or not. You can feel through the woman's body if she is feeling good or not. If the mouth is constricting, if the face has a tense expression and so on. And the expression of her eyes is very significant. Very significant. (Midwife 1)

Non-verbal communication could help the midwife to establish some contact with the woman if the midwife and the woman did not share the same language:

I think I can communicate with an immigrant woman even if I do not understand her language. My experience is that even if she does not understand what I say to her, she can give a signal with her eyes and communication takes place. (Midwife 9)

The expression of the woman's body could tell the midwife about the woman's capacity for coping with pain and if she was near the boundaries for her coping ability:

Her body expresses that, if she is tense, if she is breathing in a special way. And the eyes, especially the eyes, if you see fear in the eyes. And maybe she contacts me by her eyes and tells me that you must help me, because now it is too much for me. I cannot handle it anymore. It is obvious from her bodily expression. (Midwife 7)

According to the midwives, there were sometimes difficulties in understanding the woman's body expressions. The reason for this could be that the woman neither communicated nor understood through body expressions. Another problem was women that intellectualise and did not express themselves through their bodies:

I think the body and the soul are closely connected and influence the process of childbirth. And I think you should not intellectualise too much when you give birth. And it's comforting having some sort of control when you give birth, but not the control when you use your brain and all the time analyse everything that happens. And try to control things that you cannot control. (Midwife 4)

Although they tried their best, the midwives sometimes failed completely in understanding the woman. The midwives described women who did not express themselves with their bodies and words as examples:

And she was very introverted and I thought that she was very strong and concentrated. And if she is like that I don't do so much, just let them work. And just hold her hand and be present. I experienced that she gave birth in a very positive way. And when I talked to her afterwards she said that she had felt that she would die. It was a terrible experience for her. And I felt that I had totally failed to understand her. I thought that everything was so good and that she was handling everything but she had thought that she would die. And I can still think of this even though it is a long time ago. (Midwife 6)

To follow the woman through the process of childbirth

Finally, to be an *anchored companion* meant to follow the woman through the different phases of childbirth. Mutual trust and confidence made this process smoother. According to the midwives, time was also a key factor for this process. It was described as 'waiting for the woman':

And I can feel that we have a relationship and that she trusts me and I trust her. And the more intensive it gets the more intuitive I get. I follow the woman and become more like her. (Midwife 4)

To follow the woman through the phases of childbirth included getting information about the woman's situation from her partner. This was sometimes a problem for the midwives because of different cultural attitudes. According to the midwives, they tried to have a flexible attitude to the woman's culture and in this way establish contact with her, in order to 'follow' her and 'wait' for her:

I have learned that in some cultures the man makes the decision. And you must learn that you must not get angry with that. One needs to accept their culture. When they meet me during childbirth I cannot change that. But instead I have to enter into their culture and establish contact by first addressing the man if that's their wish. (Midwife 6)

The midwives also used their flexibility when they supported the woman to deal with pain. The midwives encouraged the woman to follow the process of pain, to feel how the pain rose and then disappeared. The midwives' intention was to give the woman the experience that the pain has its course and to take the woman further in the process. There was something happening to the woman and her body, and thus the woman could get a concept of time and a feeling for the process of childbirth. In this way, the pain has a meaning for the woman and was not just something incoherent:

You follow the pain, you feel when it comes and grows. And then she can feel that something is happening in her body and try to follow her. Then she can get a concept of time, its progress and that something is happening to her. And though it hurts a lot there is also something good. (Midwife 1)

The midwives' difficulties in following the woman could lead to an immediate reaction from the woman, for instance, problems in handling the pain:

You get an immediate reaction to your way of doing things. You can notice it in the process of labour, their eyes, their response, and their feedback. If there are any difficulties, problems with the contractions, with the fetal heart rate pattern and so on, can occur. You must try to follow the woman all the way to get a positive childbirth for her. And if you have difficulties in sensing the woman's situation adequately, you can notice a reaction, problems may arise. (Midwife 1)

According to the midwives, the task was to be sensitive to and follow the woman through the phases of childbirth, taking into consideration the woman's capacity to deal with the process and the pain. Another task was to ensure that the woman did not pass the limits of her capacity. If there were signs showing that the woman was near this limit, the midwives could, as they said, 'seize the woman', and in different ways they tried to stop this condition, by communicating more clearly. The midwives described how, at times, they could be more authoritarian and decisive if this problem occurred:

She was almost fainting and I was losing contact with her, and she was breathing very fast. And her eyes were rolling. And then you have to be distinct, you show her that 'I am here and I can help you'. And I must be more authoritarian, and react. I can't just follow her. I can't let her go. It is my duty. I get authoritarian and say, now we do this. But afterwards they have told me that they have experienced me as being very calm. (Midwife 8)

The midwives followed the woman even if there were problems during childbirth. The midwives' responsibility is the normal childbirth and if there were complications an obstetrician was called in. According to the midwives, they had no difficulties in defining their own responsibility, the normal childbirth. Sometimes they anticipated that something was not normal even before actual complications occurred. The possibility of keeping the relation between the midwife and the woman in this situation depended on the course of events and the attitude of the doctor:

Sometimes, even before the process of childbirth is disturbed, you can have a feeling that there is a problem. This is intuition. Your experience tells you that. And even if we have our new fancy equipment, it is not just about the heartbeat of the baby. Your experience can tell you even before you have problems with for example the fetal heart rate pattern, that something is not normal. (Midwife 3)

And we have doctors that are very humble and only do their job and leave things to us afterwards. But they vary. But I have no problems with my responsibility and I know when I should contact a doctor. (Midwife 6)

Discussion

This study was undertaken with a small group of midwives from two University hospitals in Sweden. We cannot claim that the midwives in this study are representative of all midwives in Sweden, let alone all midwives. It is possible that bias was introduced by asking the head midwives to select the midwives as they may have wished to give 'good examples' of the midwifery profession. However, there are some lessons that can be learnt from these findings.

The main finding from this study is that the midwives' approach when encountering the woman and her pain during childbirth can be described as being both *anchored* and a *companion*. The midwives' role as a companion is fundamental for midwifery. The word midwife is derived from the old English 'with woman' (Kaufman, 1993). According to Kaufman (1993), this means physical, psychological and emotional presence, and a relationship built on mutual trust and confidence. This is verified by the findings from this study, which show that the establishment of a trusting relationship is crucial for the companionship between the midwife and the woman. According to the midwives in this study, a trusting relationship means that the woman should be able to trust both herself and her ability, and the midwife. A trust in the midwives' authority is also important for the development of good relationships, according to McCrea and Crute (1993). In this study to be a *companion* also means to be available to the woman. Availability means confirming the individual's suffering just as it is and not explaining it away or destroying it, but to make it a part of life (Eriksson, 1993). This is confirmed in this study by the midwives in terms of their listening to the woman and following her through the phases of childbirth. This process, the midwife following the woman through the phases of childbirth, has been described as a journey (Page, 1993; Halldorsdottir & Karlsdottir, 1996b). Sensitivity and listening to the wishes and needs of the woman are important when the midwife follows the woman through the process of childbirth. This is verified by Flint (1993) and Page (1997) who argue that sensitivity and making each woman feel that she is unique are required for good midwifery practice. If verbal contact is hindered the midwives reported that they can obtain information about the women's situation from their bodily expressions. The most important signals come from the eyes, but also the face, the breathing, and expression of the whole body are important signals to the midwife. This knowledge can be deepened by the study of the philosophy of Merleau-Ponty (1964). He argues that the own living body is not a thing, but instead it is the subject that performs all actions. In this meaning, one's own body is the incarnated subject that we never alienate from, and never fly away from (Bengtsson, 1988). According to Merleau-Ponty (1964) we can get information about another person by the expression of the body 'I cannot know what you are thinking, but I can suppose it, guess at it from facial expressions, your gestures, and your words – in short from a series of bodily appearances of which I am only the witness' (p.114). Non-verbal communication can help the midwife to establish contact with immigrant women, as well as women who in some phases of childbirth do not want to talk. But this does not mean that the midwife should avoid talking verbally to immigrant women via an interpreter if needed. Non-verbal communication needs further investigation. It would be interesting to ask women about this matter.

To be a companion is also, according to the midwives, to share the responsibility of childbirth. Paterson and Zderads (1976) argue that a relationship also demands responsibility. The midwives in this study reported that many women do not want to be responsible and active during childbirth. Instead, they want the midwife to take all the decisions. This is interesting; do we act in such a way that we increase the opportunity for the woman to take part during childbirth? As in other countries, Sweden has problems with increasing demands from women wanting painless births with a Caesarean section. Is this the result of the lack of participation and responsibility by the woman? The attitude in society is to be dependent upon experts according to the midwives. Giddens (1990) argues that the modern organisation of maternity care leads to a high degree of expert-dependence for women during childbirth, leading to decreased participation and personal responsibility. An organisational form that emphasises both responsibility and participation for women is birth centre care (Waldenström, 1993). Evaluation from this type of care shows that women's level of satisfaction in such care is much higher than in standard care. These findings indicate that women want to be responsible if they have an opportunity. Another organisational example emphasising participation and responsibility, is woman-centred care in the UK (Department of Health 1993).

Continuity is a key factor in such care which would give the midwife the opportunity to 'get to know the woman' before childbirth (Flint, 1993) and prepare her for participation and responsibility.

According to the findings from this study the midwife's role, as a companion should be combined with being *anchored*. To be anchored is to respect the woman's ability limits. The woman is in a special state of mind during childbirth (Brudal, 1985). This can also be described as a 'transition to motherhood' (Schumacher & Meleis, 1994). The challenge for the midwives as described in this study, was to encourage the woman to be in this transition and special state of mind, but not to pass the limits of her capacity. According to the midwives, this can sometimes be a problem when contact between the midwife and the woman is disturbed. A philosophical concept describing this process is 'boundary situation'. A boundary situation is a situation that in some way expresses the contradictions of being. Hereby, forces that are included in the thrust of being, meaning and growing, are being developed (Jaspers, 1963). The developing of forces in a boundary situation is verified in this study by the midwives, through their expression of how the experience of childbirth can strengthen the woman.

To be anchored is also to respect professional limits. The professional limit for midwives in Sweden is to provide care in normal pregnancy and childbirth. The concept of 'normal' birth is not well defined. What we call normal birth can vary over time and in different cultures (WHO, 1996). An analysis of the concept normal birth is important for midwifery practice as the medicalisation of childbirth increases (Gould, 2000). Due to the problems in defining normal birth, WHO (1996) as well as The Swedish National Board of Health and Welfare (2000), have summarised the state of knowledge, with practical recommendations for maternity care. It is interesting that the midwives in this study have no problems with defining their professional limits even though normal birth is not well defined. Maybe experienced midwives have a clear understanding of this concept, embedded in practice and long tradition.

In summary, the findings from this study show that the midwives were acting with a desire to be both a *companion* and to be *anchored* when encountering the woman and her pain during childbirth. Several studies have focused upon the relationship between the midwife and the woman during childbirth from the woman's perspective (Berg et al,1996; Halldorsdottir & Karsldottir, 1996a; Fraser, 1999; Hodnett, 1999; Seibold et alm, 1999; Walsh, 1999). Studies also show that stress and burnout is a problem in midwifery today (Sandall, 1997; Mackin & Sinclair, 1998). It is possible that an imbalance between being a companion and being anchored could be one explanation of the problem of burnout in midwifery. This means telling the midwife about her important role as a companion without focusing her role as anchored, by not focusing the professional limits and the limits of the woman's ability. According to the midwives in this study there is a risk of burnout if the midwife takes on all the responsibility for the childbirth. If we really want to meet women's needs during childbirth we must organise maternity care in a way that gives midwives an opportunity to be anchored companions for the women. This could be done by emphasising listening to the woman, participation, responsibility, a trusting relationship, and a clear understanding of the professional limits as well, as the limits of the woman's ability.

REFERENCES

Bengtsson J 1988 Sammanflätningar. Fenomenologi från Husserl till Merleau-Ponty (Phenomenology from Husserl to Merleau-Ponty). Daidalos, Göteborg

Berg M, Lundgren I, Hermansson E et al.1996 Women's experience of the encounter with the midwife during childbirth. Midwifery 12: 11-15

Bergum V 1997 A child on her mind. The experience of becoming a mother. Bergin & Garvey, Westport

Brudal LF 1985 Födandets psykologi (The psychology of childbirth). Natur och Kultur, Vällingby

Dahlberg K, Drew N, Nystrom M 2001 Reflective lifeworld research. Studentlitteratur, Lund

Department of Health 1993 Changing Childbirth, report of the expert maternity group. HMSO, London

Eriksson K 1993 Möten med lidanden (Meeting suffering). Åbo Akademis tryckeri, Åbo

Flint C 1993 Midwifery teams and caseloads. Butterworth-Heinmann Ltd, Oxford

Fraser DM 1999 Women's perceptions of midwifery care. A longitudinal study. Birth 26: 99-107

Giddens A 1990 The consequences of modernity. Polity Press, Cambridge

Giorgi A 1997 The theory, practice, and evaluation of the phenomenological method as a qualitative research procedure. Journal of Phenomenological Psychology 28: 235-260

Gould D 2000 Normal labour: a concept analysis. Journal of Advanced Nursing 31: 418-427

Halldorsdottir S, Karlsdottir S 1996a Empowerment or discouragement: women's experience of caring and uncaring encounters during childbirth. Health Care for Women International 17: 361-379

Halldorsdottir S, Karlsdottir S 1996b Journeying through labour and delivery: perceptions of women who have given birth. Midwifery 12: 48-61

Hemmiki E, Virta A-L, Koponen P et al.1990 A trial on continuous human support during labour: feasibility, interventions and mothers' satisfaction. Journal of Psychosomatic Obstetrics and Gynaecology 11: 239-250

Hodnett ED 1999 Caregiver support for women during childbirth. The Cochrane library, Issue 1, P.1

Hofmeyr GJ, Nikodem VC, Wolman et al.1991 Companionships to

modify the clinical birth environment: effects on progress and perceptions of labour, and breastfeeding. British Journal of Obstetrics and Gynaecology 98: 756-764

Jaspers K 1963 Introduktion till filosofin (Introduction to philosophy) Alb. Bonniers boktryckeri, Stockholm

Kaufman KJ 1993 Effective control or effective care? Birth 20: 156-158

Klaus MH, Kennel JH, Robertson SS et al.1986 Effects of support during parturition on maternal and infant morbidity. British Medical Journal 293: 585-587

Lavender T, Walkinshaw SA, Walton I 1999 A prospective study of women's views of factors contributing positive birth experience. Midwifery 15: 40-46

Lundgren I, Dahlberg K 1998 Women's experience of pain during childbirth. Midwifery 12: 105-110

Mackin P, Sinclair M 1998 Labour ward midwives' perceptions of stress. Journal of Advanced Nursing 27: 986-991

McCrea H, Crute V 1993 Valuing the midwife's role in the midwife/client relationship. Journal of Clinical Nursing 2: 47-52

McCrea BH, Wright ME, Murphy-Blach T 1998 Differences in midwives' approaches to pain relief in labour. Midwifery 14: 174-180

Merleau-Ponty M 1964 The primacy of perception. Northwestern University Press, Evanston

Merleau-Ponty M 1976 Phenomenology of perception (translated by C.Smith).The Humanistic Press, New Jersey

Niven, C 1994 Coping with labour pain: the midwife's role. In: Robinson S, Thomson AM (eds) Midwives, research and childbirth, Vol.3. Chapman & Hall, London

Page L 1993 Redefining the midwives' role: changes needed in practice. British Journal of Midwifery 1:21-24

Page L 1997 Evidenced based maternity care: science and sensitivity in practice. New Generation Digest 20: 2-3

Paterson JG, Zderad LT 1976 Humanistic nursing. Wiley, New York

Sandall J 1997 Midwives' burnout and continuity of care. British Journal of Midwifery 5: 106-111

Schumacher KL, Meleis Afaf I 1994 Transitions: a central concept in nursing. Journal of Nursing Scholarship 26: 117-125

Seibold BA, Miller M, Hall J 1999 Midwives and women in partnership: the ideal and the real. Australian Journal of Advanced Nursing 17: 21-27

Simkin P 1992 Just another day in a woman's life? Part II: nature and consistency of women's long-term memories of their first birth experiences. Birth 19: 64-81

The Swedish National Board of Health and Welfare 2000 Normal birth – state of the art document (Socialstyrelsen 2000 Normal förlossning – state of the art document) Stockholm

Waldenström U 1993 Föda barn på ABC (Giving birth at an ABC-unit). Team Offset, Malmö

Waldenström U, Borg IM, Olsson B et al.1996 The birth experience, a study of 295 new mothers. Birth 23:144-153

Waldenström U 1999 Experience of labour and birth in 1111 women. Journal of Psychosomatic Research 47: 471-482

World Health Organization 1996 Care in normal birth. Report of the Technical Working Group Meeting on Normal Birth 25-29 March, Maternal Health Safe Motherhood Programme, Geneva

Walsh D 1999 An ethnographic study of women's experience of partnership caseload midwifery. The professional as a friend. Midwifery 15: 165-176

Zhang J, Bernasko JW, Leybovich E et al.1996 Continuous labour support from labour attendant for primiparous women: a meta-analysis. Obstetrics and Gynaecology 88: 739-744

Midwifery 2002; 18: 155-164

Normal birth
– does it matter?

Belinda Phipps

With the Caesarean rate over 20% (Thomas, 2001) and the number of births that take place without medical intervention below 25% (Downe, 2001) perhaps we as a society have concluded that normal birth doesn't matter. If it did matter, surely our maternity services would be set up to maximise the opportunity for normal birth. But what do mothers think? The National Childbirth Trust is in touch with hundreds of thousands of new mothers each year. Many women write their birth stories and send them to the charity. A short questionnaire sent to NCT branches resulted in a very rich and passionate range of responses.

One question that was asked was 'does birth matter?' These quotes illustrate how much it matters. Women saw their births as at the same level of importance as the death of a close relative or their wedding day. There were some who saw their birth as less important as time went by, and from the submitted stories these comments came from those who had a Caesarean birth or a highly medicalised birth. Perhaps there is a connection between the perceived importance of birth and the mode of birth. Perhaps it's time we looked at the importance of birth, and the manner in which it occurs, from a woman's point of view.

'It ranks as number 1 in my great moments – the way a woman gives birth can affect the whole of the rest of her life – how can that not matter – unless the woman herself doesn't matter'

'It's something you never forget and it does mark a huge transition in your life'

'Incredibly important'

'Nothing can compare to the experience of giving birth and holding your child for the first time. It definitely altered my relationship with my partner – for the better.'

'Life changing – more meaningful than all other experiences'

'Birth experiences strike at the very heart and soul of you, they touch new emotions not experienced before and bring a whole new perspective to life'

'I think birth is very important if it is a recent experience and then as other things take over in your life then it becomes less important'

The terminology used for birth is also a matter of debate. The NCT favours 'birth' over 'delivery' (babies are born, pizzas are delivered!) because it gives the active role to the woman who gives birth rather than her carers. 'Normal birth' is often used, and definitions have been published and discussed. But because the opposite is abnormal birth it is deeply offensive to those women who had necessary medical support including those who had a Caesarean.

The NCT firmly believes in providing support and information to all women, without discriminating over their mode of birth. 'Normal' has the potential to be divisive. 'Physiological birth' is a commonly used term but for women without any medical grounding 'physiological' is a meaningless and frighteningly complicated word.

The NCT itself has used 'natural birth' in its distant past. This phrase appears to be a value judgement, and those who need medical support feel excluded. 'Natural' also gives some journalists the opportunity to create an image for the NCT as Pollyannas who recommend birth in a bender with suffering and risk thrown in for good measure.

The naming debate has been particularly lively within the NCT as we develop a birth policy to guide the charity's future work. Our interchanges are leading us to use the term 'straightforward vaginal birth'. For women this is a meaningful, plain English term. There are also a number of value-free opposites to choose from, such as 'complicated vaginal birth'. Straightforward vaginal birth is, however, not very media friendly. Journalists would rather their teatime broadcasts did not contain the word 'vaginal'.

What do women think about 'straightforward vaginal birth'? Interestingly, the most positive comments about 'straightforward vaginal birth' came from those women who had experienced both a complicated birth and a

Table 5.3.1 Questions asked to stimulate thinking and generate a fuller response

What about the issue of so-called 'normal birth' – what does that mean to you – what is normal?

How much does having a vaginal birth matter?

What about the various medical procedures – vaginal examination, sonicaid monitoring, electronic fetal monitoring, having your membranes ruptured, having a drip to accelerate your labour, forceps/ventouse, having an episiotomy etc?

What do you think about the various pain control/relief methods – from a warm bath to epidural?

Does having a live and healthy infant make up for any level of unpleasant/frightening birth experience?

Some obstetricians think that all labours should be kept to less than 12 hours – how do you see it?

Where did you get your views on birth from – your mum, your friends, the TV? Did they change after you had given birth?

Did you change after having given birth? If yes, how did you change?

If you could choose entirely the manner of your giving birth, what would you choose and why?

How important were your birth experiences to you, to your relationship with your child and your partner? Relative to other experiences in your life (such as the death of someone close to you, your first experience of sex, your wedding) were they more or less important?

straightforward vaginal (often home) birth. Perhaps those who have had only straightforward births take for granted the feelings of ecstasy, empowerment, fulfilment and achievement described by those with a wider range of experience.

'It would have been everything to me – but I was robbed by a C-section'

'I was fairly open to either way before the birth – but I did feel a sense of achievement at having given birth vaginally'

'When I was expecting my second child I was desperate for a vaginal birth simply because I could not see how I cope with a toddler and a newborn after such a major operation'

'Overall I felt very cheated that I had not had a vaginal delivery'

'Having a vaginal birth did mean a lot to me. I'd made it through the rite of passage'

'I firmly believe the way I gave birth made a huge impact on my view of myself and my baby'

'I was elated, I had managed to give birth naturally'

'My second birth experience, my homebirth, was the most significant, empowering and important experience of my life'

'The birth of my second child was a wonderful experience for my family and me'

'My personal experience really makes me believe that birth matters and has implications throughout the child's life'

'It matters a hell of a lot!'

'It was totally life changing for the positive. It enabled my husband and I to deal with the pain and anguish of the first labour. The birth of my second child brought healing and reconciliation'

'We felt like the happiest family in the world'

'Having a vaginal delivery, knowing that I could actually give birth to a baby, rather than having it extracted from me like a tooth, did wonders for my confidence. Just that feeling, that your body has done what it was designed to do, is great'

We know astonishingly little from the woman's point of view about the effect that birth has on her, and we have little understanding of women's internal experience of birth. Researchers focus on whether this or that intervention has this or that effect on the length of the baby, the APGAR score of the baby etc. If anyone remembers to ask women about their experience, crude satisfaction scores are reported almost as an afterthought.

'Straightforward birth' may need some defining. What exactly constitutes straightforward? Rather than answer this with a list of interventions that are OK and a list which are not, understanding of the accumulation of interventions is useful. One paper by Sarah Clement et al, describes the weight of interventions as experienced by women (Clement et al, 1999). Adding up the scores for what you might have thought was a fairly straightforward birth is an interesting exercise. The cumulative effect can be very large from apparently routine interventions like vaginal examinations. It may be more useful to think of birth on a continuum from 'straightforward non-intervened' in vaginal birth to 'complicated birth with many medical interventions'.

From the rich seam of birth stories available to the NCT our conclusion is that birth matters – it matters very much. It is a life changing event and it has the power to strengthen a woman and empower her as a woman, a lover and a parent. What is most disturbing is that we don't actually know what effect birth has.

We now know more and are continuing to find out more about the physical and mental health benefits of breastfeeding for both the mother and her baby in the short term and in the long term. We know enough to be able to calculate the financial cost to the health service of those mother-baby pairs that are using artificial formula. Policy makers need information to be presented in this way. It is only when a clear case is made that action (albeit slow action) is taken. The breastfeeding rate is rising as a result of concerted effort backed by hard numbers. Do we have this for birth – can we say with certainty that a 'straightforward' birth has mental and physical health benefits for mothers and babies in the short and long term? Although there are anecdotal indicators and some research, we do not have all the information pulled together with a plan to fill the gaps. So will policy makers take 'straightforward birth' seriously? Not until we can put hard numbers against it and show a cost to the health service of our failure to be effective in supporting women to have a 'straightforward vaginal birth'.

REFERENCES

Clement S, Wilson J, Sikorski J. 1999. the development of an intrapartum intervention score based on women's experiences. Journal of Reproductive and Infant Psychology, 17(1), 53-62

Downe S, McCormick C, Beech BL. 2001. British Journal of Midwifery, 9(10), 602-6

Thomas J, Paranjothy S. RCOG Clinical Effectiveness Support Unit, 2001. National Sentinel Caesarean Section Audit Report. London: RCOG Press

The Practising Midwife 2002; 5(2): 23-24

Action: promoting normal birth

Gill Skinner

We all know that the Caesarean section rate is rising – it is a national emergency! As with any national emergency, we need to do what we do best – pull together and change the world!

The Sentinel Audit (Thomas & Paranjothy, 2001) has given us some hard facts and some insights into why there are more Caesarean sections than ever before. This is, of course, very interesting. However, this audit, like any audit, is useless without action. We must all – that is, midwives, obstetricians, women, professional organisations and the NHS – commit to that action.

Many people have already pledged to 'prevent unnecessary Caesarean sections' and there are good examples of action such as external cephalic version clinics and policies for vaginal birth after Caesarean section. That is great, but 'preventing unnecessary Caesarean sections' feels negative and medicalised. Let us start bv changing the action to 'promoting normal birth' – say that loud and let the positivity and passion wash over you!

Let's look at women's expectations of birth in this century. Women have stopped believing in their bodies' ability to give birth without drama, drugs and damage – the 3 'D's! This is fuelled by the media (have you ever seen a calm, normal birth on TV?). How can we influence the media – or how can we give the message to women that normal birth is not a drama? That's why it is never seen on TV: it wouldn't attract the viewers. What is shown is not real life.

This generation's mothers are the daughters of high-tech conveyer belt obstetrics. They have few role models to learn from. So their expectations demand a service that is still high-tech, and instant. How do we influence this, and the next generation of mothers? How do we ensure that today's women have enough confidence in their bodies to allow nature to do its stuff? The answer would appear to be one midwife – one woman – one doula! Extra support from doulas really works: look at the evidence.

We could also challenge traditional antenatal care, and ensure that information and labour preparation become the priority. Information influences women when the relationship with the midwife is good. We all know a midwife who simply tests urine, takes a blood pressure, checks for growth and asks if the bag is packed! How much time does she spend on building a trusting relationship with the woman?

The relationship the midwife has with the woman is key to the woman's confidence for labour and birth. Building that relationship does not happen in one or two visits. You have to know the woman you care for very well, and she needs to know you. You need to understand her thoughts and feelings on birth, and what has influenced her (for example, the woman next door, who has had three sections and loved them!). You need to understand her social situation, and see if there are issues you can address, or put her in touch with someone else who can help, so that preparing for birth becomes her priority, not all the other problems she faces.

We need a variety of avenues for care and information open to us. We may have to let go of the traditional things that we do and increase support to women using new methods of working. Let us challenge the professional boundaries within our everyday world and work together with GPs, health visitors, doulas, care assistants, social workers and all other parties concerned with maternity care. Then we will be able to maximise an individual programme of care, support and information for each pregnant woman and her family. The aim is simple: to make sure that everybody involved in the woman's care bolsters her confidence in her ability to give birth.

Midwives, there is so much we need to do to reverse the upward trend in Caesarean birth. We are achieving a lot already. Midwifery education has changed drastically over the last five years. New midwives know and understand the evidence to underpin practice. Their training is based in normality. What happens when they qualify? Do they consolidate their experience in normal midwifery? Do they work in a community setting? Do they hold their own caseloads? Do they experience the fascination of watching an expert at work – a midwife at a home birth? If you can answer yes to all of these, we are winning. Consolidating normal midwifery practice must be a priority after qualification before the accumulation of high-tech skills, IV drugs, scrubbing in theatre, CTG interpretation. These skills are important, but not first. We need to ensure that the art of midwifery is not lost forever.

My view is that midwives who work within a community setting should be the focus of our action. They can keep birth normal already. It is ridiculous to make them come into the delivery suite for 'updating' – updating skills such topping up epidurals and CTG interpretation. Surely it should be the other way around – hospital midwives should go and update their midwifery practice in the community to remind themselves of what constitutes a normal birth.

The environment for birth is also an area for action. A busy delivery suite is not conducive to a calm birth experience. Let's change it. Set up birthing rooms in a quiet place, open birthing centres, encourage home birth. Keep the delivery suite for women who need that level of care. However, remember that women with problems need supportive midwifery care too. They should not be able to distinguish between low tech or high-tech except for the odd drip or two!

I would be wrong not to recognise that some women have genuine problems in pregnancy, labour and birth, that need skilled detection and care from a highly-trained team of midwives and doctors. Obstetricians and midwives who are skilled in this area of care need to concentrate on developing even better services than we already have. They do not need to interfere in normal midwifery practice. Be brave, let go, encourage obstetricians and your midwifery colleagues to focus on their area of expertise – women and babies with problems need them.

Let's challenge and change our world together. Stop fitting women to the service you provide. Fit the service to them. The right information, care and support in the right environment create confidence. Say no to drama, drugs and damage and say yes to confident women, confident midwives and promoting normal birth.

REFERENCES

Thomas J and Paranjothy S, 2001. RCOG Clinical Effectiveness Support Unit. The National Sentinel Caesarean Section Audit Report. London: RCOG Press

The Practising Midwife 2002; 5(3): 4

Hong Kong Chinese women's experiences of vaginal examinations in labour

Chit Ying Lai, Valerie Levy

Objective: to explore women's experiences during vaginal examinations in labour.

Design: qualitative with phenomenological approach. Data were collected by tape-recorded open-ended interviews during the early postnatal period.

Data analysis: phenomenological hermeneutic analysis based upon Riceour's interpretation theory.

Participants: a purposive sample of eight women post-delivery who had given birth vaginally and were able to speak and read Chinese.

Setting: a maternity unit of a University-affiliated District General Hospital in Hong Kong.

Key findings: women accepted the necessity for vaginal examinations, but expressed the need to be able to trust that the examiner would respect them as individuals and try to maintain their dignity, perform the examination skillfully and communicate the findings to them. Pain and embarrassment were frequently experienced during vaginal examination. Women wanted to be supported during the examination by someone they knew and trusted; they appreciated practitioners who tried to minimise their physical and psychological discomfort. Some women felt embarrassed when examined by a male doctor, but the attitude and approach of the examiner was generally found to be more important than gender.

Implications for practice: practitioners should be continuously aware of the need to show respect and consideration for the dignity of a woman undergoing vaginal examination in labour. Although this seems an obvious statement to make it is reiterated because some practitioners display insensitivity in this regard. Each woman should be treated with courtesy and respect, and her modesty protected by minimal exposure and examiners/examinations. Findings from the examination should be discussed with her. Practitioners should be aware of the cultural influences that may lead a woman to hide her pain during examination and should be alert for signs of this.

Introduction

Vaginal examination is a common procedure carried out by midwives during which progress in labour may be assessed, and procedures, such as artificial rupture of membranes, performed. Vaginal examination is performed digitally, and/or instrumentally by speculum. It is often performed when a women is admitted in labour, and may be repeated during labour, the frequency depending upon institutional policies as well as clinical indications (O'Driscoll & Meagher 1986, Gibb 1991, Lefeber & Voorhoeve 1998).

Despite the probability that many hundreds of thousands of vaginal examinations during labour are carried out daily throughout the world there appears to be surprisingly little literature that has explored women's experiences and feelings during this procedure. Three strategies were used to access the relevant literature. Firstly, midwifery and obstetric textbooks locally available in university and hospital libraries were consulted. Secondly, a computer search was conducted using medical literature on-line (MEDLINE), cumulative index to nursing and allied health literature (CINAHL), and the Cochrane Database. The English language literature was searched, using key words such as vaginal and pelvic examinations, women's feelings and/attitudes, and touch. Thirdly, personal communication was attempted between the first author of this study and possible authors of relevant work, via midwifery research Internet mailing lists. Despite these strategies, there appeared to be a surprising paucity of studies focusing on the feelings of women regarding vaginal examination during labour. Fourteen publications were obtained which pertained to pelvic examinations, but none of these specifically investigated women's feelings regarding examinations during labour, focusing instead upon women's preferences regarding the gender of the examiner, observational studies of examiners' behaviours, rectal versus vaginal examination, or women's experiences of examinations in gynaecological rather than labour situations. Five of these publications comprised personal descriptions or brief literature reviews of pelvic examination in various settings rather than accounts of empirical enquiry. However, throughout the literature, there was a general acceptance that pelvic examinations were a source of anxiety, discomfort and embarrassment to women. For example, in a study comparing the reactions of women towards rectal and vaginal examinations during labour Murphy et al. (1986) noted that women described vaginal examinations as intrusive and embarrassing, and Bergstrom et al. (1992) commented that women's expressions of pain were sometimes ignored during vaginal examination. The focus of this latter study, however, was on the behaviour of caregivers during the second stage of labour, rather than upon labouring women's feelings and perceptions. To reduce women's anxiety, Magee (1975) suggested that the examiner should introduce himself/herself first before the examination starts while the woman is sitting upright and clothed. Swartz (1984) and Henderson and Jones (1997) advocated that the woman should adopt a semi-sitting position during the examination to decrease any feelings of vulnerability; eye contact and communication could then, they suggested, be maintained more easily. The gender of practitioners during vaginal examinations has been shown to influence the feelings of women.

Alexander and McCullough (1981) found that female health professionals were preferred by 70% of women. Elderen et al. (1998) concluded that female family doctors were perceived as showing significantly more caring behaviours particularly during consultations and vaginal examination; women examined by a male doctor tended to feel more anxious and embarrassed (Moettus et al. 1999). To summarise, a variety of search strategies have revealed few studies on vaginal examinations, particularly examinations during labour, and no empirical study has been found which has explored women's experiences of these examinations in depth. It appears to be generally accepted, however, that vaginal examinations are often perceived as embarrassing and stressful.

In view of the apparent scarcity of studies exploring women's experiences and feelings about vaginal examination in labour, it was decided to conduct this present study, which was carried out in the first author's place of work, a major Obstetric Unit in Hong Kong.

Background to the study

The study was carried out in the postnatal ward of a consultant obstetric unit in Hong Kong. Over 96% of women giving birth at this hospital are Chinese. According to the hospital labour ward protocol, vaginal examination is performed four hourly during the latent phase of labour and two hourly during the active phase. The unit is part of a university teaching hospital and women may be examined by a supervisor as well as a midwifery or medical student.

There are total of 14 beds in the delivery area. Four beds are located in two private rooms. In each room, these two beds are separated by a wall and there is also a curtain at each bed end. These rooms are mainly reserved for private patients. The other ten beds are separated by curtains to provide some privacy. In an emergency, these curtains can be removed to give a larger working space. However, the situation is far from ideal, and privacy is often compromised especially during busy days when staff may walk hurriedly between curtains.

Method

A qualitative research design based upon hermeneutic phenomenological methods was used as this is considered useful for studying phenomena or events about which little is known (Field & Morse 1985). Hermeneutic phenomenology aims to understand and interpret individual's feelings about events or situations. Hermeneutics can be loosely defined as the theory or philosophy of the interpretation of meaning (Bleicher 1980). A Heideggerian hermeneutical approach was chosen, as the basis for this lies in the belief that interpretation is necessary in the attempt to understand how individuals perceive an event or situation, rather than relying upon pure description (Cohen & Omery 1994). This was considered important in this study, in which it was planned to interview several women about their experiences, and to interpret their comments, in order to identify clusters of data relating to particular aspects of the overall experience of vaginal examination in labour.

Sampling and recruitment

The target sample were women who had had experiences of being vaginally examined in labour. Both speculum – as well as digitally – examined women were included since speculum examination was used to confirm rupture of membranes during the early stage of labour. Purposive sampling was used in order to recruit information-rich cases for in-depth study (Coyne 1997). Eight women post-delivery were invited to participate as, upon initial contact between the first author and the women, they appeared articulate, reflective, and willing to share their perceptions with the interviewer. Women who had undergone elective Caesarean section were not included, because they were unlikely to have experiences of vaginal examination in labour.

Those who could not speak and read Cantonese were also excluded as this (the local Chinese dialect of Hong Kong) was the language of the interviews. Women whose babies needed special or intensive care also were excluded from the study as it seemed unkind to request their participation at such a stressful time.

Formal approval was given from the Research Ethics committee of the Chinese University of Hong Kong. A full explanation of the purpose of the study was given verbally and written consent to participate was obtained from each woman before the research interview. Anonymity was guaranteed in that the woman's identity did not appear in the research data. Names were not used in tapes or transcripts, women being addressed by the neutral term 'tai tai' which is a courteous and acceptable mode of address between Chinese women. The interview was conducted in a single room of the postnatal ward to ensure privacy.

Data collection

Recruitment and interviews took place in the postnatal ward at a time convenient to participants, at least 24 hours post-delivery when prospective participants felt sufficiently rested to take part. The ward staff cared for the baby during the interview. Each interview lasted between 30 minutes and one hour. Unstructured interviews were carried out, offering the researcher flexibility in gathering information (Polit & Hungler 1999). The first author carried out the interviews, starting by asking 'Please tell me your experience during vaginal examination', encouraging the woman to tell her story in a naturalistic, narrative fashion. Probing questions were also used such as 'What does this mean to you?'; 'Can you tell me what you thought at that point?'; 'Can you explain this more?'

Data analysis

All interviews were audio tape-recorded and transcribed, initially using the Cantonese language. The decision was taken to translate relevant passages into English before data analysis ('relevant passages' comprised any data pertaining to the experience of

vaginal examination). The reason for this decision was that if the study were to be published in an English language journal (midwifery journals written in Chinese have an extremely limited circulation), translation at some point would be required. Furthermore, translation relatively early in the analytic process enabled the second, non-Cantonese speaking author to advise on the data analysis. Efforts were made to facilitate accurate translation. With the help of another fluent Cantonese/English speaking midwife, passages of translated text were cross-checked against the tapes for accuracy of transcription and translation. Random passages of the translated English scripts were also back-translated to Cantonese to check for accuracy and reliability.

The transcribed data were interpreted according to a phenomenological hermeneutic method inspired by Ricoeur (1976), which comprises three main systematic stages: naïve reading, structural analysis and comprehensive understanding (described by Hildingsson & Haggstrom 1999). Hallgren et al. (1999) used different terms to describe the same processes: understanding the whole, exploring the parts and understanding the whole text once again. 'Naïve reading', or 'understanding the whole', involves reading the data in order to gain an initial, basic understanding of its meaning and what it is expressing. During 'structural analysis' or 'exploring the parts', the data are studied in more depth, guided by the purpose of the study (in this case, the experiences of women during vaginal examination in labour) and impressions from the naïve reading. Patterns in the data are sought which describe this experience, and these are developed in a dialectic process involving interpretation and abstraction in order to verify or refute understanding gained during the naïve reading and to help develop categories. This leads to 'comprehensive understanding', when insights into women's experiences during vaginal examination may be articulated.

The data and emerging categories were scrutinized and discussed by the two authors using this dialectic process in order that personal bias during analysis could be reduced as far as possible, and so that the categories would accurately and meaningfully reflect the participants' experiences of vaginal examination. All passages of text referring to the experience of vaginal examination were considered relevant and were incorporated into the analysis.

Findings and discussion

When undergoing vaginal examinations in labour, women appeared to experience some degree of conflict between accepting that the examination was a necessary part of labour and yet resisting it (if only passively) because of the pain and embarrassment they perceived it would cause. This conflict was the underlying storyline; in order to resolve it women needed to have confidence both in the examiner and the examination. Four categories were identified that accounted for these needs, a woman needed to be able to:

- trust in the examiner's respect for her as an individual and that the examiner would maintain her dignity;
- trust that the examination would be performed skillfully;
- trust that the findings would be accurate and communicated to her;
- trust that she would be supported.

The examiner could be trusted to respect the woman as an individual and to maintain her dignity

Traditionally, the Chinese perceive touch as offensive and impolite (Giger & Davidhizar 1991). A study of Hong Kong women's perception of support from midwives during labour (Holroyd et al. 1997) revealed that women ranked 'praised me', 'kept me informed about my progress', 'instructed me in breathing/relaxing', 'answered my questions truthfully', 'provided a sense of security' as the top five supportive behaviours, whereas supportive behaviours involving touching were ranked the lowest.

The practice of digital examination and intimate touching was viewed by several women as unnatural, constituting an intrusion of the woman's integrity. At the same time, however, women either accepted the medical view that vaginal examination was necessary during labour, or were unwilling to challenge the powerful medical system:

I can tolerate it... there is no other way round, labour is like this' (Yee)

I know every pregnant woman will have the examination... since I am pregnant, I don't care too much. Once you are pregnant, you get less shy (Ling)

This is a very natural and normal event... it is OK and I can accept this. (Oi)

This acceptance may have been influenced by Chinese Confucian values of obedience, proper conduct, control of impulses, and the acceptance of social obligations, whilst a relative lack of emphasis is given to independence, assertiveness, and creativity (Bond 1996). As a result, women suppressed their distress or discomfort during vaginal examination in order not to lose face by offending the caregiver, or being labelled as a problem patient.

Women commonly said they felt embarrassed during the examination. They felt a loss of dignity by exposure in the modified or full lithotomy position they were required to adopt. Embarrassment at exposing intimate areas of the body is not, of course, confined to Chinese women and has been noted in several studies (Murphy et al 1986; Bergstrom et al, 1992; Larsen & Kragstrup, 1995). Obviously, such exposure should be minimised and this is not difficult to do with a little thought and consideration by the examiner. Embarrassment leads to feelings of helplessness and vulnerability (Jarvis, 1992) and at such a time the woman particularly needs to have confidence in the examiner. If the examiner has not shown a basic care and respect for the woman's dignity by such simple means she is unlikely to feel much confidence in the examiner's concern for her integrity. By succumbing to a vaginal examination, the woman's traditional values such as modesty and respectability, particularly important in Chinese culture, may be compromised. This confrontation, together with feelings of relative powerlessness when required to comply with hospital and obstetric procedures prescribed by powerful medical professionals, may reinforce feelings of helplessness and vulnerability, possibly leading to feelings of shame. For example, Ling thought that she may have vulval lesions and worried that these would lead to the examiner labelling her as sexually promiscuous:

I don't know how they view me . . . if my skin condition is not so good, or if the area has a lesion. I don't know how they view me after they have discovered I have a lesion or poor skin condition.(Ling)

The presence of attendants who were not involved in the examination could give the woman the impression that she was being exposed unnecessarily. During some vaginal examinations theatre staff were present because they wanted to know immediately the outcome of the examination and whether the theatre should be prepared for Caesarean section. As Man said:

It was embarrassing when there were many people around and watched my examination... it will be better if there was nobody except the examiner.(Man)

Being examined by different people in one single examination, or being used to demonstrate the procedure of vaginal examination, could also lead to embarrassment. Ling's comment demonstrates this; she was not asked beforehand for her permission to be examined in this way:

There were a group of doctors, including medical students... I guess. They were male doctors. Also some nurses were there. The doctor did the examination and he showed the students how to do. I think it is quite embarrassing. I was not accustomed to it therefore I curled up once they touched me. (Ling)

Curtains provided only a flimsy assurance of privacy, and people could walk in on an examination with little prior warning. On some occasions, domestic workers were allowed to intrude during the examination, to clean the floor. Women were not informed of the reasons for these people's presence, nor was their consent sought. Indeed, it was highly unlikely that consent would have been given willingly in these circumstances:

If the curtain is not fully screened and people suddenly dropped in, privacy is not always guaranteed... the ward attendants do their cleansing work. But I think if they can wait until my examination is finished...(Wah)

Wah described her feelings of humiliation that the ritual of cleansing work was seen as more important than her privacy. The importance of sensitivity towards women's feelings during vaginal examinations cannot be underestimated, and it is possible that the gender of the examiner may have some effect here. For example, Elderen et al. (1998) suggested that, since female doctors were themselves female, they were more likely to be sensitive to women's feelings. Some women found being examined by a female less embarrassing (an observation concurring with that of Alexander & McCullough 1981):

If the examiner is a female doctor, I am less tense. If he is a man, then it is very embarrassing. (Ling)

However, on the whole there seemed to be a general feeling that the women would rather have a kind, considerate, experienced and skillful examiner no matter his or her gender:

No difference... as long as the doctor is experienced enough. (Yee)

One woman was examined on different occasions by a female and then a male obstetrician. She perceived that, whereas the female obstetrician was hurried and abrupt, the male doctor was gentle and showed concern for her feelings:

It was done by a male doctor, he did it very gently... he informed me of every step... the female doctor just started the procedure once she came in. She did not explain anything to me during and after the examination. (Wah)

Any differences in attitudes between genders may be attributed more to personality, or perhaps to a wish on the part of male examiners that their own wives and daughters would be accorded similar sensitivity when undergoing vaginal examinations. Another explanation may concern medico-legal issues in that men are far more prone to accusations of sexual misbehaviour during intimate examinations, particularly if the woman had perceived a disrespectful attitude on their part.

Women expressed strong wishes to be respected. They indicated that a sincere attitude on the part of the examiner, shown by adequate emotional and informational support, formed the elements of respect. This helped women to gain a feeling of control over the situation. They also wanted to know and feel familiar with the midwife who cared for them so that they felt less insecure:

Midwives were nice... they left a good impression on me... I feel deeply impressed...(Yee)

Before the examination, I hoped that the midwives would inform me and introduce themselves. Then I can ask her whenever I need help. There were so many people who I didn't know. I felt insecure. (Ping)

Some women commented that they would have liked the same midwife or doctor to perform the vaginal examinations. Although it was recommended for successive examinations to be carried out by the same people (O'Driscoll & Meagher 1986), shift changeovers sometimes made this impossible. This was not always perceived to be the reason for discontinuity of examiner, however:

...staff changed not because of the handover... they treated me as routine, they think whoever does the examination is OK...(Wah)

The examination would be conducted skillfully

Every woman remarked that the examination, whether instrumental or digital, had caused a certain degree of discomfort, even pain:

The speculum is harder, colder.(Man)

The speculum is big. I felt very uncomfortable when they put it inside. Fingers are better. (Ping)

. . . the feeling was different and unnatural. Although they wore gloves, everyone's finger is of different size. The pain was psychological, the feeling was really weird, I don't know how to describe it (Oi)

Some women described the vaginal examination as more painful if the examiner performed it too vigorously or had explained the procedure inadequately beforehand. Pain is a subjective experience of physical, psychological, or spiritual experiences and can be modified by neurochemistry, cognition and sensory and socio-environmental factors (Weber, 1996). If the woman is naturally tense, she will cope less well with stress than one who is relaxed and confident. In such a situation she needs extra care and empathy. As caregivers, we may never experience another person's pain, but can gain some information about it through the sufferer's behaviour, physiological responses and reports of pain (Lundgren & Dahlberg, 1998). Screaming or crying out during labour or birth is shameful according to Chinese culture; birth is believed to be painful but women are expected to tolerate the pain (Lauderdale, 1999), and so it may not be immediately apparent that the woman is experiencing pain. Midwives should be highly sensitive to each woman's feelings and tailor appropriate care for her. Several women expressed their appreciation of the care given to them by midwives:

Midwives were very good. They were professionals. They

talked to me, smiled at me even if they didn't talk. I feel it is really good. (Oi)

...if they asked me 'are you OK?' any discomfort? I will know they are not only carrying out a procedure but also taking care of me. (Wah)

Some women indicated that unskilled technique during examination had added to the pain. One woman said she could identify the examiner's inexperience by the time taken and the gentleness of the examination:

One was abrupt in starting it, she didn't say what she was going to do, it was quite painful... she took quite a long time to check... I felt quite a lot of discomfort... those who were experienced did it very quickly... maybe some midwives and doctors were so young, they did not know the examination was actually very painful. (Ping)

Several women commented that their pain was more psychologically induced than physical, which accords with Bevis' (1996) findings. Expressions of pain or discomfort during the examination can be an individual's response to the fear and anxiety rather than actual trauma. Women's impression of the examination partly depended on what she encountered. If the midwives were friendly and considerate, women felt cared about and their anxiety about the examination was reduced.

The findings were accurate and would be communicated

Apparently, inconsistent findings between examiners were a source of distress to some women, and resulted in a loss of confidence in their attendants:

One midwife told me that I was 4 cm dilated. A doctor told me I was 5 to 6 cm... I don't think there is any consistency in the examination finding... too many different opinions, I don't know who to believe. (Yee)

Yee revealed later in the interview that the doctor had done the examination 30 minutes after the midwife. After the interview it was explained to her that further cervical dilatation was possible even within such a short period of time. This explanation could easily have been given at the time of the second examination, which would probably have reduced her anxiety considerably. Women commented that explanation about the procedure lessened their fear and anxiety, and they expected midwives to tell them the findings after the examination. Excluding a woman from discussions of her progress relegates her to a powerless position, resulting in a less fulfilling birth experience (Green et al, 1990; Mckay & Smith ,1993). As Wah said:

They chat among themselves... It was not so good...they should have more communication with me...I know they are talking about my examination findings. They should involve me. (Wah)

Being supported

According to current practice in this hospital, only the woman's partner is permitted to accompany her in the labour ward. However, owing to the partitioning of the labour beds by curtains, the visit of the partner depends on the ward situation in order to preserve the privacy of other labouring women; if the labour ward is busy he may not be permitted to be with her. To some women this was a disappointment, they would have appreciated the reassuring presence of their partner during labour, and during vaginal examinations.

Ling said she wanted her husband to be present to ensure he would not feel jealous when she was being examined by another man; she was able to validate his words of reassurance by watching his facial expression during the examination. She explained that she would never expose her 'private area' to others except her husband or a gynaecologist, stating that her body belonged to her husband, and she worried about his true reaction if it was exposed to another man. Respect is a central tenet of many Chinese relationships (Bond 1996), and a wife shows respect to her husband by being loyal to him. Exposure of private areas of her body to another man would constitute possible disloyalty to her husband and she wanted to be sure that he did not regard the exposure as such.

Summary

This study is limited by several factors. As this was a phenomenology which studied a small group of women cared for within a particular context and circumstances unlikely to be found elsewhere, generalisation is not possible. Because of the translation of the data there was a danger that subtle shades of meaning may have been lost or changed (Twinn, 1997). Two strategies were adopted to try to reduce this. Firstly, a second fluent Chinese/English speaker checked random passages of the tapes against the translation and very few disagreements arose. When they did, they were minor and easily resolved. Secondly, after the data analysis and interpretation the tapes were listened to again to check that the sense of the women's feelings and perceptions, as expressed in Chinese, had remained intact throughout the interpretation process. The requirement for translation may have limited the study; nevertheless, the findings have revealed several issues.

Women generally found vaginal examination in labour to be an uncomfortable and embarrassing procedure, although they accepted its necessity during labour. Women valued highly the support given by midwives and others during examinations. The gender of the examiner was mentioned by a few women, who said that, generally, although they preferred to be examined by a woman, it was not a must. They wanted a kind, considerate, experienced and skilful doctor irrespective of his or her gender. One woman said she thought the male obstetrician who had attended her had been more caring and concerned for her feelings than women professionals. This is in contrast to previous findings (Elderen et al, 1998), which maintained that female attendants are more sensitive to women's issues as they are of same sex.

Respect in terms of providing privacy, information and companionship was appreciated, whereas perceived uncaring and unsupportive behaviours were resented. This resentment, however, had not been expressed by any woman at the time of the examination. Although women said they often felt discomfort and embarrassment, none of them said they had protested at the time of the examination, saying they felt they had to tolerate vaginal examinations as it was an integral part of labour. They felt powerless to control when and how the examination was conducted, referring to the dominance of medical and midwifery professionals in such decision-making in Hong Kong. The voice of women regarding childbearing issues in Hong Kong is still almost silent. In some hospitals (home birth is almost unknown in Hong Kong) women still labour in multi-occupied rooms, separated from each other only by curtains. Privacy is consequently difficult to maintain, and in these situations the presence of partners is discouraged. In many maternity units, however, single rooms for labouring women are the norm, although it seems ironic that the increasing provision of single rooms for labour is, at least in part, being influenced by men's demands to be present at the birth of their babies, rather than the acknowledgment that women need to be afforded privacy and dignity in labour. Chinese women, even when exposed to Western culture, tend to follow and reinforce hierarchical structures and are reluctant to challenge powerful medical hegemonies. In Hong Kong, as elsewhere, it is the better educated, more affluent women who are sufficiently articulate and assertive to demand, for example, privacy during labour and these are the women who are more likely to seek private medical care where such provisions are the norm. It is hoped that these standards may percolate gradually throughout the less advantaged community of women, and that the general attitude of Chinese women towards medical and midwifery professionals will become more assertive (bearing in mind, of course, that all midwives in Hong Kong are female and the great majority Chinese and subject to medical dominance as are their clients). For example, The Patients' Charter (Hospital Authority 1993) has outlined the rights and responsibilities of 'patients' as well as patients' rights of access to information which relates to their condition and treatment. These rights should pertain to sensitivity towards the needs of women in labour, including the provision of explanations and information regarding vaginal examinations, so that women are empowered to make informed choices regarding examinations and the management of their labour, should they wish to do so.

Acknowledgements

The authors would like to thank the midwifery colleagues in the postnatal ward for their co-operation in facilitating the interviews. We also wish to thank Ms Chu Yuet Wah (Department Operation Manager) and Ms Sandra Wong (Ward Manager) for their support of the study. Gratitude also goes to the midwives' counterparts who have been helping the author in searching relevant literature via the electronic mail.

REFERENCES

Alexander K, McCullough J 1981 Women's preferences for gynecological examiners: sex versus role. Women and Health 6(3/4): 123-134

Bergstrom L, Roberts J, Skillman L et al 1992 You'll feel me touching you, sweetie: vaginal examinations during the second stage of labor Birth 19(1):10-18

Bevis R 1996 Pain relief and comfort in labour. In Bennett VR, Brown LK (eds) Myles Textbook for Midwives. Churchill Livingstone, Edinburgh

Bleicher J 1980 Contemporary hermeneutics as method, philosophy and critique. Routledge and Kegan Paul Ltd, London

Bond MH 1996 The handbook of Chinese psychology. Oxford University Press, Hong Kong

Cohen MZ, Omery A 1994 Schools of phenomenology: implications for research. In: Morse JM (Ed) Critical issues in qualitative research methods. Sage, Thousand Oaks, CA

Coyne IT 1997 Sampling in qualitative research. Purposeful and theoretical sampling; merging or clear boundaries? Journal of Advanced Nursing 26:623-630

Elderen T, Maes S, Rouneau C et al. 1998 Perceived gender differences in physician consulting behaviour during internal examination. Family Practice 15(2):147-152

Field AP, Morse JM 1985 Nursing research. The application of qualitative approaches. Croom Helm, London

Gibb D 1991 A practical guide to labour management. Blackwell Scientific Publications, London

Giger JN, Davidhizar RE 1991 Transcultural nursing: assessment and intervention, 12th edn. Mosby, St Louis

Green J, Coupland V, Kitzinger J 1990 Expectations, experiences, and psychological outcomes of childbirth: a prospective study of 825 women. Birth 17:15-24

Hallgren A, Kihlgren M, Forslin L et al. 1999 Swedish fathers' involvement in and experiences of childbirth preparation and childbirth. Midwifery 15: 6-15

Henderson C, Jones K 1997 Essential midwifery. Mosby, London

Hildingsson I, Haggstrom T 1999 Midwives's lived experiences of being supportive to prospective mothers/parents during pregnancy. Midwifery 15: 82-91

Holroyd E, Lee YK, Wong PYL et al. 1997 Hong Kong Chinese women's perception of support from midwives during labour. Midwifery 13: 66-72

Hospital Authority 1993 Patients' Charter Public Affairs Division Hong Kong, Hong Kong Hospital Authority

Jarvis C 1992 Female genitalia in physical examination and health assessment. W.B. Sauders Company, Philadelphia

Larsen SB, Kragstrup J 1995 Experiences of the first pelvic examination in a random sample of Danish teenagers. Acta Obstetric Gynaecologic Scandivania 74: 137-141

Lauderdale J 1999 Childbearing and transcultural nursing care issues. In Andrews MA, Boyle JS (eds) Transcultural concepts in nursing care. 3rd edn. Lippincott, Philadelphia

Lefeber Y, Voorhoeve HWA 1998 Indigenous customs in childbirth and childcare. Van Gorcum, Van Gorcun, Assen

Lundgren I, Dahlberg K 1998 Women's experience of pain during childbirth. Midwifery 14: 105-110

Magee J 1975 The pelvic examination: a view from the other end of the table. Annals of Internal Medicine 83(4): 563-564

Mckay S, Smith SY 1993 'What are they talking about? Is something wrong?' Information sharing during the second stage of labour. Birth 20(3):142-145

Moettus A, Sklar D Tandberg D 1999 The effect of physician gender on women's perceived pain and embarrassment during pelvic examination. American Journal of Emergency Medicine 17(7):635-637

Murphy K, Greig V, Garcia J, Grant A 1986 Maternal consideration in the use of pelvic examinations in labour. Midwifery 2: 93-97

O' Driscoll K, Meagher DC 1986 Active management of labour. WB Saunders, London

Polit DF, Hungler BP 1999 Nursing research principles and methods 6th edn. Lippincott, Philadelphia

Ricoeur P 1976 Interpretation theory: discourse and the surplus of meaning. Texas Christian University Press, Texas

Swartz WH 1984 The semi-sitting position for pelvic examination. Journal of the American Medical Association 251(9): 1163

Twinn S 1997 An exploratory study examining the influence of translation on the validity and reliability of qualitative data in nursing research. Journal of Advanced Nursing 26: 418-423

Weber SE 1996 Cultural aspects of pain in childbearing women. Journal of Obstetrics, Gynaecologic, and Neonatal Nursing 25(1): 67-72

Midwifery 2002; 18: 296-303

The rhombus of Michaelis

A key to normal birth, or the poor cousin of the RCT?

Sara Wickham with Jean Sutton

Midwives often talk about how we can re-collect the kinds of knowledge which were held by our predecessors who attended births before they were taken over by medicalisation and moved out of the home environment. Occasionally, somebody discovers knowledge which is both 'old' and 'new', recognises its implications, and this becomes their passion. Such is the case with Jean Sutton and the rhombus of Michaelis, an area of the lower back which plays a key role in physiological birth. Much of this article is based on a discussion/interview with Jean which took place during August 2002; her words are in italics.

Before we get into the finer details of what Jean affectionately calls 'the rhombus', I should add that part of the point in writing about this is that this is the kind of knowledge that some midwives will see as very obvious; they will have read about it in The Practising Midwife (Sutton, 2000) before, heard Jean speak or be independently aware of this feature of birthing bodies. They might be surprised that anyone feels the need to write about it again. Yet others will not have heard of the rhombus of Michaelis or of the difference that their knowing about this can make to the women they attend. Such has been my experience in talking to midwives about this kind of experiential/physiological knowledge or, as Jean calls it, 'women's wisdom'. What seems obvious to one midwife will be news to another.

So where is this rhombus, and what does it do?

The rhombus of Michaelis (sometimes called the quadrilateral of Michaelis) is a kite-shaped area (Figure 5.6.1) that includes the three lower lumber vertebrae, the sacrum and that long ligament which reaches down from the base of the skull to the sacrum. This wedge-shaped area of bone moves backwards during the second stage of labour and as it moves back it pushes the wings of the ilea out, increasing the diameters of the

Figure 5.6.1

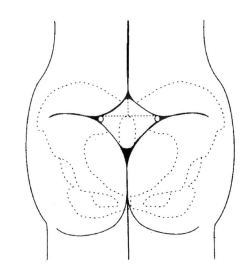

pelvis. We know it's happening when the woman's hands reach upwards (to find something to hold onto), her head goes back and her back arches. It's what Sheila Kitzinger was talking about when she recorded Jamaican midwives saying the baby will not be born 'till the woman opens her back' (Kitzinger, 1993). I'm sure that is what they mean by the 'opening of the back'.

The reason that the woman's arms go up is to find something to hold onto as her pelvis is going to become destabilised. This happens as part of physiological second stage; it's an integral part of an active normal birth. If you're going to have a normal birth you need to allow the rhombus of Michaelis to move backwards to give the baby the maximum amount of space to turn his shoulders in. Although the rhombus appears high in the pelvis and the lower lumbar spine when it moves backwards, it has the effect of opening the outlet as well.

When women are leaning forward, upright, or on their hands and knees, you will see a lump appear on their back, at and below waist level. It's much higher up than you might think; you don't look for it near her buttocks, you look for it near her waist. You can also feel it on the woman's back, it's a curved area of tissue that moves up into your hand, or you may suddenly see the mother grasp both sides of the back of her pelvis as the ilea are pushed out and she is suddenly aware of those muscles that have never been stretched before. Normally, the rhombus is only out for a matter of minutes, it comes out just as second stage starts, and it's gone back in again by the time that the baby's feet are born, in fact sometimes more quickly than that.

As a student midwife, I spent a lot of time holding and rubbing woman's backs for them, and the first time I heard Jean speak about the rhombus, I realised that this is what I had felt moving. At the time, I always assumed it was the baby's head pushing the sacrum backwards. (Now I am wondering if I was unwittingly interfering with the physiology of these women's labours!) I also recalled women in labour raising their hands just before their baby was born. In one hospital, they would grab the 'monkey bars' which had been provided for the women who had epidurals. I learned to see these bars not as a negative reflection of the degree to which technology prevailed in hospital birth, but as a potentially important and useful tool in the birth room.

In some birth centres and forward thinking hospitals, you can find gymnasium-type bars on the wall or brightly coloured ropes hanging from strengthened parts of the ceiling (Figure 5.6.2). These act as supports for women needing something to hold while their pelvis moves. It is interesting that, in the UK, we tend to be focused on getting women off the bed and onto the floor, with our sales pitches for beanbags, birth balls and padded mats which offer knee protection to the crawling woman and her midwife. While I know of a few exceptions, we do not seem to have become as aware as our European and American colleagues of the need for aerial as well as ground-based equipment in the birth room.

Hindering physiology

Jean cites a number of examples of ways in which the rhombus can be effectively prevented from helping the pelvis to open:

- *If women are on their back with their legs up, then their strong gluteal muscles prevent the rhombus from moving backwards.*
- *If a woman has her hands behind her knees and is pulling her legs up towards her tummy, the rhombus is also prevented from moving.*
- *If she's got an epidural in, the nerve supply is interfered with so that the impulse for it to happen is obstructed.*

So what do women need to know?

We need to tell women that if they want to have a short second stage of labour and they don't want to have to spend ages pushing, then they need to make sure that their pelvis will open to make enough space for the baby. And that this is perfectly safe as long as they have something to hold onto and that it will be gone back into place as soon as the baby is born. More importantly, they need to know that they shouldn't let anyone else move their legs while they are in second stage labour because, while they themselves will feel if they are moving them incorrectly, it is possible for an attendant to put the leg down so that the pelvis goes back in the 'wrong place' – this isn't a very technical way of saying it but at least women understand what you mean.

I think we need to get women to understand that, although epidurals are great for pain relief, they actually get in the way of a spontaneous second stage and vaginal birth. In many cases, the reason they've got an epidural is that the baby wasn't in the best position when it started, and the baby in the less suitable positions needs all the space he can get to turn around in. The OP baby needs the rhombus of Michaelis to move backwards so he has room to turn round so he can come out as an OA baby. The woman should then get out without having her pelvic floor damaged. Pelvic floor damage is a major worry for women, but if they can be in an upright position with their weight well forwards so that the rhombus is free to move, very little damage is done to their internal anatomy.

Figure 5.6.2

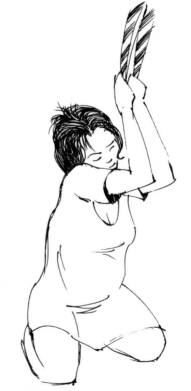

Gathering midwifery knowledge

So there it is: free, simple, helpful information. While Jean's articles and books go into slightly more depth, you know almost as much about the rhombus of Michaelis as she does right now. Which is part of the problem.

Jean hasn't been able to find an anatomy textbook which assigns any role to the rhombus, although many draw and identify it. It was identified in the literature as early as the 1930s, when a New Zealand obstetrician called Corkill (1932) asserted that there is 16cm of space in the outlet of the pelvis during the second stage of labour. It appears not to have occurred to anyone to explore the difference between this assertion and the received midwifery textbook 'wisdom' that the diameter of the outlet is 13cm. The only other possible link to this area that Jean has identified is in Michel Odent's work on the fetus ejection reflex (Odent, 1987).

Jean feels sure that 'there must be some seriously large nerve plexus that triggers it off'. She has proposed that this could be linked with the Ferguson reflex, or that the plexus might be the G-spot, identifying parallels between the actions of women (and men) during orgasm and the second stage of labour. Thus far, although a couple of midwives have become interested in researching this area, it has not attracted the level of interest which might be expected of something so potentially important to the physiology of labour.

One of Jean's hopes in preparing this article is that midwives who have observed the rhombus in action will contact her, as she would like to collate records of the actions of the rhombus during physiological second stage. My interest is also in what we can learn by thinking about the different types of knowledge which we access as midwives, and noticing what we can about the relative emphasis which is put upon these.

Given the lack of research and the minuscule quantity of discussion in midwifery and medical literature about the rhombus, you never can tell whether common sense wisdom is really that common. While Jean asserts that an understanding of this area can lead to a vastly increased chance of a woman having a physiological vaginal birth, I can only find six references to this on the Internet and in midwifery journal searches, and at least half of these are written by Jean herself. By contrast, when I looked for information on the Canadian Term Breech Trial last week, I found over 100 web pages discussing this listed on just one Internet search engine.

I know that a comparison of these two examples may bring accusations of contrasting apples and oranges, but it being the season of goodwill and all, I am hoping I might be forgiven! Which of these is the more useful source of information for women and midwives? Is it the one which was generously funded, feted, dramatically stopped, cited around the world and which has changed hospital practice (and limited women's choice) overnight, despite a number of serious methodological and philosophical concerns? Could it be that those who lead the way in generating knowledge through large-scale research are asking loaded questions, putting money into certain high-profile areas and ignoring the kinds of knowledge that could make a real difference to women?

Or maybe it doesn't matter. We don't really need an RCT to see if the rhombus of Michaelis makes a difference. We just need to talk about it more amongst ourselves; spread the word to women and other midwives; email Jean so she can do something useful with our observations; think more about how we can re-collect knowledge as women and midwives. All of which are low-cost and reasonably pleasurable.

And as it is the holiday season and I feel compelled to end on a positive note, it seems only fair that Jean, being (marginally) less prone than me to 'rant' about these sorts of things, should get the last word:

If midwives want to be assisting women to have as many normal births as possible ... to be able to promise women that birth is quite manageable ... that they don't need to have the interventions ... that it's simple and it's safe, as long as it follows the process, then having the back open is just part of that process. If we can understand this, we'll be getting back part of our midwifery skills.

Jean Sutton can be contacted at jeansutton@xtra.co.nz She is also very happy to be contacted by anyone who would like to take this area on as a project!

REFERENCES

Corkill TF. 1932. Lectures on Midwifery and Infant Care. Whitcombe-Toombs, New Zealand

Kitzinger S. 1993. Ourselves as Mothers. Bantam, London

Odent M. 1987. The fetus ejection reflex. Birth 14 (2):104-5

Sutton J. 2000. Birth without active pushing and a physiological second stage of labour. The Practising Midwife 3 (4): 32-34

The Practising Midwife 2002; 5(11): 22-23

Cardiotocography versus intermittent auscultation

Using pinards and Dopplers in low risk women

Jennifer Wrightson

Why are midwives using cardiotocography (CTG) for low risk women when multiple randomised controlled trials have found no evidence relating to the validity of external fetal monitoring for women with low risk pregnancies (Goodwin, 2000)? This paper will review the historical aspects relating to the introduction and acceptance of cardiotocography for low risk women by midwives. An evaluation and comparison of the clinical effectiveness of cardiotocography with intermittent auscultation using pinards and Doppler devices in low risk women is included. The evidence related to cardiotocography versus intermittent auscultation is reviewed and discussed as well as the implications for women and midwifery practice.

Historical review

Audible heart sounds were described as early as 1650 by Marsac and likened to the 'clapper of a bell'. The first heart sounds were crudely auscultated in 1818 by Mayor placing an ear on the abdomen. This was replaced by the use of a wooden stethoscope in 1821 by Kergadac (Chez, Harvey, Harvey, 2000). This method does not seem far removed from the current practice of using a pinards stethoscope. Following these first early attempts to hear the fetus's heartbeat a revolution in monitoring has occurred. Has it been to the advantage of the mother and baby? The idea of external fetal monitoring using cardiotocography was thought about as early as 1833, however electronic fetal monitoring was not developed until 1958 by Hon and was not made available until the 1960s (Flood, Harvey, Harvey, 2000). Midwives were encouraged to use cardiotocography by hospital protocols which advocated the use of cardiotocography when caring for women during pregnancy and labour in order to bring about a reduction in perinatal morbidity and mortality. Cardiotocography was heralded as an essential step in fetal heart rate auscultation: for the first time midwives would have a quantifiable method of assessing the fetal heart beat. Midwives were told that information would be present that was not readily obtainable by auscultation (Chez, Harvey, Harvey, 2000).

Cardiotocography spread quickly in the 1970s when commercially available (Hoerst, Fairman, 2000). Medical technology was taking over and induction rates were increasing. Midwives became blinded by the concept of technology and the initial promises of reduced perinatal mortality and morbidity if they used cardiotocography. Despite a profound lack of evidence to support these promises cardiotocography was welcomed by midwives – after all, midwives wanted the very best for women and this new technology appeared to herald a new era in midwifery care.

Acceptance of fetal monitoring

Fetal monitoring became accepted even for normal women. One reason for this could have been short staffing, which meant that midwives often cared for a number of women during labour. The use of continuous cardiotocography during labour enabled midwives to see the fetal heart rate trace at any time. Midwives thought that this would increase the safety of caring for the fetus and prevent litigation. However there were costs associated with the rapid introduction of cardiotocography. The number of CTG machines within midwifery doubled between the 1970s and 1980s, causing concern for midwifery managers (Spencer, 1994). Training of all carers challenged managers, the cost of study days and study time impacted on the practice environment. The medicalisation of childbirth and increased operative delivery had an impact on the use of all resources. Costs to management included:

- Training of all midwives and doctors
- New CTG machines

- Employment of technicians
- Paper for monitoring
- Increased medicalisation and operative delivery.

Thacker and Stroup (2001) described the rapid rise in the use of cardiotocography (CTG) in labour in the United States and suggested that by 1992 73.7% of normal women were monitored using this method. However, figures within the United Kingdom were unreliable at this time due to a lack of sufficient documentation by staff. Wide variations existed between units related to the application and use of cardiotocography in women. Inconsistencies were evident in the recognition of maternal risk factors and the need for CTG. The management of normal labour varied between units – some used CTGs, others did not (Parer & King, 2000). It was recognised by Parer and King (2000) that this had an impact on the reliability and validity of randomised controlled trails that were conducted on the use of CTGs.

Midwives became concerned over the lack of evidence for the use of cardiotocography and the increased medicalisation of normal childbirth. They recognised that women who had normal pregnancies were being denied choices during childbirth related to their care. Cardiotocography restricted movement and reduced ambulation, which led to increased interventions and a risk of Caesarean section. This view was supported by Thacker, Stroup & Chang (2001) who analysed nine randomised controlled trials from all over the world including the UK and found that there was still a statistically significant rise in the rate of Caesarean and operative delivery in women who had CTG monitoring, particularly in low risk women. Further concerns were raised by midwives related to their own skills and competencies: they acknowledged that skills may be lost in the use of the Pinnards stethoscope. Debate over the value and cost of CTGs raged for over a decade. However, in the 1990s the arguments mainly surrounded the lack of evidence for the use of cardiotocography.

Evidence

Promises of reduced perinatal mortality and morbidity in babies given to midwives in the 1960s were not supported by valid evidence. Randomised controlled trials (RCTs) were not introduced by researchers until 1976, when they were used to examine the evidence related to intermittent auscultation using Pinnards versus cardiotocography in high risk and low risk women (Parer & King, 2000). However, despite the use of RCTs to evaluate the use of CTG and its effect on the fetus, researchers had problems with validity and reliability. According to Crozier & Sinclaire (1999) generally one-to-one midwifery care was used when trials were carried

Table 5.7.1 Evidence for and against CTG

Evidence against CTG
- False positives in term babies
- No reduction in the incidence of cerebral palsy occurring during labour
- No proven reduction in perinatal mortality and morbidity in low risk women
- No proven benefits of CTG versus the use of Pinnards for auscultation in low risk women
- Increased invasion of the woman's autonomy
- Increased interference and medicalisation of childbirth in women leading to complications: LSCS, forceps, ventouse

Proven benefits of CTG in low risk women
- A reduction in neonatal seizures
- A reliable healthy trace in the term neonate where concern related to fetal wellbeing.

out, creating a Hawthorne effect. Midwives were aware that they were participating in the studies and this may have led to the midwife providing more care for the woman and fetus, creating bias in the results. Researchers had further problems when completing randomised controlled trials. They were unable to prove cause and effect due to problems with variables including inconsistent application and interpretation of cardiotocography. Inability of healthcare professionals, including midwives, to interpret CTGs led to confounding of the research evidence. A lack of National Standardisation led to interobserver inconsistencies in interpretation. Indication for the use of cardiotocography also varied between units and documentation was incomplete, creating further problems with variables (Parer & King, 2000; Chez, Harvey, Harvey, 2000; Feinstein & Sprague, 2000). Inconsistencies still exist according to Sprague & Trepanier (1999) related to interpretation, application and documentation of CTGs. As many as 99.8% false positives for fetal depression can occur in fetal heart rate traces in the term baby following wrong interpretation. This will lead to increased interventions which are not necessary, and will also have an impact on the birth experience for both parents and the baby. The problem of inconsistency and interobserver reliability has been partially addressed with the introduction of annual mandatory updates and study days on cardiotocography. Electronic packages have also been introduced in delivery suite areas in order to improve consistency (Crozier & Sinclaire, 1999; Thacker & Stroup, 1999; Simpson & Knox, 2000).

Further reviews of 12 world wide randomised trials which include Europe failed to demonstrate the superiority of CTG versus hand held devices for auscultation in the fetus (Chez, Harvey, Harvey, 2000). There was no direct relationship between the use of CTG and fetal outcome. Perinatal morbidity in low risk pregnancy was unaffected by the use of CTG. Further doubts relating to the benefits of cardiotocography

Table 5.7.2 Benefits of auscultation using a hand held device

Autonomy is enabled
Choice, comfort and control regained
Improved contact with the midwife
Avoids the use of increased interventions related to the use of CTG
Avoids increased operative delivery related to the use of CTG

Table 5.7.3 NICE Guidelines: NICE (2001) recommends continuous fetal monitoring where the following risk factors are present:

Maternal risk factors
– Previous Caesarean section
– Pre-eclampsia
– Post term pregnancy (>42 weeks)
– Prolonged rupture of the membranes (>24 hours)
– Induction of labour
– Diabetes
– Antepartum haemorrhage
– Other medical disease and maternal risk factors

Fetal risk factors
– Fetal growth restriction
– Oligohydramnios
– Abnormal Doppler artery velocimetry
– Multiple pregnancy
– Meconium liquor
– Breech

Intrapartum risk factors
– Induction or augmentation of labour with oxytocins
– Deviations from the normal heart rate (<110, >160)
– Vaginal bleeding in labour
– Maternal pyrexia
– Fresh meconium liquor
– Evidence on auscultation of any deceleractions
– Epidural

versus auscultation using a Pinnards arose. The Royal College of Obstetricians and Gynaecologists (1989) stated that the use of external fetal monitoring and intermittent auscultation for fetal assessment were equal, and a statistical difference in the perinatal outcomes did not exist. This statement did not appear to affect the use of fetal monitoring in the United States according to Haggerty (1999) with the use of CTG in low risk women rising to 83% by 1996. The use of CTG did not affect the rate of cerebral palsy: 1-2 babies per 1000 develop cerebral palsy of which only 10% will occur during labour (Simpson & Knox, 2000). However one benefit was found: a reduction in neonatal seizures in 1995 directly related to the use of cardiotocography was proven during an extensive review of twelve large scale randomised controlled trials (Thacker & Stroup, 1999). Was this finding significant, as not all seizures are associated with long term consequences?

In summary, research has not proved that the use of CTG prevents perinatal mortality or morbidity but has proved that its use could reduce seizures in the neonate. However, in the low risk woman an increase in medicalisation and operative delivery occurs when CTGs are used to monitor the fetus, creating many costs for women related to their childbirth.

An increase in medicalisation not only puts the woman at risk, it reduces maternal autonomy during labour. Choices are restricted relating to ambulation and choice of position. Maternal comfort and satisfaction will be reduced, which may result in anxiety and increased need for analgesia (Feinstein, Sprague, Trepanier, 1999). It is proposed that this will lead to an increased use of operative interventions in low risk women when CTG is utilised which casts doubt on the long term benefits for the baby and mother.

In contrast, Simpson & Knox (2000) highlight that cardiotocography can produce a reactive healthy trace in a term baby which may reassure the midwife where there is concern related to fetal wellbeing. For example, if the mother has concerns related to reduced fetal movement, a thorough examination of the mother and assessment of fetal condition which includes the use of CTG may reassure both the midwife and mother that all is well. Alternatively, the midwife may order further assessment of the fetus in order to prove wellbeing.

NICE (2001) guidelines recommend that CTG is not used in low risk women as its use is not supported by the current evidence. Policies and protocols within all delivery suite areas should reflect the recommendations of NICE 2001. However we need to examine the evidence related to auscultation using hand held electronic devices and Pinnards.

Evidence related to intermittent auscultation

Intermittent auscultation is not without problems relating to validity and reliability. According to Parer & King (2000) evidence relating to the effectiveness of auscultation is scarce. Inconsistencies exist in practice between practitioners related to auscultation using a Pinnards or Doppler device and competence in use varies. However this could be due to a lack of use which will reduce competence and consistency. It is essential that midwives and student midwives use all types of devices for auscultation regularly to maintain skills. Midwives generally have the auditory ability to determine the rate, rhythm, spontaneous accelerations and decelerations of the fetal heart on auscultation using either a Pinnards or an electronic device; however, there is no available evidence to support the recognition of variability (Feinstein, Sprague, Trepanier, 2000). Despite not being able to determine variability there is no difference in fetal outcome using CTG versus hand held devices for auscultation.

Clear guidelines have been produced by NICE (2001) which will address the problem of maintaining consistency in auscultation; however, mandatory study days should cover all types of auscultation rather than just CTG in order to improve consistency in practice. They should include knowledge related to all aspects of auscultation of the fetus, a competency based skills component and an assessment which would give the practitioner opportunity to utilise all types of auscultation in a range of situations. A competency based educational approach which includes comprehensive coverage of the NICE (2001) guidelines is essential for all midwifery staff. Many midwives who do not have the opportunity for rotational posts who need to maintain their practice in the area of auscultation of the fetus would benefit from this opportunity. Study days should also include clear pathways where there is cause for concern and examine local and national guidelines for auscultation.

Earlier in this paper the lack of valid evidence relating to a reduction in perinatal morbidity and mortality when CTG is used in low risk women has been highlighted. However, the advantages for the woman of having a midwife auscultate the fetus using either a Pinnards or a Doppler device rather than direct use of CTG is evident in improved outcomes for women as well as reduced medicalisation of childbirth. Improved midwifery contact will enhance the relationship that the midwife has with the woman during labour.

Comfort and control are regained by the woman: the woman can adopt any position she wants without being restricted in choice by belts and monitors. Further choices can be enabled related to the use of either the Pinnards or the hand held Doppler. Many women prefer to hear their baby throughout labour, however anxiety can be caused if an abnormality in rhythm is audible and this may challenge the midwives' communication skills in the area of maternal support. The benefits to the mother of intermittent auscultation are clearly evident. Midwives may also benefit if low risk women regain their control over labour, with job satisfaction being improved.

Unreliable technology causes more harm than good

The overwhelming acceptance of the use of CTG for low risk women has led to a reduction in choice for women. Confinement to bed has led to increased operative intervention, Caesarean section and loss of control for women related to their labour (Thacker & Stroup, 1999). Some midwives have successfully changed their practice, however other midwives have been restricted in some areas of the country due to rigid medicalised protocols which include routinely using CTG on admission for low risk women. Prior to the production of the NICE (2001) guidelines a survey was carried out in the UK on the use

electronic fetal monitoring, with 79% of units studied carrying out a routine CTG on admission for women, even if they were deemed low risk (CESDI, 2002). Unfounded concerns related to litigation, according to Symon (1998), has led midwives to accept the use of CTG on admission and intermittently during labour in order to feel reassured that the baby is well. However, inappropriate use of CTG will lead to litigation. CESDI (1998) raised concerns over fetal surveillance, particularly related to the delay in reporting evidence of fetal depression. An example of this is where midwives have utilised CTG when they have been too busy to stay in the room with the woman in the misguided belief that this would protect them from litigation. Instead, this may have added to their risk of litigation where there was evidence of fetal compromise on the trace, particularly where there was a delay in recognising and reporting the incident. New guidelines are available from NICE (2001) which contradict the use of CTG in low risk women. Midwives should empower women through providing informed choice relating to the use of intermittent auscultation using hand held devices and prevent the unnecessary use of CTG with subsequent risks to the mother and fetus.

Recommendations for practice

New guidelines produced by NICE 2001 clearly indicate a path that midwives can take related to fetal auscultation and discuss the use of intermittent auscultation using hand held devices versus CTG. They suggest that providing women are healthy, with an uncomplicated pregnancy, they should receive information from their midwife which will enable informed choice relating to the use of intermittent auscultation using hand held devices versus the use of CTG. Admission CTG is not recommended in low risk women due to the absence of evidence related to its benefits compared to intermittent auscultation using Pinnards or hand held Dopplers. Healthy women should be offered and recommended intermittent auscultation during labour. There should be simultaneous palpation of the maternal pulse to ensure that you are monitoring the fetus and not the mother. According to NICE (2001) guidelines the fetal heart rate should be auscultated for a minimum of sixty seconds immediately following a contraction. Intermittent auscultation using a hand held device should take place a minimum of every fifteen minutes during the first stage of labour and five minutely during the second stage. During the active phase the heart rate should be monitored after each contraction. In order to carry out these guidelines it would appear that one-to-one care is essential: it would be impossible for the midwife to care for another woman due to the required frequency of auscultation of the fetus during the active phase of labour.

Midwives may still be using policies related to auscultation which do not reflect the NICE (2001) guidelines and this may be due to staffing levels which would not provide one-to-one care for low risk women. In practice, all women should have the provision of one-to-one care and the shortfall of midwives should be addressed. Further reasons contributing to a lack of implementation of the guidelines may be barriers including a fear of litigation if CTGs are not used; however, litigation may increase if CTGs are used inappropriately, particularly when there is a delay in reporting concerns related to CTG traces. When there is concern related to the fetus there should be clear policies and guidelines, with documented pathways relating to the immediate actions required and communication between all carers (CESDI, 1998). Midwives should sign, date and consistently document any events that take place during labour which may affect the fetus, and work within their policies and guidelines. This should reduce risks to the mother, infant and midwife. Clear national guidelines (NICE, 2001) exist in relation to documentation and the use of intermittent auscultation. Local policy and guidelines should reflect these and should be developed by midwifery teams in order to foster a consistent approach to auscultation of the fetus. Previous research has been confounded by inconsistencies in practice and the adoption of a clear national policy will help to overcome this. Further consistency will be fostered by the review of mandatory study days on CTG. All types of auscultation should be covered, in a range of circumstances (e.g. antenatal clinics, antenatal day units, delivery suites and community midwifery care), and competency based packages that include the use of hand held devices should be developed. Audits should be regularly carried out in order to monitor closely standards of care related to auscultation of the fetus and policies adjusted appropriately.

Table 5.7.4 Implications for midwifery practise

Midwives need to maintain their skills in intermittent auscultation using hand held devices.
Educational packages on auscultation should include the use of hand held devices and be competency based.
Interdisciplinary protocols need to be critically examined and developed where there is cause for concern. Action pathways and communication should be clear.
Midwives need to actively develop and update protocols for the use of all types of auscultation within their teams, not just the use of CTG.
Midwives need to take part in active strategies to promote the use of intermittent hand held devices for auscultation in low risk women both on admission and during labour.
Midwives should provide consistent evidence based information related to all types of fetal auscultation for women in order to facilitate choice.
Midwife researchers are required to examine the views of women on the use of CTG versus hand held devices for auscultation.
Practice audits should be regularly carried out which evaluate the use of auscultation and change should be made where necessary to protocols.

Further research is needed, particularly in the area of intermittent auscultation where randomised controlled trials are scarce. Maternal views of the use of cardiotocography in labour versus intermittent auscultation using hand held devices and their effect on labour also need to be researched in order that midwives can meet women's needs.

Midwives should actively promote women's choices by providing evidence-based information on all types of auscultation. Midwives also need to question the use of CTG when used inappropriately in practice. Midwives and women need to actively participate in the production of policies which do not advocate the use of CTG for low risk women either on admission or during labour, in order that low risk women can regain control and have the autonomy that they so rightly deserve.

REFERENCES

Chez BF, Harvey MG, Harvey CJ. 2000. Intrapartum fetal monitoring: past present and future. Journal of Perinatal Neonatal Nursing, 14(3), 1-18

Confidential Enquiry into Stillbirths and Deaths in Infancy. 1998. 7th Annual Report www.cesdi.org.uk

Confidential Enquiry into Stillbirths and Deaths in Infancy. 2002. Executive Summary of the 8th Annual Report www.cesdi.org.uk

Crozier K, Sinclair M.1999. Birth technology: electronic fetal monitoring. RCM Midwives Journal, 2(5), 160-4

Feinstein N, Fischbeck, Sprague A, Trepanier M. 2000. Fetal heart rate auscultation: Comparing auscultation to electronic fetal monitoring. AWHONN Lifelines, 4(3), 35-44

Goodwin L. 2000. Intermittent auscultation of the fetal heart rate: A review of general principles. Journal of Perinatal and Neonatal Nursing, 14(3), 53-61

Haggerty LA. 1999. Continuous electronic fetal monitoring: contradictions between practice and research. Journal of Obstetrics Gynecology Neonatal Nursing, 28(4), 409-16

Hoerst BJ, Fairma, J. 2000. Social and professional influences of the technology of electronic fetal monitoring on obstetrical nursing. Review. Western Journal of Nursing Research, 22(4), 475 -91

National Institute For Clinical Effectiveness. 2001. The use of electronic fetal monitoring. London: NICE

Parer JT, King T. 2000. Fetal heart rate monitoring: is it salvageable? American Journal of Obstetrics and Gynecology, 182(4), 982-7

Simpson KR, Knox GE. 2000. Risk management and electronic fetal monitoring: Decreasing risk of adverse outcomes and liability exposure. Journal Perinatal Neonatal Nursing, 14(3), 40-52

Spencer JAD. 1994. Electronic fetal monitoring in the United Kingdom. Birth, 21(2), 106-7

Sprague A, Trepanier MJ. 1999. Charting in record time: Setting guidelines for documenting FHR enhances care for labouring women. AWHONN Lifelines, 3(4), 35-40

Symon A. 1998. Is using CTG defensive? British Journal of Midwifery, 6(9), 568-70

Thacker SB, Stroup D, Chang M. 2001. Continuous electronic heart rate monitoring for fetal assessment during labour. Review. The Cochrane Library http://cochrane.athens.ac.uk

Thacker SB, Stroup DF. 1999. Continuous electronic fetal heart rate monitoring versus intermittent auscultation for assessment during labour. Oxford: The Cochrane Library

The Practising Midwife 2002; 5(7): 35-39

Reflecting on labour and birth

• How would you define "normal birth"? Do your colleagues and the women you work with define this the same way? Does your definition of this affect the way you practise midwifery?

• Look at the general themes that arose in Chit Ying Lai and Valerie Levy's research (respecting women, conducting examination skilfully, accurate and well-communicated findings, offering support). Do you feel your practice would meet the needs of the women they interviewed? Do you feel that one or two of these areas are more important than the others? How would you feel about being examined by someone who practised just like you?

• Have you ever seen the rhombus of Michaelis? Do you use your observation of this phenomenon in your practice? Have you noticed any other changes in women's bodies (apart from the obvious ones!) when they are in labour or giving birth? We already have a few other examples, such as the purple line (discussed in volume 1 of this series) and I was recently told that there are apparently changes in women's feet during labour, although I haven't yet seen or experienced this, and I am sure that there must be other signs and changes still waiting to be observed by eagle-eyed midwives!

If you feel like writing…

• Think about your own experiences of being with women in pain, how it makes you feel, what issues it brings up for you, what you think about when you are with women and write about your experiences.

If you feel like taking action…

• What can we do to promote normal birth? Which of Gill Skinner's suggestions are already being carried out in your area? Are there any that you and your colleagues could take on as a project?

SECTION CONTENTS

Care in labour in the event of perinatal death

Rosemary Mander

In this paper I plan to present a picture of the care of the woman in labour and her partner in association with the 'loss' of a baby. The term 'loss' is sometimes avoided in this context because of the way that it may imply some degree of carelessness. I use it here, however, to indicate a wide range of experiences which happen when the woman faces grief for one of a number of reasons. These experiences may be associated with death, or they may take some other form in which the woman's hopes and aspirations of childbearing have not been achieved.

In the latter part of the twentieth century the care of the grieving mother was transformed. A healthier understanding of bereavement in childbearing became established, due to increasing knowledge of the psychological processes of pregnancy and the early postnatal period. This improved understanding resulted in more sensitive forms of care being offered. In order to facilitate healthy grieving the mother is encouraged to be involved in the creation of memories of the one who is 'lost'. These memories serve as a focus around which her grief may move forward. The memories which are created also help the mother to understand and recognise the reality of her motherhood. Although the research evidence relating to the benefits of these more sensitive forms of care remains ambiguous, it seems that that care really has become more empathetic (Chambers & Chan, 2000).

The picture of midwifery care which I present is based on certain crucial issues which underpin the midwife's care at this time. Alongside each of these five crucial issues I present a small number of examples of specific aspects of midwifery care which serve to illustrate relevant points. I have chosen these examples because of their relevance and, as far as possible, their research base.

Issue 1: Decision-making

Some carers may assume that by relieving a woman of

the need to make choices they are making her experience less painful; this may not be the case. In the research which I undertook on the midwife's care of the mother who does not have her baby with her, the locus of decision-making emerged as important (Mander, 1993). The main reason for its significance is the potentially conflicting expectations of the mother and the midwife. Obviously, such interpersonal conflict may seriously impair the mother's healthy grieving. It is crucial that the midwife should recognise the woman's need to assume some degree of control over what may seem to be an uncontrollable event. To study the woman's need for control Gohlish (1985) interviewed 15 mothers of stillborn babies and asked them to identify the 'nursing' behaviours which they considered most helpful and least helpful. The mothers clearly wished to be able to decide such matters as when to talk about the dead baby, how long she should stay in the maternity unit after the birth and where she should be accommodated.

In contrast, my own research showed that the midwife is reluctant to burden the grieving mother with what appear to her to be relatively mundane decisions. The midwife has a very clear perception of the decisions which should be taken by the mother, such as what contact to have with her baby. The midwife also has a clear picture of which decisions should be taken by the midwife, such as whether the mother should have any company during her hospital stay.

Example: Place of labour

The place where the woman labours may be a matter of limited choice in view of the health risks associated with giving birth to a baby who is dead. There may, however, be some room for manoeuvre even within a maternity unit or a labour suite. The research by Hughes (1986) suggests that there is also some flexibility regarding where postnatal care should be provided. She found that the woman may not be averse to sharing a room, and other mothers may not be averse to sharing a room with a bereaved mother.

Example: Induction of labour

Induction may be recommended, because of the risk of infection and hypofibrinogenaemia. As I was informed during my research (Mander, 1994), in this case the woman may realise that the timing of the birth of her baby may be her decision, rather than the medical practitioner's.

In this discussion of the onset of labour, I am obviously making the assumption that the woman will labour, as opposed to giving birth by Caesarean section. McDonald (1996: 94) recounts how in her experience as a midwife she has been asked by women whose baby has died in utero why it is necessary to labour and why a Caesarean is not possible? The logic of this question is clearly apparent. The rationale for going through labour for a baby who is not alive would not be immediately obvious. Without spelling out the recognised health risks involved in the birth of such a baby by Caesarean, McDonald suggests that every midwife should prepare herself to handle this question sensitively.

Example: Pain control

Medication in very large amounts may sometimes be recommended for the mother who does not have a live baby; the rationale being that there is no risk of neonatal respiratory depression. This form of care is reminiscent of the days when maternity staff sought to obliterate the birth from the woman's memory, rather than help her to work through her loss. The woman should, as with other aspects of her experience, be encouraged to make the decisions about what level of pain she wishes to feel. It may be that the experience of some pain would help the woman to accept that, even though she does not have her baby with her, she really is a mother. In a large retrospective epidemiological study in Sweden, the more traditional rationale prevailed (Rådestad et al, 1998). Of the 380 mothers who had given birth to a stillborn baby, 41% (n=130) were administered epidural analgesia, whereas only 18% (n=59) of the 379 controls used that method.

Example: Lactation inhibition

Lactation inhibition using powerful medication such as bromocriptine, may be deemed necessary for the bereaved mother. It has been suggested, however, that allowing the breasts to lactate may comfort the mother by reassuring her that, had her baby survived, she would have been well-nourished (Lewis & Bourne, 1989). Rådestad and colleagues also suggest that non-

pharmacological methods of lactation management may facilitate grieving for this woman by helping her to confront the reality of the death of her baby (1998: 116). These researchers go on to draw attention to the number of bereaved mothers who encounter adverse side effects from the use of pharmacological methods of lactation inhibition. Although these researchers do not suggest it, it is necessary to question whether such complications may have adversely affected the woman's healthy resolution of her grief.

Example: End of life decision-making

End of life decision-making is a problem facing neonatal staff more than labour ward midwives. The withdrawal of pointless life-prolonging treatment is a contentious issue that may be disturbing for staff. As well as the need to draw up best practice guidelines, the involvement of parents in such decision-making is fiercely debated (McHaffie, 1998). The research by McHaffie and Fowlie (1998) sought to address these problems by interviewing a total of 176 nursing and medical personnel. Conflict and tension were identified by staff as probably being inevitable. These researchers suggest a range of strategies which may be implemented by the individual and by the team in order to overcome the areas of conflict. These strategies may be summarised in terms of mutual understanding of and respect for team members and their views in a culture of honesty and trust.

Issue 2: Communication

As with many aspects of care, that which is ordinarily important becomes absolutely crucial in the care of the grieving mother. The aspects of communication which the midwife needs to address include:

- her own and other professionals' communication or information-giving to the parents
- the opportunities made for the mother to articulate her feelings and to be actively listened to
- the encouragement of effective communication both between the couple and with other family members
- communication between carers relating to this woman's care.

Based on her qualitative study of different forms of loss in pregnancy, Moulder (1998: 228) emphasises that good communication is fundamental to individualised care. She goes on to explain that, to be effective, communication involves imparting complex and distressing information in a short time in a comprehensible, clear and sensitive manner. Such communication also requires the ability to hear, recognise in other ways and then handle the emotional component of the situation. Moulder's study suggests that care providers are comfortable with the information-giving aspects of communication. She maintains, however, that the more human and interactive skills, such as listening and responding appropriately, may still need some careful attention.

Example: Breaking bad news

Breaking bad news is a task which is not relished by those who have to do it, which may be the reason why it is so often done so badly (Kirk, 1984). Carers tend, in their anxiety, to resort to jargon or at least technical terms, which has the effect of compounding the hearer's incomprehension.

Requiring the mother to wait pending the arrival of a supportive partner before imparting bad news has been criticised as cruel and unusual, as it also serves to raise anxiety to a counterproductive level (Statham & Dimavicius, 1992). On the basis of their study involving the relatives of trauma victims, Jurkovich et al (2000) found that clarity, privacy and the possibility of getting questions answered are crucial in imparting bad news. This survey found that touching, in the form of a hug, hand-holding or a handshake, could be either a help or a hindrance. Thus, such non-verbal communication should be used with caution.

Example: Documentation

Documentation, as with all aspects of communication, assumes even greater significance in the case of the grieving mother. It is essential that each midwife providing care should be able to learn from the mother's records about decisions and actions that have already been taken.

The statutory documentation relating to a baby who dies is specific to each of the countries of the UK (McDonald, 1996). Details of the registration documentation, the forms necessary for burial or cremation and the other requirements in each of the four countries of the UK are provided in the websites listed with the references at the end of this article.

Example: Checklists

Checklists are one form of communication between carers which is frequently recommended to ensure that all the necessary aspects of care have been addressed. It is necessary to recognise that if a multiplicity of carers are involved, or if a woman's labour extends over one or more changes of shift, or if relatively inexperienced staff are involved, such a method of communication becomes invaluable. Obviously, such care is far from ideal: it

might even be appropriate to suggest that care of such a low standard should not be offered to a woman who is as vulnerable as the bereaved mother. If any woman is likely to benefit from the much-vaunted 'continuity of carer' it is the grieving mother.

As Leon (1992) identifies, though, such lists are not without their problems. He suggests that they may hinder the carer's 'emotional engagement' with the grieving parents. Additionally, Curtis warns of the 'routinised approach' which may have been introduced with recent protocols (2000: 530) and which may serve to deny the uniqueness of the mother's experience as well as the circumstances surrounding it.

Issue 3: Support

As mentioned already, the more empathetic care which has become standard focuses on providing good psychosocial support to facilitate the healthy grief of the bereaved mother (Chambers & Chan, 2000). There tends to be an assumption that a maternity unit is not a good place to grieve, but the research by Rajan (1994) suggests that this may not be so. She found that in the 'community' those around the grieving mother were so concerned about their own reactions to the loss that they were unable to offer support to the mother. The extreme form of this inability was found in those family members who actually called on the grieving mother for support, thus preventing her from completing her grief work.

Certain groups of mothers have been identified as being at particular risk of incomplete or morbid grief. It would be appropriate, therefore, to focus supportive activities on mothers who are socially isolated or those who lack effective social support (Forrest et al, 1982; Lake, 1987; Rajan & Oakley, 1993).

Example: The partner's needs

The partner's needs, as well as his role, should be recognised. The father of the baby is likely to have been socialised into believing that his role comprises 'being strong' for his womenfolk. With this background he is unlikely to be able to recognise that he needs to grieve the loss of his child. In the absence of healthy grieving he may resort to a range of other, even less healthy, behaviours which may provide a temporary distraction from his unmet needs. These unhealthy responses may aggravate tensions which arise within the couple's relationship due to the fundamentally different patterns of grieving adopted by women and by men.

Example: Support groups & counselling

The midwife's role relates not only to providing the

support which the woman needs, but also to ensuring that the woman is later able to find that support herself. This means that she should be encouraged to contemplate the sources of support which are likely to be available to her. As well as the informal sources of support mentioned already, there are a number of formal support mechanisms. In other countries, telephone support systems have become established (Mittelstaedt et al, 2000) and other more highly structured programmes have been evaluated (Murray et al, 2000). In the UK, some midwifery staff have developed a role focussing on the support or possibly the counselling of the bereaved parents (Horsfall, 2001). More frequently, though, a self-help group, such as the Stillbirth and Neonatal Death Society (SANDS) may be available to provide support.

Example: Staff support

Support of staff may not be a priority in a working environment that is as stressful as a labour ward. Additionally, overworked staff may give their own coping strategies meagre attention. It has been argued, however, that the midwife, as well as others who work in challenging environments, has her own specific needs. These needs should be taken into account, if not actually addressed by those who organise the service. On this basis the following recommendations have been made:

- Genuine and meaningful engagement at a fundamental level is encouraged
- Peer supervision and support is implemented to ensure emotional health
- Grieving parents are involved in a more collaborative form of care
- Assessment of the midwife's current coping ability is necessary before she is allocated to an emotionally challenging situation.

Although it is fortunately a situation which most midwives will never have to face, my own research has shown the importance of speedy and effective support for staff involved in the death of a mother (Mander, 1999). The fact that it happens so infrequently in the UK, and the general belief in the healthiness of childbearing, make it difficult for the midwife to accept that this tragedy may occur, and more difficult for her to cope if and when it does.

Issue 4: Information and consent

The importance of the mother's active involvement in decision-making has been mentioned above. This involvement can only be fully autonomous if the mother has been able to assimilate the information on which to base her decisions. Although research evidence is not yet available to inform all midwifery activities, attempts are being made to provide the mother with such evidence as exists. The use of research evidence is no less important in the care of the grieving mother. It goes without saying that for any woman to be treated as an autonomous being is a fundamental human right. This autonomy requires that she should be given full information in advance of any intervention. On the basis of this information she may consent to or refuse the intervention.

Example: Creating memories

As well as consent obviously being required for interventions such as surgery, consent also needs to be sought for less invasive activities. Many of these are the activities which are crucial to the care of the grieving parents and have been entitled the 'creation of memories' (Rådestad et al, 1996). While taking a photograph or cutting a lock of hair may seem to be relatively benign and non-invasive activities, parental consent is still needed if the midwife is to intervene in this way.

Example: Post mortem

In the hope of preventing a future loss, the parents may be advised that the baby should have a post mortem examination and their permission sought. This raises many difficult issues for parents, who may consider that their baby has suffered enough already. In the UK the information given to bereaved parents has recently attracted considerable media attention. Because of this, the guidelines about the information given to the parents prior to seeking their consent for the post mortem have recently been redrafted. These new guidelines aim to prevent certain abuses, such as the retention of body parts, which have in the recent past caused anguish to some bereaved parents (DoH, 2000; Dimond, 2001).

Issue 5: Long-term care

As the midwife who attends women in labour is well aware, the effects of her care do not end with the birth of the baby: there are long-term implications. This is equally true of the care of the woman in labour who is bereaved. The midwife is able to help the woman to look ahead to the sources of information and support which will be available to her.

Example: Follow-up

The follow-up is intended mainly to provide information

for the parents, although this should be provided in a supportive environment (Kohner, 1995). It may be appropriate for the midwife who attended the birth to participate in the follow-up appointment. As well as ascertaining that the woman is recovering from the birth, information will be provided about any investigations, such as the post mortem or chromosomal or bacteriology laboratory tests. The importance of this meeting should not be underestimated as the information provided is fundamental to the woman's emotional health (Rådestad et al, 1998). This information may also comprise the basis of the couple's subsequent childbearing decisions. These researchers found that approximately one third of the women in their study did not have an explanation of the reason for the baby's death. This figure is contrasted with the figure of twelve percent with no identifiable cause which these researchers quote as the standard.

Example: Care in a subsequent labour

The care in a subsequent labour is another way in which perinatal loss may make demands on the midwife in the birthing room. The next labour featured in Hense's study of the woman's experience of giving birth after having a stillborn baby (1994). Her study summarises the complexity of the woman's feelings as she approaches the labour and the birth. An element of replacement of the lost baby was a prominent component of the women's feelings. The women were keen to protect their unborn babies and, thus, to prevent a recurrence of their previous loss. These manoeuvres involved the parents in attempting to avoid attachment to the baby. Hense found that the stillborn baby was not completely 'acknowledged' (1994: 193) until, after the subsequent birth, the mother was able to form a relationship with her new baby.

Conclusion

To sum up the message of this paper, I must emphasise

Table 2.5.1 Websites about registration and other statutory documentation of a stillborn baby

England & Wales
www.statistics.gov.uk/nsbase/registration/registering_still_birth.asp
Scotland
www.gro-scotland.gov.uk/grosweb/grosweb.nsf/pages/groreg
Northern Ireland
www.belfastcity.gov.uk/bdm/howto3.htm

the importance of two principles in the care of the bereaved woman in labour. The first principle is that the woman's care should be sensitive to the point of catering for her needs as an individual. The second principle is that her care should be of the highest standard possible. While these twin principles should apply in the care of every woman in labour, those of us who inhabit the real world know that shortcomings and omissions may sometimes occur. Because of their potential for serious long-term damage, shortcomings and omissions have no place in the care of the grieving mother.

This standard of care should never fall below the standard necessary for the woman to recover healthily from her experience of perinatal loss. The standard to which the midwife should seek to aspire is the standard spelt out to me by a wonderful midwife who participated in my research on mothers who do not have their babies with them. This midwife, who I called 'Annie', explained to me how she provided care which did not impede the woman's grieving. This is the standard which I have been discussing. Annie took her care a stage further, though. Building on this basic standard, she sought to work with the woman in labour to achieve an experience of which the woman could be proud. This meant that the woman would be able to look back on her labour with a sense of having done it right for her dead baby. Thus the midwife has the potential to convert what could be an emotional disaster for the woman into a positively life-changing, even life-enhancing, experience.

REFERENCES

Chambers HM & Chan FY. 2000. Support for women/families after perinatal death. Cochrane Database of Systematic Reviews. Update Software Issue 2

Curtis P. 2000. Midwives' attendances at stillbirths: an oral history account. MIDIRS Midwifery Digest, 10(4), 526-30

Dimond B. 2001. Alder Hey and the retention and storage of body parts. British Journal of Midwifery, 9(3), 173-6

DoH. 2000. Organ retention: Interim guidance on post mortem examination. London: Department of Health http://www.doh.gov.uk/pm2.htm

Forrest GC, Standish E, Baum JD. 1982. Support after perinatal death: a study of support and counselling after perinatal bereavement. British Medical Journal, 285(20), 1475-9

Gohlish MC. 1985. Stillbirth. Midwife, Health Visitor and Community Nurse, 21(1), 16

Hense AL. 1994. Live birth following stillbirth. Chapter 5 in: Field PA & Marck PB (Eds). Uncertain Motherhood: Negotiating the risks of the childbearing years. Thousand Oaks: Sage

Horsfall A. 2001. Bereavement: Tissues, tea and sympathy are not enough. RCM Midwives Journal, 4(2), 54-7

Hughes P. 1986. Solitary or Solitude: Views on the management of bereaved mothers. University of Wales, Unpublished DipN Dissertation

Jurkovich GJ, Pierce B, Pananen L, Rivara FP. 2000. Giving bad news: the family perspective. Journal of Trauma-Injury Infection & Critical Care, 48(5), 865-70

Kirk E. 1984. Psychological effects and management of perinatal loss. American Journal of Obstetrics and Gynaecology, 149, 45-61

Kohner N. 1995. Pregnancy loss and the death of a baby: Guidelines for Professionals. London: SANDS

Lake M, Johnson TM, Murphy K, Knuppel RA. 1987. Evaluation of a perinatal grief support team. American Journal of Obstetrics and Gynaecology, 157, 1203-6

Leon IG. 1992. Commentary: Providing versus packaging support for bereaved parents after perinatal loss. Birth, 19(2), 89-91

Lewis E & Bourne S. 1989. Perinatal Death. In: Oates M (Ed). Psychological Aspects of Obstetrics and Gynaecology. London Baillière Tindall

Mander R. 1993. Who chooses the choices? Modern Midwife, 3(1), 23-5

Mander R. 1994. Loss and Bereavement in Childbearing. Oxford: Blackwell Scientific

Mander R. 1999. Preliminary Report: A study of the midwife's experience of the death of a mother. RCM Midwives Journal, 2(11), 346-9

Mander R. 2000. Perinatal grief: Understanding the bereaved and their carers. Chapter 3 pp 29-50 in: Alexander J, Levy V & Roth C. Midwifery Practice: Core Topics 3. London: Macmillan

McDonald M. 1996. Loss in Pregnancy: Guidelines for midwives. London: Baillière Tindall

McHaffie HE. 1998. Ethics: Withdrawing treatment from neonates – a review of the issues. British Journal of Midwifery, 6(6), 384-8

McHaffie HE, Fowlie PW. 1998. Ethics: Deciding when to stop treatment – interpersonal conflicts. British Journal of Midwifery, 6(7), 466-70

Moulder C. 1998. Understanding Pregnancy Loss: Perspectives and issues in care. London: Macmillan

Mittelstaedt E, Bice-Stephens WM, Russell M. 2000. Perinatal grief support: developing a telephone follow-up pathway. Mother Baby Journal, 5(4), 32-6

Murray JA, Terry DJ, Vance JC, Battistutta D, Connolly Y. 2000. Effects of a program of intervention on parental distress following infant death. Death Studies, 24(4), 275-305

Rådestad I, Nordin C, Steineck G, Sjögren B. 1996. Stillbirth is no longer managed as a non-event: a nationwide study in Sweden. Birth, 23(4), 209-17

Rådestad I, Nordin C, Steineck G, Sjögren B. 1998. A comparison of women's memories of care during pregnancy, labour and delivery after stillbirth or live birth. Midwifery, 14(2), 111-7

Rajan L & Oakley A. 1993. No pills for the heartache: the importance of social support for women who suffer pregnancy loss. Journal of Reproductive and Infant Psychology, 11(2), 75-88

Rajan L. 1994. Social isolation and support in pregnancy loss. Health Visitor, 67(3), 97-101

Statham H & Dimavicius J. 1992. Commentary: How do you give the bad news to parents? Birth, 19(2), 103-4

The Practising Midwife 2002; 5(8): 10-13

Bereavement, grief and the midwife

Barbara Burden, P. Cynthia Stuart

Support and caring for women are fundamental components of the role of the midwife. In the majority of cases, this care is provided to support women and their families through a joyous event. However, in some cases the process culminates in a stillbirth, neonatal or maternal death. This outcome is traumatic and devastating to the family, who require support and counselling from their midwife. The severity of the grief and the period of bereavement vary between individuals. The process of caring for the woman and her family can be extremely intense and stressful for a midwife. Midwives are human and subject to the same emotions and feelings as others. They often develop a relationship with the woman that equates to a strong friendship with both the mother and her baby. When the birth outcome results in a death then the midwife is exposed to feelings of loss and bereavement leading to a state of grieving. As part of this grieving process, midwives need to be able to access appropriate support and care for themselves, so they are able to reflect and debrief on the experience and thus work through the grieving process so that it does not impinge on the care they provide to other mothers. This article explores the literature in relation to grief and bereavement and the effect this has on the midwife.

Grief and bereavement

In the course of everyday living, we do not usually dwell on the possibility of imminent death, as the fear and anxiety that this creates is too stressful. Following the introduction of media approaches to presenting world affairs, we are now exposed daily to dramatic and horrifying scenes of death and destruction, bringing death into the home of every individual. Although there may be an immediate display of concern, often this is displaced with a feeling of relief that the deceased are not, themselves, friends or relatives. Death is therefore seen as being a great distance away, as an unfortunate event that happens to other people and purposely kept at that distance.

Death and the fear of death are universal. Historically, Becher (1973) described the phenomenon of 'the terror of death', arguing that this terror is as old as time itself. As death is classed as the ultimate 'terror' then the process must be painful (Becker, 1997). Close associates are portrayed as being 'left behind' following a death, in a state of grieving pain perpetuated by a fear of the unknown and the loss of a loved one. The classic definition of bereavement derives from an old English word 'reafian' meaning to rob or take away by force. However, there are certain cultures that have a belief that welcomes death as a significant continuation of the process of life (Raphael, 1995). In the Western World, death is still a taboo subject shrouded by mystery and despair. Whatever the cultural stance on death, the huge impact death has on an individual is indisputable, resulting in grief and feelings of bereavement and loss (Parkes et al, 1997). Expression of grief is often frowned upon within society, being deemed a weakness. Grief is something to be expressed in private so that others are not compromised in having to acknowledge or deal with the outcome (Gunzburg, 1993); it is easier to conceal grief than to expose it. This inability to accept grief results in a society that pretends not to be affected by it and subsequently results in a scarcity of interpersonal support (Lendrun & Syme, 1992).

The period of bereavement that follows death varies from individual to individual (Kubler-Ross, 1997). It is during the very early stages of this period that the midwife is often called upon to support the woman and her family. It is during this time that the midwife needs to utilise skills in listening, counselling, reflection and diagnosis to support the family. When there is a death, close members within that relationship go through their own process of bereavement. The situation requires support to be given to relatives and friends by someone who is able to function effectively at this difficult time and assumes that health professionals, and particularly midwives, are trained to cope and deal with issues of death. In order to offer this care and retain compassion the midwife needs support and relief from an excessive caseload, in order to prevent her becoming cold and insensitive towards mothers and their families.

Grief affects not only the physical, cognitive and behavioural aspects of our lives, but also our emotional and social wellbeing. Grief itself is not an illness: although it is often defined or discussed in terms of symptoms, there are no descriptions of the intensity of these feelings or symptoms (Cowles and Rogers, 1991). The important aspect of grief is that it is a normal reaction to a loss, part of the experience that needs to be worked through so that both physical and psychological healing can take place. Any member of the family or healthcare personnel associated with bereavement can experience grief, particularly where a close relationship has occurred. The intensity of the relationship between mothers and midwives can result in midwives feeling personally responsible for the death, even where there is no evidence to support this. The symptoms of sadness and guilt can be borne silently by a midwife without anyone else being aware of the situation. The midwife in the professional role as carer and clinician may well feel that the care of others supersedes her own needs and feelings. These feelings of sadness and guilt can be carried to other clinical cases. If this is the case there may be significant repercussions for the midwife's behaviour and functions and therefore competence, following bereavement in practice. Midwives, therefore, need to care for themselves and grieve in their own way if they are to give effective emotional support to other women in their care. If they do not care for themselves they stand the likely risk of suffering burnout, stress or an inability to cope with other bereavement situations.

Various physical symptoms of grief have been described over the years. Although there are several dramatic examples, such as tightness in the chest, shortness of breath, and a feeling of choking, there are others, such as a sense of panic and gastrointestinal disturbances. Identified symptoms of grief include sad and lonely feelings, physical distress, preoccupation with the image of the deceased, guilt, hostile reactions and disruptions in patterns of conduct (Lindemann, 1994). Imagine the disruption to the care of a client and the other team members if a grieving colleague were to suddenly become indisposed at a crucial moment when caring for a client. This could result in the midwife feeling guilty at letting down both clients and colleagues.

The tasks of grieving are described as accepting the reality of loss, working through the pain of grief (to bypass this task could led to unresolved grief), adjusting to the new environment (the changes) and dealing with emotionally relocating the deceased, and moving on with life (Worden, 1991). These tasks must be accomplished for equilibrium to be re-established in the body, and also for the process of mourning to be completed. If the tasks are not achieved, the bereavement is incomplete and grief will therefore be unresolved. Grief that is not resolved is neither good personally, nor of benefit to the NHS at large.

Stress relating to grief is not unique to the healthcare professions. The concept is linked to professions allied to medicine, such as paramedics and fire officers. It was also identified in the police force following the publication of the Taylor Report (HMSO, 1990) addressing the Hillsborough Stadium disaster where police officers were directly involved in the results of traumatic grief, both for themselves and the public. This was the first incident that confirmed that professionals were able to grieve and face bereavement without having to accept it as part of their job. Employers are now required to take notice of the effects of stress in the workplace and act to reduce the incidence.

Effects on professionals and their clinical practice

There are various research studies assessing the impact of death and dying on healthcare professionals, most of which agree that the close relationship that staff have with their clients results in feelings of loss and inadequacy at their death. The Western influence perpetuates the idea of death as something to be feared, with death being concealed from children in the hope of protecting them from the realities of dying. This perpetuates the image of hospitals as places were people go to get well, rather than to die. The studies of Hurtig and Stewin (1990) and Lyons (1988) on death education in nursing showed that fear of death, or of the dying patient, must first be overcome before the nurse is able to help someone who is dying. Both students and midwives are dependent on the support of others within the clinical environment to enable them to develop the necessary skills to deal with dying clients. It is the first experience of caring for someone at this time that develops the individual's attitude to subsequent experiences. Time should therefore be spent on supporting students and midwives throughout this initial period to make this a meaningful experience. However, in reality, practitioners are themselves often inadequately prepared to offer this support. If practitioners are to develop a caring attitude then they have to learn to be open and share their feelings with others. This same openness without adequate support can cause the practitioner to experience emotional hurt and subsequent burnout. Loftus (1998) explored the experiences of third year student nurses caring for dying patients in a range of healthcare settings. This phenomenological study reviewed student nurses' lived experiences of the sudden death of their patients. Informal interviews produced narrative accounts of the student's experience. The themes emerging from the study included the sudden death experience, vulnerability of the student and support required. The results outlined the students' sense of 'letting down' the patient by not providing care that resulted in life, of being unable to act as advocate and of the distress felt by the students when death occurred. However, the students identified that they had also learnt from the experience of caring for an individual who was dying, developing the necessary skills to aim for competence in this area of practice.

The emotional experiences of nurses when their patients died have also been studied (Beck, 1997). These emotions included fear, sadness and frustration. The process of death, dying and bereavement can be extremely stressful for midwives and students involved, particularly where both mother and baby die. Davies et al (1996) noted that when nurses were aware that a child in their care was dying the nurses became distressed, and used various ploys to manage this distress. These included the practitioner leaving the client unattended at the point of death, avoiding entering the room or selectively undertaking other tasks to delay caring for the client. Caring for the dying reminds practitioners of their own mortality and when faced with this scenario they implement defence mechanisms to blur the reality of having to cope with the stress of this event. This can involve avoiding a discussion with the client regarding their death (Field and Kitson, 1986) or incorporating a language of avoidance to delay the discussion (Lyons, 1988).

Health professionals are expected to cope with traumatic events often without appropriate support or, in some instances, appropriate education and training. Of interest are the thoughts of an unknown author (Anonymous, 1993: 30). Anonymous was a senior student nurse who experienced a distressing event regarding a child's death on the ward on which she was working. She vividly describes the death of a little girl who was the victim of a road traffic accident. The author commented:

'I found myself in the ward kitchen, crying uncontrollably, almost hysterically.'

and

'The staff in that trauma ward could not have given more support to Laura's mother, yet not one of them seemed to realise that they also had a student with a problem.'

Midwives who care for grieving families need to be educated on how to support the client, relatives and others. Any programme of education must consider the life experience of the midwife or student, to take account of the professional's own needs. Regular time to listen to each other and share feelings and concerns ensures that debriefing and refuelling takes place. Thomas (1995) describes the concept of socialised training support for midwives. Central to this activity is the need to allocate time to discuss the practitioner's needs and feelings, including their reactions to the event, in order that the individual can assess and comprehend their strengths and limitations. Discussing the event and coming to terms with the outcome enables midwives to understand the special role they play in supporting families who are grieving.

Support mechanisms

Professionals, because of the strong identification they develop with their clients, may need considerable support from others when a client dies; this maybe from family members or colleagues alike (Raphael, 1995). If the professional is to maintain compassion and empathy, social support is necessary. It can be argued that any professional who is not able to share the burden of pain and sorrow of bereavement may develop a defensive behaviour. This behaviour results in poor interpersonal relationships, and having a cold attitude towards colleagues and clients. In extreme cases the professional may even suffer the risk of burnout and resort to self-consoling behaviours such as alcohol abuse.

Communication plays a significant role in counselling situations, especially the use of therapeutic communication where clients are enabled to utilise self-expression to promote health, understand the client's problems and assist in the identification and resolution of problems (Fertig-McDonald, 1996). Empathy is an important quality in this approach and necessary to the success of the relationship between carer and client, and between midwife and midwife. Other techniques enhance communication such as:

'...silence, support and reassurance, giving information, interpretation, restating, reflecting, clarifying and role playing' (Fertig-McDonald, 1996: 167).

Communication helps lessen the post-bereavement morbidity that can occur following bereavement. There is a need to talk over the events with someone, especially if that person has experienced a similar event. Conversing with someone helps the bereaved develop a new perception and behavioural skills, enabling progression through grief. Communication encompasses other skills such as listening, enabling, verbal and non-verbal interaction, which are necessary in counselling situations and central to enable individuals to share painful feelings and experiences (Burnard, 1999).

Listening is an integral part of communication. This is demonstrated not only with verbal behaviour but also non-verbal signals. A person in grief needs to communicate with others to ease the pain of bereavement; therefore the listener owes a duty of care to the bereaved person to listen to what is said. Listening needs to be an active process and, if not carried out effectively, can cause the listener to miss vital pieces of information or clues. Weinstein (1997: 7-9) describes this listening role as:

'simply to sit alongside the mourner on the edge of the abyss and to bear witness to that individual's pain.'

He continues:

'We also need to hear the story – however endless this can seem to us'.

SANDS (1995) recommend that all professionals who care for bereaved parents should have an open, supportive atmosphere in which to share feelings and problems. A recommendation was also made that opportunities should be made available for staff to see a bereavement counsellor confidentially, and that strategies for alleviating stress should be employed. SANDS (1995: 85-6) clearly considered the care of the professionals in its report. The organisation interviewed professionals following bereavement incidents, and noted regular use of certain phrases, such as:

- *'painful findings...'*
- *'a sense of having failed...'*
- *'findings of helplessness and frustration'*
- *'stress and exhaustion'*
- *'heightened awareness of personal fears'.*

The use of a 'time-out' room and debriefing after traumatic events helps reduce the stress of the practitioner's work. The allocation of a mentor or friend as advocate to ensure that a period of reflection and listening takes place could facilitate effective review of the case, ensuring that grieving can take place. Examples of good practice are present within other professions; for example, paramedic teams each have an experienced senior officer who acts as mentor. This person organises debriefing meetings when the team returns from a bad incident, so that members are able to come and talk to their colleagues to share their experience. The situation is similar in the police force, where police stations include a room where officers can go to report the incident and reflect on their experience with colleagues. The training officer can also refer staff involved in difficult cases to the Occupational Health Department.

Hodgkinson et al (1993: 201) outlined the support required by the bereaved that could be applied to the process of helping the midwife come to terms with the loss of a client. The authors state that:

- *'the helper views the body and is able to give preliminary feedback'*
- *'the bereaved and the helper view the body together'*
- *'there is a debriefing, in which any questions about the reason for the state of the body are addressed.'*

It is possible to hypothesise that the process of discussing the events and care with the client's relatives enables the practitioner to discuss with another person the process of death. This in turn helps the practitioner come to terms with the event and enables them to grieve for the person, where necessary. Telling the story or talking about events is a significant part of coping with grief. Empathy communicates to another person your understanding of his or her experiences or feelings. Once the bereaved person feels that the listener is empathic and is therefore prepared to listen to their story, the speaker is encouraged to talk and relive the story.

Conclusion

The close relationship that a midwife develops with women and their babies, and often other members of the family, is similar to that experienced between close friends. Where the outcome of birth results in death the midwife is exposed to the processes of bereavement and grieving. Developing skills to enable support of students and midwifery colleagues is an important component of the practice of midwifery. By working together as a family, midwives are able to offer strength and support to colleagues and, in turn, develop these skills in student midwives in their care. This in turn enables midwives to offer expert care and support to others while reducing the stress and anxiety that bereavement of a mother or child in their care may bring.

REFERENCES

Anonymous. 1993. A cry for help. Nursing Times, 89(4), 29-30

Becher HK. 1973. Non-specific forces surrounding disease and treatment of diseases. Journal of American Medical Association, 179(6), 437-40

Beck CT. 1997. Nursing students' experiences of caring for dying patients. Journal of Nursing Education, 36(9), 408-15

Becker E. 1997. The Denial of Death. New York: Free Press

Burnard P. 1999. Counselling Skills for Health Professionals. 3rd Edition. London: Stanley Thomas Publishers Limited

Cowles KV, Rogers B. 1991. The concept of grief: A foundation for nursing research and practice. Research in Nursing and Health, 14(2), 119-27

Davies B, Clarke D, Connaught S et al. 1996. Caring for dying children: Nurses' experiences. Pediatric Nursing, 22(6), 500-7

Fertig-McDonald S. 1996. Principles of Communication. Cited in: Fortinash KM, Holoday-Worret PA. Psychiatric Mental Health Nursing. London: Mosby

Field D, Kitson C. 1986. Formal teaching about death and dying in UK nursing schools. Nurse Education Today, 6(6), 270-6

Gunzburg J. 1993. Unresolved Grief: A practical, multicultural approach to health. New York: Singular Publishing Group

Hodgkinson PE, Joseph S, Yule W, Williams R. 1993. Viewing human remains following disaster: helpful or harmful? Medical Science and Law, 33(3), 197-202

HMSO. 1990. Taylor Report: The Hillsborough Stadium Disaster. London: HMSO

Hurtig WA, Stewin L. 1990. The effect of death education and experience on nursing students' attitude towards death. Journal of Advanced Nursing, 15(1), 29-34

Kubler-Ross E. 1997. On Death and Dying: What the dying have to teach doctors, nurses, clergy and their own families. London: Scribner

Lendrum S, Syme G. 1992. Gift of Tears: A Practical Approach to Loss & Bereavement Counselling. London: Routledge

Lindemann E. 1994. Symptomatology and management of acute grief. American Journal of Psychiatry, 151(6), 155-60 (Supplement)

Loftus L. 1998. Student nurses' lived experiences of the sudden death of their patients. Journal of Advanced Nursing, 27(3), 641-8

Lyons G. 1988. Bereavement and death education – a survey of nurses' views. Nurse Education Today, 8(3), 168-72

Parkes CM, Laungani P, Young B. 1997. Death and Bereavement across Cultures. London: Routledge

Raphael B. 1995. The anatomy of bereavement. London: Routledge

SANDS (Stillbirth and Neonatal Death Society). 1995. Pregnancy loss and the death of a baby: Guidelines for Professionals. London: SANDS

Thomas J. 1995. The effects on the family of miscarriage, termination for abnormality, stillbirth and neonatal death. Child Care Health and Development, 21(6), 413-24

Weinstein J. 1997. Looking into the Abyss: A gestalt model of working with bereavement. Managing Clinical Nursing, 1(1), 7-10

Worden JW. 1991. Grief Counselling and Grief Therapy: A handbook for the mental health practitioner. Second Edition. London: Routledge

The Practising Midwife 2002; 5(8): 14-17

Women, men and stillbirth

How do they cope?

Barbara Kavanagh

The loss of a baby through stillbirth is such a devastating event, but has often been considered by our society as a lesser form of bereavement. Parents may be regarded as being unable to have established a meaningful bond with their child.

The purpose of this article is to provide midwives with some insight into the coping process that may take place between the parents following this occurrence. A basic understanding of this will therefore allow health professionals to support the bereaved more effectively.

Parents do not expect to outlive their children, this is not the natural order, children are their link with future generations. The death of a child cuts off all expectations and future hopes and dreams are thrown into turmoil (Golding, 1991). Not only is there a loss of the person whom the parents have helped to create, there is a loss of future aspirations and ambitions. They have loved, nurtured and built a future around the baby. When deaths occur during pregnancy or childbirth, parents are stunned, because death is not the expected outcome of pregnancy. In many ways, life will never be the same for these families (de Montigny, Beaudet & Dumas, 1999). People may think because the baby never lived that it had no real existence or designated place in society. This can be extremely difficult for the parents to endure. Parents undergo intense grief reactions following the death of their baby; these feelings are very similar to any other form of bereavement.

In 'A Grief Observed' (1966), CS Lewis wrote:

'No one ever told me that grief felt so much like fear. I am not afraid, but the sensation is like being afraid. The same fluttering in the stomach, the same restlessness. I keep swallowing.'

This baby had been very much alive to its parents: when something goes wrong, it comes as a shattering blow. There are often so few tangible memories for them to hold onto, and most of these are shared only by the parents themselves.

Rituals

Death has no place in the process of birth, the natural order of things is turned upside down. Instead of welcoming new life into the world, there is a funeral to prepare for. Over the years, a funeral is almost all that remains to help the bereaved to grieve publicly. This ritual is a farewell, giving the bereaved permission to grieve and eventually redirect their lives. Rituals mark transitions in life, confirming our identity within our social and cultural group and regulating human interaction (Dyregrov, 1996). They provide bereaved people with a shared spiritual meaning for death which they can integrate within their own belief system. In our society, there has been a gradual loss of rituals. Due to this, present generations now find that they have fewer means available to help them to express their feelings caused by ever-increasing pressures and varieties of loss. The freedom to mourn is important following any death: there is nothing new about this fact, but what has altered is the attitude to those in mourning. Mourners are rarely comforted for long, and are frequently shunned (Boston & Trezise, 1988).

Parents of stillborn babies are one group of people who find their need to grieve goes unrecognised. Stillbirth has been described as a traumatic 'non-event' (Stewart & Dent, 1994). Mothers in particular do have a deep need to mourn the loss of the child that has lived inside them.

In our culture, the attempts not to know about death, and not to be reminded about it, are predominant. There seems to be a general conspiracy that death has not occurred (Pincus, 1997). Lily Pincus observed in 'Death and the Family' that we lack those 'rites of passage', the rituals which allow for psychological transition, to assist the bereaved to adjust to their new status and to those around them. Our society does not afford a climate in which grief and mourning are accepted, supported and valued. There is a need to mourn a loss, and if this is not made possible there is a likelihood of suffering, either psychologically or physically, or both (Roose-Evans, 1994).

Studies of bereavement in the 1960s showed that the majority of British people were without adequate guidance as to how to treat death and bereavement. It appears that there is little evidence to show that social behaviour has changed significantly since then. Society often compounds the pain and isolation of bereaved mothers through people's reluctance to speak of the death of the baby. The closeness of the mother to the child, as well as the roller-coaster ride of the physical and emotional changes can make this time extremely difficult to deal with (O'Neill, 1998).

Attachment theory

The psychoanalyst Bowlby (1997) developed the Attachment Theory. This concerns the strong bonds of affection that human beings make with others, and the powerful emotional reaction that occurs when those bonds are threatened or broken. Bowlby's thesis asserts that these attachments develop early in life. They come from a need for security, safety and survival of the social group, and are usually directed toward a few specific individuals, and tend to continue throughout a large part of the life cycle. Close, intimate relationships between individuals can be thought of as attachments. Love is invested in a relationship from which we reap safety and security, and the subsequent loss of that attachment results in grief (Powell, 1997). Bowlby's study generated ideas relating to phases of grief in bereavement.

A woman's feelings of attachment to her unborn baby are probably much greater than a man's, because of the physical and emotional closeness of a pregnancy. It places her in much closer contact than the father, who does not have the same chance of this early bond. The bonding of mother to growing fetus may account, in part, for evidence suggesting that mothers appear to grieve more deeply and for longer than fathers (Dyregrov & Matthiesen, 1991).

Although the experience of grieving is personal and intense, it is a normal, healthy response to loss. Grief does, however, invite differing responses from different individuals (Moules & Amundson, 1997). Many studies undertaken in the past assumed that men and women responded similarly to loss. It now appears that there are differences between men and their partners in terms of the nature, intensity, duration and expression of grief (Murphy, 1998). There are cultural expectations within our society for men to behave appropriately following any death. In the case of stillbirth men appear to recognise that they should suppress their own feelings in order to support their partner. Traditionally they are seen as the protector, a male role that fits comfortably. Following a stillbirth, a man may experience a feeling of powerlessness and helplessness when seeing the person he loves in pain. The often unspoken devastation and confusion men feel when faced with loss through death can accentuate the anger and guilt which often forms part of the normal grieving process (Roberts, 2000). Differences in the ways men and women express their emotions may cause tension in the relationship. It is important for men to be open about their feelings, so that partners understand that they too have suffered a loss. Studies by Hughes and Page-Lieberman (1989) aimed to describe the experience of 51 fathers who had experienced perinatal loss. These men described the need to keep their feelings of sadness, loss and anger suppressed in order to support their partners. They also felt that the intensity, duration and expression of their grieving was different and less than those of their partners, who were so obviously distressed by the experience.

Such feelings were also reported by Murray Parkes (1998). Men are less likely than women to seek psychiatric help following all types of bereavement, and they often see themselves as having responsibility to contain their own grief in order to look after their wives. Thomas and Streigel (1998) studied 26 couples who had lost a baby by stillbirth, and concluded that mothers and fathers grieve differently:

'Mothers grieve for their babies, fathers grieve for their wives.'

Difficulties arise when trying to use and fit traditional methods in helping men grieve. Women are more co-operative and explore feelings, whereas men find it a struggle to identify feelings other than anger, and recoil from the intimacy of sharing (Roberts, 2000).

Dual process model of coping with bereavement

Research undertaken by Stroebe and Schut (1999) has shown that traditional theories about effective ways of coping with bereavement have many shortcomings. Contemporary researchers differ in their conclusions about the efficacy of working through grief in coming to terms with loss. Therefore they have proposed a revised model of coping with bereavement, the Dual Process Model.

This model identifies two types of stressors, loss and restoration orientation. It also goes on to talk of a dynamic, regulatory coping process of oscillation, whereby the grieving individual at times confronts, at times avoids the different tasks of grieving (Stroebe & Schut, 1999).

Coping efforts are needed by the bereaved to deal

Table 6.3.1 A dual process model of coping with loss

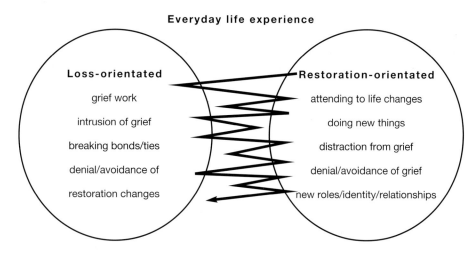

with these stressors. However, it is evident that coping does not take up all of a bereaved person's time. There are occasions when time is taken off from grieving, for example when watching television or attending to everyday tasks.

Loss-orientation

This refers to dealing with the loss experience itself, particularly with respect to the deceased person. There is an attempt to try to make sense of the loss. Freud, cited in Murray Parkes (1998) identified a theory of 'grief work', an activity used in preparing bereaved individuals for a full acceptance of their loss. Many emotions are present, and range from concentration on the circumstances and events surrounding the death, yearning for the deceased, crying and painful longing. Stroebe and Schut do not propose a model with a sequence of stages, but more 'a waxing and waning', an ongoing flexibility over time. In early bereavement, loss-orientation dominates.

Restoration-orientation

This second bereavement stressor focuses on the needs of the bereaved and how they are dealt with. Newly bereaved people are not only faced with the death of a loved one, but they also have to adjust to the changes that are a secondary consequence of the loss. For example, in the case of parents of a stillborn baby, they move from the role of 'parents to be' to 'parents of a deceased baby'. This added stress together with the sorrow already felt by the parents causes extreme anxiety and confusion.

Cook and Oltjenbruns (1999) see the death of a child as not changing household role structures, but instead

affecting household communication patterns. Men and women handled their grief very differently, which, they concluded, resulted in redirection of negative emotions towards the spouse. Escalation of problems due to miscommunication or lack of communication could then result.

There are many similarities between the restoration-oriented dimension and Worden's Four Tasks of Mourning Model (2000). However, Stroebe and Schut identified additional tasks to be undertaken. Worden's First Task is to accept the reality of the loss. They saw it as necessary to accept the reality of the changed world. Task Two is to experience the pain of grief. They argue the additional necessity to take time off from the pain of grief. The Third Task is to adjust to an environment in which the deceased is missing, referring to external, internal and spiritual adjustments. Here, Stroebe and Schut add the need to reconstrue the environment itself. The Fourth Task is relocation of the deceased emotionally, and moving on with life. Stroebe and Schut add the specification that bereaved persons need to develop new roles, identities and relationships.

Oscillation

Oscillation is regarded by Stroebe and Schut as the central element of the Dual Process Model. This refers to the interchange that takes place between loss- and restoration-oriented coping, the process whereby there is confrontation and avoidance of different stressors associated with bereavement. At times, the bereaved are confronted by their loss; at other times they will avoid it, either by distraction or through having to attend to normal everyday things such as earning a living or caring for children (Stroebe & Schut, 1999).

Stroebe and Schut see this as a 'dynamic, back and forth process'. It is assumed that this oscillation is necessary for the most favourable adjustment over time. Murray Parkes (1998) also recognised that bereaved people oscillate back and forth between grieving and the other demands of life – eating, sleeping, caring for surviving children and so on. For bereaved parents to immediately accept their loss would involve a number of changes in their identities. These cannot take place quickly: it takes time. Oscillation is part of a gradual process of realisation that they have lost a baby.

Stroebe and Schut view their model to be descriptive of the way men and women grieve. Recent evidence has shown bereaved mothers to be more loss-oriented than fathers following the death of their child (Stroebe & Schut, 1999). As already mentioned, there are gender differences in the way that men and women express themselves. Stroebe and Schut maintain that 'if a mother's grief over the loss of a child is more loss-oriented, a father's more restoration-oriented, this discordance in ways of coping may, at times, be mutually unconducive. It would be easy for a mother to make the attribution that 'he is grieving less than I am', rather than what might be the case, that 'he is grieving differently from the way I am.'

Further research into gender differences by Stroebe and Schut suggest that levels of distress can be lowered when bereaved couples learn how to cope in ways often adopted by the opposite sex, i.e. men need to be more emotion-oriented and women more problem-oriented.

Conclusion

There is evidence that bereaved people undertake certain coping strategies to enable them to come to terms with their loss, and avoid severe health problems. Whereas, others assume strategies that can be detrimental to their health. With the aid of this model, midwives may be able to identify different reactions that could be taking place between parents. This will give them a valuable insight into the coping process each individual adopts following the death of their baby.

Midwives are not expected to counsel bereaved parents without the adequate training and support required, but if a problem has been identified they can refer couples to the appropriate professional help available, i.e. bereavement counsellors.

It is worth remembering that a bereaved mother, or couple, may appear or want to be coping, but this could be part of the process of oscillation, which changes almost daily in the early days of bereavement.

Acknowledgement

The Child Bereavement Trust Ellen Poll Scholarship was awarded to the author, enabling her to complete the Bereavement Counselling Diploma. The author wishes to thank Jill Poll and her family.

REFERENCES

Boston S & Trezise R. 1988. Merely Mortal. London: Methuen
Bowlby J. 1997. Attachment and Loss. Volume 1. London, Boston: Faber & Faber
Cook AS & Oltjenbruns KA. 1999. The bereaved family. In: Cook AS & Oltjenbruns (Eds). Dying and Grieving: Lifespan and family perspectives. Forth Worth: Harcourt Brace. Cited in Stroebe M & Schut H. The Dual Process Model and coping with bereavement: Rationale and description. Death Studies, 23, 197-224
De Montigny F, Beaudet L, Dumas L. 1999. A baby has died: The impact of perinatal loss on family social networks. JOGNN Clinical Studies, 28(2), 151-6
Dyregov A & Matthiesen SB. 1991. Parental grief following the death of an infant: A follow-up over one year. Scand J Psychol, 193-207
Dyregov A. 1996. Childen's participation in rituals. Bereavement Care, 15(12)
Golding C. 1991. Bereavement. Wiltshire: Redwood Press Ltd
Hughes CB & Page-Lieberman J. 1989. Fathers experiencing a perinatal loss. Death Studies, 13, 537-56
Lewis CS. 1996. A Grief Observed. London: Faber & Faber
Moules N & Amundson J. 1997. Grief – An invitation to inertia. A narrative approach to working with grief. Journal of Family Nursing, 3(4), 378-93

Murphy F. 1998. The experience of early miscarriage from a male perspective. Journal of Clinical Nursing, 7, 325-32
Murray Parkes C. 1998. Bereavement Studies of Grief in Adult Life. London: Penguin
O'Neill B. 1998. A father's grief: Dealing with stillbirth. Nursing Forum, 33(4), 33-6
Pincus L. 1997. Death and the Family. London, Boston: Faber & Faber
Powell A. 1997. Grief and the concept of loss in midwifery practice. Professional Care of Mother and Child, 7(2), 37-9
Roberts J. 2000. Let the cry come. Community Care, 24
Roose-Evans J. 1994. Passages of the Soul. Dorset: Element Books Ltd
Stewart A & Dent A. 1994. At A Loss. London: Baillière Tindall
Stroebe M & Schut H. 1999. The Dual Process Model and coping with bereavement: Rationale and description. Death Studies, 23, 197-224
Thomas V & Striegel P. 1998. Stress and grief of a perinatal loss: Integrating qualitative and quantitative methods. Omega, 30(4), 299-311. Cited in: Murray Parkes C. Bereavement Studies of Grief in Adult Life. London: Penguin
Worden W. 2000. Grief Counselling and Grief Therapy. London: Routledge

Teaching grief and bereavement

Involving support groups in educating student midwives

Mary Mitchell, Gill Catron

The death of a baby poses many difficulties and challenges, not only for parents but also for the professionals who care for them. Supporting parents whose baby has died is a crucial aspect of a midwife's practice and student midwives need preparation to fulfil this role. Involving support groups in educating professionals about death is one strategy that is recommended in the literature. This article presents an account of the experiences of students when this educational strategy was adopted to facilitate the preparation of student midwives in caring for bereaved parents. It also includes the views of one bereaved parent who has made significant contributions to this preparation.

Preparing student midwives to care for bereaved parents

Preparing professionals to deal with death is a complex and sensitive issue (Papadatou, 1997). Western culture views the subject of death as morbid and a topic to be avoided. This is particularly the case with death around the time of birth. Thus, many midwifery students have little or no experience of death. Indeed Cavanagh and Snape (1997) found that student midwives reported dealing with death to be a significantly stressful experience. This may also be an issue for educators. Whittle (1997) in her research on death education uncovered that only a small self-selected group of children's nurse teachers were happy to teach about death. Given the lack of research and discussion in midwifery literature this may also be the case for midwifery teachers. Both parents and professionals still report inadequacies in the care given when a baby dies (Moulder,1998; Rådestad, 2001) yet we know that the care parents receive around the time that a baby dies can have a significant effect on how they cope.

Kohner and Henley (2001) argue that education should enable professionals to have a better understanding of parent's experiences and needs surrounding the time of their baby's death. Over the years, practices surrounding the care of bereaved parents have changed. Support and pressure groups such as the Stillbirth and Neonatal Death Society (SANDS) have contributed greatly to the professional's understanding of parents' needs when they experience the death of a baby. Involving bereaved parents and support groups in educating professionals is recommended in the literature as a way in which this can be achieved (Attig, 1992; Heuser, 1995; Whittle, 2002). This was the rationale for inviting members of SANDS to contribute to preparing student midwives to care for bereaved parents. The following presents the views of a bereaved parent and the students in relation to this strategy.

A bereaved parent's view

My first child, Chester, was stillborn at 38 weeks. I felt that the midwife that delivered him had no training or preparation for the delivery and just drew the short straw by being in the delivery suite with us. My husband was obviously very upset too, when we arrived at hospital to be told there was no heartbeat during labour. Our midwife had to get on with delivering him. She was obviously very stressed, not really knowing how to treat us or what to say. She disappeared promptly (for about 11/2 hours in total), obviously upset and awkward, and leaving my husband, particularly, very angry. In the hours that followed we subsequently had help from another midwife who did treat us properly and we are ever grateful for her help.

I vowed in the months that followed that I would like to change things somehow for future midwives as well as bereaved families. The first time I had the opportunity to do so was about a year later when I was about 4 months pregnant with my daughter. Together with another SANDS member, I was invited to talk to a group of student midwives.

The experience of talking about what had happened to us, about my son and what could be done to make it easier to talk, made me feel that I hadn't lost my son for nothing. We gave them each a SANDS pack with our leaflets including a regrets list complied from local families who wished they had had the opportunity to do certain things with their babies.

Parents often feel isolated after losing a baby. They seem to be alone and everyone around them has a purpose with their families. They miss the baby's physical presence and no baby means a 'no mother' label. Bereaved parents feel they don't belong, and to find out about others in a similar situation is vital to their future, as a couple and as individuals. The help received from midwives is invaluable during the time of birth, immediately afterwards, and also in the next pregnancy, if there is one. This is when the fears and questions seem to arise and the midwives can really help, given special training, to alleviate the fears of the family, especially the mother.

The students seemed shocked at first, but gradually warmed to us and asked us questions, which we were only too happy to answer. Since that time, four-and-a-half years ago, feedback from bereaved parents has changed. They now seem to have so much praise for the staff around the time of delivery and afterwards and also the ancillary staff in the units. The interest from the professionals who have really taken our personal experiences to heart and helped to turn it into an experience to be remembered rather than buried away is tremendous. I also feel very strongly that being able to ask any questions in a classroom setting must make their job that much easier.

The feedback from students is very positive. We have been asked many questions about the grieving process, how they can help families and themselves in preserving memories; using special cards with hand and foot prints, locks of hair, imaginative photographs, and acknowledging that sometimes they are the only ones who have been there at the birth. In some situations the midwives are the first to realise the baby has died, the first one to hold the baby and the ones that prepare the baby before passing him or her to the parents. They are often involved with the friends and family who come to visit, and help explain what has happened. They can even help with the registration of the birth/death and smooth the administration process along, together with sorting out any medication procedures before discharging the mother.

I have been involved with lots of charity work for SANDS in recent years but being involved with student midwives particularly has shown the most benefits and really will help future bereaved parents. The experience of bereaved families in all the hospitals throughout the country seems to be 'pot luck' depending upon training, funding, facilities and staffing levels. Hopefully this important work can be extended at some time in the future to support other professionals such as GPs, consultants and general nursing staff too.

Students' views

Students felt immensely privileged to hear the parents' painful experiences of the death of a baby. They felt that the women related their stories with frankness and honestly. This approach gave them permission to ask quite emotional and probing questions which otherwise may have been difficult to ask. This gave them an insight into the emotional turmoil parents experience when their baby dies. In particular they learned about parents' responses and needs in future pregnancies.

The opportunity to openly discuss with bereaved parents how midwives can meet individual needs gave the students more confidence for practice. The students realised the potential they had to promote a positive outcome for the parents and reported feeling less anxious about what to do or say when caring for bereaved parents.

The students also gained an appreciation of the work of SANDS and the importance of a support network for bereaved parents.

Conclusion

In conclusion, the experience of involving bereaved parents in the education of student midwives has proven to have mutual benefits. For the parents, the opportunity to recount their story seems to be therapeutic. Also, by making a contribution to the education of health professionals who will be providing care to bereaved parents, they have a chance to influence and encourage best practice that meets parents' individual needs.

The students gain insight into the emotions and experiences of bereaved parents and they learn how the care received can have a significant impact. It is hoped that further discussion about death education and the involvement of support groups will be stimulated. Given the lack of research in this area, midwife teachers can gain much by the sharing of information and experiences. I would like to thank all the SANDS members for contributing to the student midwives' educational experience.

REFERENCES

Attig T. 1992. Person centred death education. Death Studies, 16, 357-70

Cavanagh SJ, Snape J. 1997. Educational sources of stress in midwifery students. Nurse Education Today, 17, 128-34

Heuser L. 1995. Death education: a model of student participatory learning. Death Studies, 19, 583-90

Kohner N, Henley A. 2001. When a Baby Dies. Revised edition. London: Routledge

Moulder C. 1998. Understanding Pregnancy Loss. London: Macmillan Press

Papadatou D. 1997. Training health professionals in caring for dying children and grieving families. Death Studies, 21, 575-600

Rådestad I. 2001. Stillbirth: Care and long term psychological effects. British Journal of Midwifery, 9(8), 474-80

Whittle. 1997. Dying to be taught. MSc Thesis. University of Bristol

Whittle. 2002. Death Education: what should student children's nurses be taught? Unpublished research. University of the West of England

The Practising Midwife 2002; 5(8): 26-27

Bereavement: learning from parents

Alison Stewart, Ann Dent

When a child dies, we lose part of ourselves as parents, part of our past and an enormous part of our future. Dreams are shattered. We miss our children physically and emotionally, minute by minute and in the following years that seem to stretch without end, as time becomes a test of endurance. We may question the spiritual beliefs we have held all our lives. The relationships we took for granted with our family and friends may change. These changes seem to pile up on that one original loss.

Bev Gatenby
1998, *whose daughter Rose died*

All parents have their own unique story to tell of their child's death, one they know and remember well, even when the event occurred many years before (Peppers and Knapp, 1980). Stories from bereaved parents, such as Bev Gatenby, provide a brief glimpse of the changes and meaning that the death of a baby holds for them. Midwives work with parents who are bereaved of a baby in different circumstances: ectopic pregnancy, miscarriage, therapeutic termination, stillbirth, perinatal/neonatal death and cot death. This article has been adapted for midwives from chapters in our recent book, *Sudden Death in Childhood: Care of the Bereaved Family* (Stewart and Dent, 2004). It uses family stories, literature and practice experiences, offering professionals 'considerations for practice' to guide them when either a child or a baby dies. Likewise, in this article we include the words of parents, which we gratefully acknowledge, to express their experiences of bereavement after the death of a baby. We make no claim that these experiences are shared by all parents, rather we emphasise that grief is diverse. It is beyond the scope of this article to discuss bereavement in detail or the experiences of infertility, ectopic pregnancy, therapeutic termination and multiple pregnancy. For further discussion of midwifery care in these situations, see Warland (2000). We begin with the story of Rose whose daughter Ruby died unexpectively nine days after birth because of a rare congenital condition.

Rose's story

At the time of Ruby's death, John and I seemed quite similar in the way we dealt with things – in the way we talked with our other two daughters and what we wanted at Ruby's funeral. However, I did notice that when friends came around to offer sympathy John would go and sit in the bedroom. After this had happened a few times I asked him why. He said he felt left out of the grief – like people seemed to focus only on me as the mother. When I thought about it I realised that it was true – maybe this only happens when it is the death of a baby. One of the things that really helped me come to terms with Ruby's death was writing poems. This was not something I had done since leaving high school but it just seemed to come out. John loved to read them and he said that they were just how he felt too. I guess they helped him a little too, just by reading them. It was a great relief for me to be able to join the Baby Bereavement Group soon after Ruby's death – having a place when it was okay to cry or get angry – no-one looked at me funnily or told me it was time to get back to normal. I believe that is one of the major differences in our coping styles. I like to talk about how I am feeling. John keeps it very much to himself. Even now, nearly 8 years later, I am happy to talk about any aspects surrounding Ruby's birth, short life and death, whereas John prefers not to talk about it at all.

When I look back at what happened during those 9 days, I can now say that I no longer feel any guilt – I know that I did everything that I possibly could to help her. I also believe that the care she received was the best that could be given. There are one or two issues centred on the time of her death, and immediately after that, which I was not happy about but I have come to terms with them now. I no longer feel angry and, because I know there is nothing I can do to change them, I can let them go. Although it seems a strange thing to say, I have had so many good things come out of the tragedy of Ruby's death. My life took a new direction and I have found great pleasure in the way my life has developed.

Parents' grief

Rose's story uncovers some of the ways in which Ruby's death has changed her life, revealing some of the challenges that she and her family faced. For many parents, pregnancy is a time of preparation for a new life, including dreaming about the future with another family member, organising a room and choosing a name. The death of a baby or a miscarriage shatters parents' worlds. In particular it is seen as 'out of sequence' in a world where parents expect to die before their children and where death is not widely experienced. As Frazer, whose son Matthew died soon after birth, commented:

'It was the first death we had ever experienced and for me, at the age of 32, that was the first time in my life that I had had death that close. I hadn't seen a dead body before Matthew died and so for us, that was a new experience that we had never had to deal with.' (Stewart, 2000)

Pain and depth of grief

One of the life-changing moments that any parent faces is hearing the news of their child's death. The reactions of health professionals at this time may remain a vivid memory for many years later. Sarah described what happened 24 hours after Matthew's birth.

'They called us into a side room and told us that he wasn't going to live because his heart wasn't formed properly. I can remember the cardiologist because he was very matter of fact – there was no emotion at all – whereas the paediatrician was kind and very compassionate. I felt sorry for the cardiologist because I thought, "he just doesn't know how to cope with this, and he's pretending it's like a sore thumb or a sore toe".' (Dent and Stewart, 2004)

Not surprisingly, many parents' first reaction to death may be disbelief. Maria recalled when her son was stillborn:

'I wanted to hold him. I wanted to avoid him, I didn't know what I wanted to do and all the time I kept looking at him and hoping he would breathe. Then he would be alright, we would go home with him and we all know that lots of babies don't always breathe immediately at birth, The time went on, the clock ticked loudly and after half an hour I knew that he would not breathe and then I knew he was really dead.' (Stewart and Dent, 1994)

After hearing the news, parents describe varied feelings such as shock, anger and guilt (Martin, 1998; Moulder, 2001; Rando, 1986). Rose mentioned that there had been several issues at the time that Ruby did which had made her angry about the care they had received in hospital. Anger may be linked to expectations that medical technology is now able to ensure the survival of pregnancies and babies. When pregnancies miscarry and babies die, parents are left with questions of 'why?' and 'why us?'. After many miscarriages, stillbirths and cot deaths the physical cause of death may not be known, causing added distress. One parent described after their baby's cot death:

'The questions were answered but I could not say that I was satisfied. This is because nobody could answer the question why our baby died.' (Dent and Stewart, 2004)

Entangled with questions of 'why,' some parents may have a sense of guilt that they did something that contributed to their child's death. Deborah Cooper described in her journal after her miscarriage:

'Lost my baby a month ago. Everyone says they're so sorry; it was meant to be; it's for the best; keep trying. But I don't know... I am sorry too, but I still wonder why. What horrible thing did I do?' (Cooper, 1997)

Many parents experience the intense pain of loss, which Anne Diamond (1995) described after the cot death of her son, Sebastian.

*'I wanted to collapse. I wanted to die. I wanted my baby back. **I wanted my baby back.** My arms felt so empty. Where had he gone? We have been robbed of our child just as cruelly as if someone had stolen into our house in the middle of the night and murdered him.'*

Particular situations where a baby dies may contribute to specific feelings and experiences. We have considered this in relation to stillbirth and miscarriage. The word 'stillbirth' still conveys the sadness, quietness and emptiness surrounding a baby born dead, a cruel contradiction to an anticipated birth. Malacrida in her work with bereaved parents described 'a special kind of pain' that occurs for women when birth and death occur at the same time. She quoted one mother:

'And I went through the birthing process, and I could feel her shoulders and her head and her arms – I could feel her toenails as she passed out of me – I could feel her being born. And I knew that, as she was being born she was dying. (Malacrida, 1998)

Death in a neonatal unit can be preceded by a roller coaster of hopes and fears, experienced amidst intensive care equipment in a setting, which is far from home-like. Rose remembered the time before Ruby's death:

'On Tuesday morning, the nurse came for me at four in the morning and said, "you'd better get down quick, she's on the way out." I got down there and I told Ruby it was OK to die. But she fought so hard and I didn't want her to suffer again. She came back again, she wasn't going to go.' (Stewart, 2000)

Such experiences contribute to the pain and distress of grief after death. Many parents, such as Rose, talk about their sadness that their babies never come home alive from hospital.

Parents together and separately

Individuals do not grieve in isolation, they grieve within a social context of which a central part may be their family (Dent and Stewart, 2004). A woman who miscarried at eight weeks described her experience:

'I felt so sad afterwards, I wanted to do nothing but cry. Ian went to work and I stayed at home. When I wanted to talk he was busy and when I cried I wanted him to cry too. When he didn't I used to go into the bathroom to cry in private because I felt he was getting frustrated with me; a watering can.'(Stewart and Dent, 1994)

Is the nature or extent of grief different between men and women? Some studies report that in the time soon after death, many fathers put their energies into practical activities and often control their emotions, rationalising the death and finding ways to divert their grief into practical activities (McGreal et al, 1997) Conversely, many mothers are described as having a greater need or willingness to recognise and talk about their feelings. However, there is increasing recognition that men's grief may be constrained by societal expectations of being strong and supportive for their partner after the death of a child or baby. (Finkbeiner, 1996; Rando, 1986; Stinson et al, 1992). In addition, their grief may be overlooked by others who ask after the baby's mother (Malacrida, 1998). Rose described in her story that John felt that other people focused on her grief. Thompson (1997) cautions against assumptions of gender-specific ways of grieving, and argues that 'it is a question of degree and emphasis rather than a simple either/or'. We believe that the stories of fathers such as Frazer and Donald (Stewart 2000) and texts such as Kohner and Henley (1995) support the view that there may be as many differences within as between gendered groups.

Because of these different ways of grieving, couples may have difficulty maintaining any closeness or understanding of each other's grief. This may sometimes lead to further tensions in an already stressful situation. Stories and studies highlight that parents' relationships may change to become distanced, separated or closer together (Kohner and Henley, 2001; Martin, 1998; Moulder, 2001). At a time when parents have to cope with their own grief they may be caring for their other children.

Parents' other children

Martin (1998) identified some of the experiences that parents encountered with their surviving children at the time of a cot death. These included:

- explaining the death and answering questions such as when the baby will be back

- coping with children's reactions, which may range from being frightened, clinging and being ill.

Some parents find that other children provide a reason to continue, as one mother described:

'Physically, I had to get up in the morning. I had to make breakfast, I had to do all those things for [the other children], and in turn, it was I think, getting me through the steps maybe a little faster.' Martin, 1998)

Similar experiences are apparent in the comments of parents who have had a miscarriage or stillborn baby.

The support of family, friends and health professionals can guide parents in answering the questions of the surviving siblings, recognising their needs, and deciding whether to take them to the funeral. Rose reflected on this:

'I ring Mum every day – that's the way we are. I mean I can just ring up Mum when I feel sad and when I feel happy and I know she remembers all the days that are hard for me...And she keeps my feet on the ground. When I moan about the girls she says to me, "You've got to be a bit more understanding" because sometimes I forget how deeply they have been affected by it.' (Stewart, 2000)

How do parents cope?

Amidst the pain of loss, parents find different ways to cope. Funerals are a ritual that can assist to maintain the reality of the death and can be part of the transition towards a life without the baby. (Dent and Stewart, 2004). They offer opportunities to create memories and can be an important event for many parents and for others in the family. For Pip, whose daughter Gracie died soon after birth, the funeral gave her the opportunity to make some choices about what happened to her child.

'We had Gracie's funeral here in the garden by the blossom tree and we just invited people that we wanted to be here. It was a really lovely day. We had Gracie down in her wee box on the table. This idea of bringing dead babies home was quite strange to a lot of people, you can imagine.'(Stewart, 2000)

Even when there is no identifiable body, such as an early miscarriage, a funeral can give parents the opportunity to create their own special farewell rituals to make the baby's death publicly visible in memorial books or by planting a rosebush (Moulder, 2001).

Feelings are only part of a reaction to loss. Memories, telling stories and thinking about the child can form part of coping with the loss of a baby. Bereaved parents move between a range of coping activities that include seeking information, being supported by others, taking direct action, retreating into or trying to control their feelings and finding ways of constructing a relationship with the deceased. Stroebe and Schut (2001) describe this as an oscillation between loss and restoration (See page 175). Rose describes moving from sadness to times of busyness.

'Sometimes I kept really busy, doing things around the house. Then at other times I would ring Mum and talk about how I felt. I went quite a bit to Ruby's grave and that helps, just to spend time thinking about her. Then it was back to cook tea and get the girls to bed.' (Dent and Stewart, 2004)

Even whilst parents may struggle to cope and feel caught in the pain of their loss, time does move on. A parent whose baby died of cot death described her experience as:

'You live everything by firsts, you know. Like the first week you go "Gee, last Tuesday I was doing this and this with [the baby]...Well, this is only a week ago, and he's not here any more. Well how weird!" You know and it was really tough, and then you go to the first month. You know, and then you go to anniversaries, birthdays...like all those firsts. You remember to the day.' (Martin, 1998)

Finding ways to live with a baby's death

Many parents are worried that they may forget their baby and the idea of 'getting over' their grief is unacceptable because it implies forgetting their baby. Instead, parents describe ways in which they maintain a link or connection (Martin, 1998) which is consistent with other writing about grief as a continuing bond (Klass, Sliverman and Nickman, 1996). Memories and mementos provide ways to maintain a connection with the baby. This means that whatever tokens of remembrance are available, such as photographs from the ultrasound scan, name bands from delivery or the blanket in which the baby was wrapped, may become important family treasures kept in memory books or boxes. Similarly, family conversations maintain the place of the baby in the family. Pip felt that *'Grandparents have a role in remembering to remember. It is the acknowledgement that is important to me.'*(Dent and Stewart, 2004). For parents who have had a miscarriage or a stillborn baby, there may be few tokens of remembrance and only a few people, such as their midwife, who knew their baby.

Parents' stories often highlight the importance of family and friends offering support in various forms, such as listening, being with or helping out (Malacrida, 1998; Martin, 1998; Moulder, 2001). However, such support may be limited when a pregnancy miscarries or a baby dies in hospital because their life and death is not known and visible to other people. Parents may grieve intensively yet their pain may not be recognised or supported by others, thus their grief is disenfranchised and intensified, as Doka (1989) discussed. One mother commented:

'It's a horrible, lonely experience. My sister's baby died the same month and she got all the family sympathy because we all knew the baby – it was real to all of us. My baby was real to me and my partner.' (Moulder, 2001)

The death of a baby has the potential to shatter lives and requires people to find a way to reconstruct a view of the world that they can live with. Rose's story illustrates that this may take years of intense thought and activity. For some parents this may include telling and re-telling the story of their baby's death to adjust to the changed reality (Malacrida, 1998; Martin, 1998). This changed view of reality is informed by previous experiences. Donald identified that the deaths of his brother, and his father, contributed to how he grieved for his daughter, Gracie.

'I think, for everybody, coming to terms with it is the big one. I mean, grief for everybody is different but it is being able to talk about it afterwards. As a family, we are getting better at grief.' (Dent and Stewart, 2004)

There have been various theories about the purpose and process of grief after the death of a significant other (Parkes, 1972; Worden, 1991) and more recently, attention has focused on the struggles that people face to reconstruct a changed view of reality (Neimeyer, 2001). Attig (2001) describes this view of grief as a *'transition from loving in presence to loving in absence. And we reweave that lasting love into the larger, richly complex fabric of our lives.'* This is apparent in the stories of many parents who ask:

- *'How do I make sense of this in my life?'*
- *'Why did it happen to me?'*
- *'What is the meaning of life?'*

Some parents, like Rose, find a meaning or a purpose for the death. Others, as Martin (1998) describes, continue to 'search for reason'. It also means that the meaning of a death will differ for individuals. For example, miscarriage can have varying meanings for parents. The meaning is linked to the parent-child relationship, which develops with varying intensity during pregnancy for most mothers and many fathers. For some parents, a miscarriage may not represent a distressing loss. One mother who miscarried at 17 weeks after 7 weeks of bleeding, described her experience:

'It was relief rather than grief. I don't think I ever grieved for it. I wasn't even aware that I was carrying a baby. I never got upset about it at all. I shed no tears and I normally cry quite easily.' (Moulder, 2001)

Finally, the meaning that parents construct around the death of their baby may shape the way in which they approach a further pregnancy. This includes whether or not to try to conceive, and the feelings of uncertainty that can remain throughout the pregnancy. Rose described her pregnancy, with Nathan, after Ruby's death:

'I had an uncomplicated pregnancy (physically), but emotionally I was torn. I really longed to have this baby but I was scared of another "failure". I often ignored the fact that I was pregnant and I often think that I short-changed Nathan by not being as involved in the pregnancy. (Dent and Stewart, 2004).

Midwives supporting bereaved parents

Parents comment positively and negatively about the support they received from health professionals at the time of their baby's death (Dent et al, 1996; Moulder, 2001; Paton, Wood, Bor and Nitsun, 1999). In addition, there may be very limited (if any) follow-up support for families after miscarriage (Moulder, 2001). The challenge facing many midwives is having both the time to provide follow-up support and, as Gardner (1999) found, gaining the knowledge and confidence to support bereaved parents.

The words from parents in this article illustrate that their grief is deep, intense, individual and long lasting. This diversity precludes having a standard approach to care since what may assist one parent to grieve may not help another. This is discussed in recent reviews (Chambers and Chan, 2004; Hughes, Turton Hopper and Evans, 2002; Radestead, Stenieck, Nordin and Sjogren, 1996).

Consequently, we believe that midwives need to listen to the stories of families, and to critically appraise research in order to consider how to plan their practice to care for particular parents, in particular circumstances at a particular time point in their grief. In Figure 1, we offer some considerations for practice.

Further reading for nurses and midwives

About death of a baby

Faldet R, & Fitton K (Eds) 1997 *Our stories of miscarriage.* Minneapolis: Fairview Press
Hey V, Itzen C, Saunders L, & Speakman M 1996 *Hidden loss.* London: The Women's Press
Hill S 1989 *Family.* (1st ed) London: Penguin
Radestad I 2000 *When a meeting is also farewell.* Cheshire, UK: Books for Midwives.

Table 6.5.1 Caring for bereaved families over time

Care and compassion are key elements. Do you have these qualities?
Offer yourself as a fellow human being, listening carefully and actively. Remember that your body language will convey what you are thinking.
Message of grief. Recognise that the pain of grief cannot be taken away; there are no instant solutions.
Plan family care with the parents to include surviving children and grandparents, where appropriate.
Arrange a case conference, if appropriate, with all the professionals involved with the death to assess and plan future care of the family.
Seek help, if possible, if you feel overwhelmed or out of your depth. Who can you go and talk to?
Supervision or workplace support should be available to you. Do you have sufficient time to debrief and learn from each situation?
Identify stressors in the family, as perceived by the parents at each visit, and work to reduce these whenever possible.
Offer regular visits and ensure that family members know where to contact voluntary bereavement agencies and mutual help groups.
Never make assumptions about the experience of bereaved family members. So avoid platitudes such as 'I know just how you feel'. (Dent and Stewart, 2004)

About parental bereavement following death of a child

Riches G, Dawson P 2000 *An Intimate loneliness: supporting bereaved parents and siblings.* Open University Press, Buckingham, UK
Rosenblatt P 2000 *Parent Grief: narratives of loss and relationship.* Brunner/Mazel, Philadelphia

Acknowledgements

We remember and acknowledge babies who have died. In particular, the babies of parents whose words we are grateful to be able to include in this article.

REFERENCES

Attig T 2001 Relearning the world: making and finding meanings. In: R Neimeyer (Ed) Meaning reconstruction and the experience of loss. Washington, American Psychological Association, 33-54
Chambers H, & Chan FY 2004 Support for women/families after perinatal death (Cochrane Review). The Cochrane Library (3). Chichester, John Wiley & Sons Ltd
Cooper D 1997 Lily in the garden: Excerpts from a journal. In: R Faldet & K Fitton (Eds) Our stories of miscarriage (pp.21-25). Minneapolis, Fairview Press
Dent A, Condon L, Blair P, & Fleming PF 1996 A study of bereavement care after a sudden and unexpected death. Archives of Disease in Childhood, 74, 522-526
Dent A, Stewart A 2004 Sudden death in Childhood: Care of the Bereaved Family. Oxford, Elsevier Butterworth-Heinemann

Diamond A 1995 A gift from Sebastian. London, Boxtree
Gatenby B 1998 For the rest of our lives after the death of a child. Auckland, NZ: Reed Books
Doka K 1989 Disenfranchised grief. Lexington, Mass, Lexington Books
Finkbeiner A 1996 After the death of a child. Baltimore, John Hopkins Press
Gardner J 1999 Perinatal death: uncovering the needs of midwives and nurses and exploring helpful interventions in the United States, England and Japan. Journal of Transcultural Nursing, 10(2), 120-130
Hughes P, Turton P, Hopper E, & Evans C 2002 Assessment of guidelines for good practice in psychosocial care of mothers after stillbirth: a cohort study. The Lancet, 360(July 13), 114-118
Klass D, Silverman S, & Nickman S 1996 Continuing bonds. New understandings of grief. (1st ed.). Washington, Taylor and Francis

Kohner N, Henley A 1995 When a baby dies. London, Pandora

McGreal D, Evans BJ, Burrows GD 1997 Gender differences in coping following loss of a child through miscarriage or stillbirth: a pilot study. Stress Medicine 13 (3):159-65

Malacrida C 1998 Mourning the dreams: How parents create meaning from miscarriage, stillbirth and early infant death. Edmonton, Qualitative Institute Press

Martin K 1998 When a baby dies of SIDS: the parents' grief and search for reason. Alberta, CA: Qualitative Institute Press, University of Alberta

Moulder C 2001 Miscarriage: women's experiences and needs 2nd ed. London, Routledge

Neimeyer R 2001 The language of loss: Grief therapy as a process of meaning reconstruction. In: Neimeyer R (ed) Meaning reconstruction and the experience of loss. Washington, American Psychological Association, 261-292

Parkes C 1972 Bereavement: studies in grief in adult life. Tavistock, London

Peppers L G, & Knapp R 1980 Motherhood and mourning. (1st ed.) New York, Praeger

Paton F, Wood R, Bor R, & Nitsun, M 1999 Grief in miscarriage patients and satisfaction with care in a London hospital. Journal of Reproductive and Infant Psychology, 17(3), 301- 315

Radestad I, Steineck G, Nordin C, & Sjogren B 1996 Psychological complications after stillbirth - influence of memories and immediate management: population based study. British Medical Journal, 312(June 15), 1505-1507

Rando T (Ed.) 1986 Parental loss of a child (1st ed) Illinois: Research Press Company

Stewart A 2000 When an infant grandchild dies: family matters. Unpublished Doctoral thesis, Victoria, University of Wellington, Wellington, NZ

Stewart A, Dent A 1994 At a Loss: Bereavement Care When a Baby Dies. London, Bailliere Tindall

Stinson K, Lasker J, Lohmann J, & Toedter L 1992 Parents' grief following pregnancy loss: A comparison of mothers and fathers. Family Relations, 41, 218-23

Stroebe M, Schut H 2001 Meaning making in the dual process of coping with bereavement. In: Neimeyer R (ed) Meaning reconstruction and the experience of loss. Washington, American Psychological Association, 55-75

Thompson N 1997 Masculinity and loss. In: Field D, Hockey J, Small N (eds) Death, gender and ethnicity. London, Routledge, 76-88

Warland J 2000 The midwife and the bereaved family. Ascot Vale, Aust.: Ausmed

Worden JW 1991 Grief counselling and grief therapy, 2nd ed. Routledge, London

From Sudden Death in Childhood: Support of the Bereaved Family. Oxford, Elsevier Butterworth-Heinemann 2004

Life after birth

SECTION CONTENTS

The question of whether 'debriefing' after birth is valuable to women has been debated in midwifery literature for a number of years, and midwives and researchers remain divided on this issue. The first two articles in this section add to this debate. Firstly, Anne Hatfield and Elizabeth Robinson outline an initiative they have been involved with, where midwives take women through their labour experiences, providing a rationale for what happened during labour and birth in an attempt to reduce stress, morbidity and complaints. The review by Jenny A Gamble and colleagues then looks at the research evidence in this area, demonstrating that there is still much more to be investigated about the timing, content and duration of debriefing sessions and the effect of this intervention on women. Given the inevitable tension between the desire to ensure that treatments are based on sound evidence before they are implemented and the practical reality of wanting to offer services that are perceived to be helpful even in the absence of studies proving their effectiveness, I suspect this debate will continue for a while to come.

Where the value of early debriefing is still being debated, the value of early examination of the newborn is rarely questioned. Since Mary Mitchell's article on this was first published, even more evidence has emerged demonstrating the value of midwifery expertise in this area, yet her article remains one of the key pieces written about midwives' involvement in the neonatal examination, discussing the various approaches to this role and the difference that midwifery involvement makes for women.

The remainder of the articles in this section focus on breastfeeding. The question of supplementation for breastfed babies has been a contentious issue for many years now, and even a decade of the Baby Friendly guidelines, one of which suggests that nothing other than breast milk should be given without medical indication, has not put a stop to this debate. Sarah Hunt gets to the heart of one of the real problems with supplementation, where babies are given a large amount of cow's milk by bottle and are then unsatisfied by their next breastfeed. She suggests that, if supplementation is indicated, we need to consider physiology when deciding what quantity of supplement should be given, yet finds there is a lack of research-based information in this area.

Liz Jones and Andy Spencer consider all kinds of issues relating to breastfeeding preterm babies in their series of three articles. The first article looks at the composition, handling and storage of milk and the effect of the mother's diet on the quality and quantity of her breast milk, while the second focuses on the expression of breast milk. Their final article looks at how we can help mothers of preterm babies establish successful breastfeeding, taking into account the differences between the term and preterm baby (for example musculature and suckling) and the emotional needs of their mothers.

Another group of women who may need extra support with breastfeeding are those who have thrush (or whose babies have thrush). Jancis Shepherd's article offers an in-depth review of this area, both in relation to the care of an individual woman and baby and a review of the research and knowledge we have in this area.

The 'debriefing' of clients following the birth of a baby

Anne Hatfield, Elizabeth Robinson

Childbirth has a significant effect on the social, psychological and physical wellbeing of women and their families (Madsen, 1994). The role of the midwife is to support women during this period of adaptation, promote health and minimise the consequences when morbidity arises. Talking and listening to women following delivery may facilitate the process. Therefore, a debriefing service was set up in 1999 at QEQM hospital with the primary aim of improving quality of care. This article intends to explore the scheme in relation to the rationale for debriefing and its suggested value to clients, the professional role of the midwife and the hospital trust.

The scheme

A system of postnatal debriefing was introduced by one of the authors as the first piece of proactive work in her new role as Supervisor of Midwives. The aim was to enhance quality of care through contributing to the short and long-term health of clients (Lavender & Walkinshaw, 1998) with other benefits to the midwives and the trust. The context of this approach is set prior to or in the early stages of labour, when the midwife is encouraged to enter the care of a woman in the form of a 'contract'. Within this framework, the woman clarifies her wishes and expectations and the midwife identifies how she will respond. The experience, therefore, is a 'coming together' of woman and midwife on a mutual and equal basis, with responsibilities highlighted by both parties.

Before the inception of the scheme, the author presented a proposal in a unit meeting to doctors and midwives, outlining the rationale for its introduction and in order to set the scene for a discussion of the interview process. The medics wanted a written structured questionnaire to be used to obtain information from the women. The midwives wanted the interview to have a less structured, 'counselling' approach, to avoid what they felt could become nothing more than a 'form-filling exercise'. The consensus was that such an approach would not achieve the objective. It was decided to implement face-to-face unstructured interviews.

Any labour experience is dynamic and may require adaptation during its process by woman and midwife. The opportunity to talk and listen about the delivery experience takes place, therefore, within hours of delivery when memories on all sides are fresh. Women with their partners/birth supporters discuss with the midwife whether or not expectations have been met, to answer any questions or simply to clarify events. This may relate to any aspect of clinical, obstetric or midwifery care. It also enables the midwife to reflect openly with her clients on all aspects of practice and professional care which essentially will involve elements of her own performance. As such, she will be able to give a direct and early response to queries and concerns.

Such an approach requires self-awareness and good communication skills; a willingness to be open, listening skills, empathy, reassurance and expert knowledge; and evidence-based information-giving. Perhaps most difficult of all, humility must grow, because the midwife may hear issues of sensitivity through a client's criticism, no matter how constructive, when reflecting on her own practice with clients.

The interview content is clearly laid down for staff. The focus must include all aspects of clinical and personal care received by the client and her partner/birth supporters during the labour. This opens discussion about the rationale for any procedures and approaches to care which were helpful, unhelpful or not understood. The woman and her partner have the opportunity to explore their feelings about the birth of their baby, the positive and negative aspects of care and how it could have been improved. Additionally, the actual mode of delivery is discussed and time is allowed for questions.

Where complications have arisen, or there has been a need for delivery interventions, clients may need more time to recover and are debriefed the following day. The strengths and limitations of the process of communication between professional staff, which include the midwife herself and the client are explored; additionally, the professionalism of the midwife. The client's notes are available for scrutiny during the debrief. Any issues of concern which involve elements of care to do with other members of staff are followed up as soon as possible, in an atmosphere of openness. It is anticipated that reflecting on midwifery practice with clients will become a developmental experience for the midwife. As such, it may be included in any discussion of midwifery supervision and may form part of the midwife's professional portfolio.

The process and outcome of the debrief is documented in the client's notes for future reference. Such an initiative could provide a useful indicator for the purposes of audit and effective risk management (Charles, 1995). It is hoped that the need for complaint will be limited and that, should complaint arise, further evidence is available which will inform an appropriate and early response. The author has observed that since the inception of this scheme fewer complaints arise at this hospital. If such an outcome is proved, it could demonstrate a positive impact on resources, since inappropriate responses to consumer concerns can lead to litigation (Symon, 1998). However, cause and effect cannot be ascertained without proper evaluation of the service.

Discussion

There are pertinent questions to ask about the value of this provision. The rationale for debriefing assumes that midwives possess the basic counselling skills to undertake a debrief (Cutts). The unstructured interview using open questions and listening skills favoured by the midwives depends largely on interview skills. At QEQM, midwives have, for some years, been encouraged to attend basic counselling skills sessions and updates with the women and children's counsellor, who is herself a midwife.

The midwife may feel 'frightened' and apprehensive about taking such direct criticism of her management from a client, or she may approve of the scheme. Some midwives at QEQM have opted not to include this approach within their own practice. On other occasions, midwives may simply forget or be unable to follow through to debrief. It is also suggested by some staff, that the safe arrival of the baby generates a 'halo' effect, so that 'happy' clients will forget their concerns or queries (Holyoake, 1996). However, it is envisaged that in a climate of a trusting relationship openness will prevail.

The 'timing' of a debrief is worthy of further consideration within any evaluation of a scheme, whether it be within hours or months following delivery.

A response close to birth, it could be argued, might reduce stress, morbidity or complaint at a later stage. Moreover, it should not be forgotten that partners can be traumatised by even apparently the most 'normal' of birthing experiences, which may need resolution (Somers-Smith). The memory of stressful events can be 'buried'. Such suppression could lead to long-term mental health consequences which could resurface in later years for either partner (Samter et al, 1993). On a simpler level, clients may benefit from recapping on events to clarify issues which may, to professionals, come within the bounds of 'normality' – this could correct misapprehensions for the future.

Current approaches to the healthcare of women in the first year following delivery do little to uncover sequelae (Glazener et al, 1995). It is well documented that women tend to under report morbidity arising from their experiences. However, it is wrong to assume that the pain and distress of childbirth are quickly forgotten once the baby is born. Experiences may affect the short and long-term health of the client and family members (Creedy, 2000). Women will bring to their current pregnancies unresolved negative experiences and trauma belonging to previous pregnancies and births (Menage, 1996). Obstetric and gynaecological procedures for routine assessment and emergency can disempower women and cause emotional pain and psychological damage to them or their birth partners (Menage, 1995). Medical interventions coupled with levels of dissatisfaction with intrapartum care may elicit trauma symptoms (Oakley, 1980). At the same time, women who undergo a 'normal' childbirth could perceive elements of their care or experience as 'very distressing'. Additionally, adults may be the survivors of child sexual assault and other forms of abuse of which they are either consciously or unconsciously aware (Rhodes & Hutchinson). Adults, younger women and girls may experience continuing abuse across the spectrum. There is also the issue that within western societies, 'pregnancy and birthing' are not learned by children (Allen, 1999). Transferred from society and conferred to the sphere of the 'professional', 'birth knowledge' possibly comes too late for the primigravida or her helper. The lack of community support invokes a societal role on the midwife or doctor, by the mother who needs someone to listen to her. Additionally, rising consumerism and materialism have raised public expectations (Rossi, 1997) and women themselves aspire to physical safety and emotional fulfilment (DoH, 2000). Financial recompense is one course of action dissatisfied clients follow if complaints are not responsively managed (DoH, 1993). This can have a detrimental effect on the resources of a service. Furthermore, the current philosophy of care within the new NHS focuses on the ethos of health promotion, prevention and partnership with clients which demands a stretch or reconfiguration of resources (Capstick, 1994).

The literature identifies the potential serious nature of some types of trauma. Debriefing could contribute to emotional health problems (DoH, 1998). Where concerns are uncovered, can they be properly resolved for clients, or has the process of 'reawakening' compounded the problem? The greater the awareness, the greater the distress, it could be argued (Small et al, 2000). It has been highlighted that psychological morbidity is not affected by debriefing in relation to current practices, although in respect of trauma, early intervention may be effective (Kenardy, 2000). Moreover, adaptation to childbearing is affected by a range of variables outside of the event itself: the pre-existence of poor mental health, the presence of persistent, on-going stressful factors, personality and coping styles, individual perception, or a tendency to deal with the 'uncomfortable' by denying its existence (Kenardy, 2000; Lewin et al, 1999).

The factors involved in adaptation to childbearing are complex for each individual. It may be difficult to ascertain cause and effect in order to give an appropriate psychological response. It is also important that all women have the opportunity to discuss their birthing experiences. Postnatal assessment and management for women should focus on 'listening and talking' and practical help with feeding and handling all aspects of baby care and relationship, as opposed to the 'postnatal check' (MacFarlane, 1988). It is innovative that midwives are 'reflecting on practice' with their clients and links to supervision can be usefully made (Alexander, 1998). Good communication facilitates empowerment and enhances satisfaction (Kirham, 2000). At the same time this is challenging for staff and it may not be helpful for all staff. Professional and patient autonomy should be equitable in areas of sensitivity. However, good communication and early intervention could resolve issues and minimise patient complaint. Whilst early intervention is recommended in some literature, there are diverse opinions as to its efficacy in the maternity services (Wesley et al, 1999; Tomlin, 2000; Raphael et al, 1995). Additionally, the terminology of 'debriefing' requires clarification. Does it mean actual psychological debriefing, reflection or discussion? (Alexander, 1998) The existing provision at QEQM warrants further evaluation in order to clarify the scope of practice for patient wellbeing, the development of midwifery practice and risk management (NICE, 2001).

REFERENCES

Alexander J. 1998. Confusing debriefing and defusing postnatally: The need for clarity of terms, purpose and value. Midwifery, 14, 122-4

Allen H. 1999. Debriefing postnatal women: Does it help? Professional Care of Mother and Child, 9(3), 77-9

Capstick BJ. 1994. Risk limitation in obstetrics. In: Chamberlain G, Patel. The future of the maternity services. London: RCOG Press

Charles J. 1995. Addressing unanswered questions: Changing Childbirth. Update, 2, 2

Creedy D. 2000. Postnatal depression and post-traumatic stress disorder: What are the links? Birth Issue, 8(), 125-30

Cutts DE. Affective care: Rhetoric or reality. Australian College of Midwives Incorporated Journal, 6(7), 439-42

Department of Health. 1993. Changing Childbirth. London: HMSO

Department of Health. 1998. Making A Difference. London: HMSO

Department of Health. 2000. NHS National Plan. London: HMSO

Glazener CMA, Abdalla A, Stroud P et al. 1995. Postnatal maternal morbidity: Extent, causes, prevention and treatment. 102, 282-7

Holyoake D. 1996. Observing nurse-patient interaction. Nursing Standard, 12(29), 35-8

Kenardy, J. 2000. The current status of psychological debriefing. BMJ, 321, 1032-3

Kirham M. 2000. Reflection in midwives: Professional narcissism or being with women. BJM, 8(4).

Lavender T, Walkinshaw SA. 1998. Can midwives reduce postpartum psychological morbidity? A randomised controlled trial. Birth, 25(4), 215-9

Lewin TJ, Webster RA, Kenardy JA. 1999. A synthesis of the findings from the Quake Impact Study. Int J Soc Psychiatry Psychiatr Epidemiol, 32, 123-36

MacFarlane AC. 1988. The longitudinal course of post-traumatic morbidity: The range of outcomes and their predictors. J Nerv Ment Dis, 176, 30-9

Madsen L. 1994. Rebounding from childbirth: Towards emotional recovery. Westpoint, Conn: Bergin & Harvey

Menage J. 1995. Post-traumatic stress disorder in women who have undergone obstetric and gynaecological procedures. MIDIRS study day: Hot topics in midwifery. Hammersmith Hospital, London, 3 July

Menage J. 1996. Post-traumatic stress disorder in women following obstetric and gynaecological procedures. Br J Midwifery, 4(10), 532-3

NICE. 2001. Risk management; Clinical audit; Clinical governance. http://www.nice.org.uk

Oakley A. 1980. Women Confined: Towards a sociology of pregnancy care. Oxford: Martin Robertson

Raphael B, Meldrum L, McFarlane A. 1995. Does debriefing after psychological trauma work? BMJ, 310, 1479-80

Rhodes N, Hutchinson S. Labour experiences of childhood sexual abuse survivors. Birth, 21, 213-9

Rossi A. Transition to Parenthood. J of Marriage and the Family, 30, 26-39. Cited in: Littlewood J, McHugh N. Maternal distress and postnatal depression: The myth of madonna. 1997. Hampshire: Macmillan

Samter J, Braudaway CA, Leeks D et al. 1993. Debriefing: From military origin to therapeutic application. J Psychol Nursing, 31(2), 23-7

Small J, Lumley J, Donahue L et al. 2000. Randomised controlled trial of midwife-led debriefing to reduce maternal depression after operative childbirth. BMJ, 321, 1043-7

Somers-Smith MJ. A Place for Partners? Midwifery, 15, 101-8

Symon A. 1998. Involvement in litigation: Emotional responses. BJM, 6(7), 439-42

Tomlin M. 2000. Enhancing communication skills with the ENB R56 course. BJM, 8(4), 228-32

Wesley S, Rose S, Bisson J. 1999. A systematic review of psychological stress debriefing interventions ('debriefing') for the treatment of immediate trauma related symptoms and the prevention of post-traumatic stress disorder. In: Cochrane Library. Issue 4. Oxford: Update Software

A review of the literature on debriefing or non-directive counselling to prevent postpartum emotional distress

Jenny A Gamble, Debra K Creedy, Joan Webster, Wendy Moyle

Background: childbirth generates powerful emotions and may lead to the development of symptoms of depression, anxiety, and trauma in some women. Debriefing and non-directive counselling have been used as early interventions to reduce the prevalence of depression and post-traumatic stress.

Methods: a review of the literature was conducted to describe the current state of knowledge on the effectiveness of a single debriefing session or non-directive counselling session to reduce depression and trauma symptoms in women following birth.

Findings: a total of three studies reported in four papers examined the use of debriefing or non-directive counselling to prevent or reduce psychological morbidity following birth. The two largest RCTs indicate that a single debriefing session with the woman whilst in the postnatal ward is of no statistically significant value in reducing psychological morbidity and may even be harmful. In contrast, women reported that an opportunity to talk with someone about the birth was helpful in facilitating recovery.

Conclusions: there is insufficient evidence to draw conclusions about the effectiveness of debriefing following childbirth, primarily because it is unclear if a standardised debriefing intervention was used. Future research should clearly describe the intervention and test alternative interventions; measure a broader range of outcomes including trauma symptoms; use inclusion criteria that acknowledge the complex contributing factors to depression and trauma; and examine the value of including the woman's partner (or significant other) in the debriefing or counselling session(s). Future studies should investigate the timing or place of the intervention, the provision of more than one opportunity to discuss the birth, and target the intervention to women who are more likely to develop trauma symptoms or post-traumatic stress disorder.

Introduction

Childbirth can be associated with short and long-term psychological morbidity including depression, anxiety and trauma symptoms. Although the incidence of postnatal 'blues' and postpartum depression following childbirth have been extensively documented, there is developing awareness that some women experience psychological trauma resulting from birth. Common symptoms associated with postnatal depression (PND) and post-traumatic stress disorder (PTSD) are discussed in this paper and the current state of knowledge regarding the use of a single debriefing session (not psychotherapy) or non-directive counselling session, to prevent or reduce depression and/or trauma symptoms following birth is discussed. Limitations in the existing literature are identified and areas for future research are suggested. Symptoms of PND may include anxiety, tearfulness, inappropriate obsessional thoughts, irritability, fatigue, insomnia, guilt, fear of harming the baby, and reduced libido (Littlewood & McHugh, 1997). Loss of self-esteem and appetite disturbances have also been reported (Boyce & Stubbs, 1994). Various theories for explaining the occurrence of PND exist, including rapid hormonal changes after the birth (Dalton, 1980), difficulties in role adjustment, lack of social support, and difficult or distressing birth experiences (Green et al, 1990; Kitzinger S, 1992; Small et al, 1994; Fisher et al, 1997). There is some variation in the reported prevalence of depression, ranging between 9% and 30% depending on the diagnostic criteria used and the time frame over which the depression is measured (Boyce & Stubbs,

1994). In Australia, Astbury et al. (1994) reported rates of depression at 15.4% at eight months. Similarly, Brown and Lumley (1998) found that 16.9% of women had scores indicating the likelihood of clinical depression using the Edinburgh Postnatal Depression Scale (EPDS) at six months postpartum.

There is significant co-morbidity of depression and post-traumatic stress and both conditions share some of the same symptoms (Ballard et al, 1995; Friedman, 2000b). Conventionally defined, trauma responses are usually associated with survivors of disasters and combat. There is, however, a growing body of evidence indicating that trauma symptoms may develop as a consequence of childbirth experiences (Wijma et al, 1997; Creedy et al, 2000) and some gynaecological procedures (Menage 1993). According to the American Psychiatric Association (APA) (1994), a traumatic event has a number of characteristics. It happens suddenly and unexpectedly, it disrupts one's sense of control, and it disrupts beliefs, values and one's basic assumptions about the world and others (APA, 1994). The stressor is usually experienced with intensity, terror and helplessness. There may be a perception of life-threatening danger, with physical and emotional symptoms. In the immediate period after the event, the person may experience numbness, emotional release, express relief, anger, loss and concern, hyperarousal and intrusion of trauma stimuli. As a result of the perceived trauma, the woman may sense a loss of control over events, feel unsupported and become distressed. A traumatic birthing experience can overwhelm a woman's normal ability to cope with stress and carries the potential risk of intensifying into PTSD. After the event trauma symptoms may include flashbacks, nightmares, numbness, irritability, sleep disturbances, anger, being easily startled, hyper-vigilance (especially regarding the baby), avoidance of all reminders of the traumatic event, panic attacks, physiological responses such as sweating and palpitations when exposed to things that remind the woman of the traumatic birth (Horowitz, 1999). A recent survey by Creedy et al. (2000) found that one in three Australian respondents (167 out of 499) reported a stressful birthing event and the presence of three or more trauma symptoms four to six weeks postpartum. Nearly 6% (n=28) of women met the Diagnostic and Statistical Manual of Mental Disorders, fourth edition (DSM-IV) criteria for acute PTSD. The diagnostic criteria for PTSD are provided in Table 7.2.1.

The prevalence of PND and trauma symptoms provide the grounds for focused attention. The symptoms of PND or trauma are distressing and debilitating at a time when a woman has the extra demands of caring for her baby. Furthermore, the consequences of postpartum emotional distress can be

Table 7.2.1 Diagnostic criteria for post-traumatic stress disorder

A. The person has been exposed to a traumatic event in which both of the following were present:
- the person experienced, witnessed, or was confronted with an event or events that involved actual or threatened death or serious injury, or threat to the physical integrity of self or others
- the person's response involved intense fear, helplessness, or horror

B. The traumatic event is persistently re-experienced in one (or more) of the following ways:
- recurrent and intrusive distressing recollections of the event, including images, thoughts, or perceptions
- recurrent distressing dreams of the event
- acting or feeling as if the traumatic event were recurring (includes a sense of reliving the experience, illusions, hallucinations, and dissociative flashback episodes, including those that occur on wakening or when intoxicated
- intense psychological distress at exposure to internal or external cues that symbolize or resemble an aspect of the traumatic event
- physiological reactivity on exposure to internal or external cues that symbolize or resemble an aspect of the traumatic event

C. Persistent avoidance of stimuli associated with the trauma and numbing of general responsiveness (not present before the trauma), as indicated by three or more of the following:
- efforts to avoid thoughts, feelings or conversations associated with the trauma
- efforts to avoid activities, places, or people that arouse recollections of the trauma
- inability to recall an important aspect of the trauma
- markedly diminished interest or participation in significant activities
- feeling of detachment or estrangement from others
- restricted range of affect (e.g., unable to have loving feelings)
- sense of a foreshortened future (e.g., does not expect to have a career, marriage, children, or a normal lifespan)

D. Persistent symptoms of increased arousal (not present before the trauma), as indicated by two (or more) of the following:
- difficulty falling or staying asleep
- irritability or outbursts of anger
- difficulty concentrating
- hyper-vigilance
- exaggerated startle response

E. Duration of the disturbance is more than one month.

F. The disturbance causes clinically significant distress or impairment in social, occupational, or other important areas of functioning.

far reaching. Children of women who experience mood disorders can have long-term disturbances to their emotional, behavioural and cognitive development (Field, 1992; Murray, 1992; Sinclair & Murray, 1998). For example, two-month old babies of depressed mothers received less appropriate and less responsive care and more negative and rejecting care than those of non-depressed mothers (Campbell et al, 1992). Depression may also result in marital problems which, if unresolved, may lead to separation and divorce (Holden, 1991; Boyce & Stubbs, 1994). Importantly, acute PTSD and PND can progress to become chronic conditions which are disabling and difficult to treat successfully (Rothbaum & Foa, 1993; Brown & Lumley, 1998; Friedman, 2000a).

The case for preventing or reducing postpartum

Table 7.2.2 Details of the studies under review

Study	Design & sample	Intervention	Outcome measures	Timing of follow-up	Relevant findings
Hagan et al. 1999	RCTsingle blind 1745 English speaking women who delivered at or near term in alarge public hospital or a privatehospital. Not under psychological care at . time of enrolment	A single structured stress debriefing interview conducted by trained research midwife within 96 hours of birth	EPDS, Beck Depression Inventory (BDI), General Health Questionnaire (GQH-28). Depression assessed by psychologist blind to the intervention status. Mothers scoring >12 on EPDS plus a random stratified sample of those scoring <13 were interviewed.	2, 6, and 12 months	282/1745 (16.2%) were depressed. No effect of postpartum stress debriefing on the prevalence of depression 134/875,15% intervention group vs148/870,17% control [RR*0.90 (95% CI 0.71,1.1)]. No differences in EPDS, BDI, GHQ-28 scores at any assessment period between the groups.
Henderson et al.1998 Australia	A cohort compromising the intervention arm of the Hagan et al.RCT (n=872) Response rate 73% (n=628)	Satisfaction with intervention. Self-report Acute Stress Disorder questionnaire and detailed items on labour, birth feelings and expectations.		Satisfaction measured 2 – 4 weeks following discharge	67% (419) found debriefing moderately to greatly helpful. 25% (155) of women were moderately to greatly distressed by birth. 81.9% (127) of distressed women found debriefing helpful. 22% (34) of distressed women found exploration of feelings helpful.16% of non-distressed women found education about what to expect when they went home and support services more useful.
Lavender et al. 1998 UK	RCT 120 women single fetus spontaneous labour at term who gave birth normally to a healthy baby. 114/120 returned questionnaires (95%)	30–120 minute unstructured interview with research midwife during postnatal stay (after Day 2)	HAD scale	Questionnaire mailed out 3 weeks after discharge	Intervention group were less likely to have high levels of anxiety (Odds ratio 13.5, CI 4.1–56.0, p<0.0001) & depression (Odds ratio 8.5, CI 2.8–30.9, p<0.0001).
Small et al. 2000 Australia	RCT 1041 women who gave birth by C/S (n=624), forceps n=353) or vacuum extraction (n=64). Response rate 88.1% (n=917)	Debriefing session during postnatal stay conducted by trained research midwife	Maternal depression (EPDS), physical, mental and social health status (SF-36 subscales) measured via postnatal questionnaire	6 months postpartum	No difference in mean scores on EPDS or SF-36 sub-scales except for role functioning – emotional where women in debriefing arm fared worse, mean scores 73.32 v 78.98, t=72.31, 95% CI,10.48 – 0.84. Women reported that the debriefing was helpful 237/467 (50.7%) or very helpful 200/467 (42.8%).

* RR = relative risk

emotional distress is compelling yet in Australia most women are not routinely assessed for PND or psychological trauma resulting from birth (Webster et al, 2000) and many go untreated. The strategies used to prevent or minimise postpartum emotional distress have used social support, non-directive counselling, or debriefing (Holden et al, 1989; Oakley et al, 1990; Small et al, 2000). Because the terms debriefing and counselling have been used loosely in the literature to date, a description of the meaning of these terms is included in this review.

Debriefing describes a structured intervention that is intended to act as primary prevention to mitigate, or at least inhibit acute stress reactions not specifically related to birthing. Debriefing was developed separately by Mitchell (1983) and Dyregov (1989) and more informally by Raphael (1986). Mitchell's technique was called Critical Incidence Stress Debriefing (CISD) and Dyregrov (1989) referred to psychological debriefing. These two debriefing schedules were similar and in 1993 Mitchell and Dyregov jointly detailed a seven phase debriefing protocol designed to take place as a single group session within 24 to 72 hours after the event. The seven steps are as follows:

1. Establishing the ground rules of the debriefing session.
2. Establishing the facts of the event with individuals presenting the event from their own perspective.
3. Describing thoughts about what happened.
4. Discussing the emotions.

5. Reviewing the signs and symptoms of distress.
6. Providing information on stress reactions, the normal nature of the stress reactions the woman is experiencing, and specific techniques which may help to reduce acute stress reactions.
7. The "re-entry phase", in which participants raise questions, address issues in more depth or raise new issues. This phase can include future planning and advice on where to obtain further help if needed.

Debriefing has also been applied more flexibly in relation to the timing of the intervention in relation to the potentially traumatising event (Armstrong et al, 1991) and the number of sessions included in the intervention (Robinson & Mitchell, 1993). It is also commonly used with individuals as well as groups (e.g. Hobbs et al, 1996; Lee et al, 1996) or used as part of a package of interventions such as Critical Incident Stress Management (CISM) (Everly & Mitchell, 1997). Sometimes the term 'debriefing' is used loosely to describe a range of postbirth discussions and this has caused some confusion about the purpose and effectiveness of this intervention (Alexander, 1998). For the purpose of this review the term 'debriefing' means a structured intervention using the steps outlined above.

Non-directive counselling is sometimes referred to as 'listening visits' and has been used for both the treatment and prevention of psychological sequelae of childbirth (Holden et al, 1989; Charles & Curtis, 1994; Lavender & Walkinshaw, 1998). Non-directive counselling or 'listening visits', seem to consist of providing the woman with an opportunity to discuss her birth experience. It is led by the woman and is unstructured in nature. The counselling approach or responses of the midwife/professional are rarely explained in the literature. In this review, non-directive counselling is taken to mean an unstructured, participant-led discussion which is initially centred on the woman's perception of the birth. Active listening, reflection, and empathetic responses are skills used in the counselling sessions but it does not involve providing information or advice.

Methods

A search of the major databases (Cochrane, Pubmed, Cinahl 1982-2000, Embase, Sociofile, Psychlit) was undertaken to retrieve English language publications using search parameters that were specified at the outset of the review.

The search parameters were combinations of key words by which the relevant studies might be indexed. The key words used were childbirth or postpartum with post-traumatic stress disorder, anxiety, depression, trauma, stress, debriefing and counselling. Reference lists of all relevant articles obtained were checked and

additional potentially relevant articles retrieved. Informal contact with some experts and authors in this area assisted in retrieving conference proceedings.

Studies using any method of debriefing or nondirective counselling that was administered as a single session in the early postpartum period with the intent of preventing psychological morbidity postpartum were included in the review. The goal was to retrieve all research articles meeting these criteria that used any type of formally planned research.

We considered including in the review, research relating to other potentially distressing psychological events involving women, such as rape or gynaecological procedures. Although this research may have some applicability we were concerned that the larger volume of information on sexual assault would overwhelm the intent of the paper which is to focus on preventive treatments for emotional distress following childbirth. Studies into women's satisfaction with maternity services were also excluded if they did not measure postpartum symptoms of depression or trauma.

The material was critiqued by two researchers, summarised, assessed for content and tabulated using the following headings; study design and sample, intervention, outcome measures, timing of follow-up and relevant results.

Findings

Using these methods nine papers were retrieved. Of these, four articles that reported on the use of debriefing or counselling following childbirth were excluded. These excluded articles described innovative services that offered women the opportunity to discuss their birth experiences rather than evaluate an intervention (Charles & Curtis, 1994; Allott, 1996; Smith & Mitchell, 1996; Westley, 1997). They provide some evidence that women valued the service but were excluded because women's psychological morbidity was not measured and the women were seen at any stage postnatally, even years later. Therefore the intervention does not meet the criteria of being preventive of psychological morbidity. A study by Mauthner (1997) used a thematic analysis of the views of women who identified themselves as being depressed or recently recovered from depression to determine the helpfulness or otherwise of various factors. This study was also excluded because psychological morbidity was not measured and the study did not have a preventive focus. A study by Hagan et al. (1996) was also excluded because it provided more than one session and used a cognitive-behavioural therapy intervention (i.e. psychotherapy).

Three randomised-controlled trials that were reported in four papers were included in the review. Participants in the Hagan et al. (1999) study had their perceptions of the intervention reported separately by Henderson et al. (1998). Details of these studies are shown in Table 2. These three studies used a midwife to facilitate an intervention referred to as debriefing. In all three studies, the debriefing intervention was conducted while the women were in hospital following childbirth (Lavender & Walkinshaw, 1998; Hagan et al, 1999; Small et al, 2000). Outcome measurement was conducted variably at three weeks postpartum (Lavender & Walkinshaw, 1998), six months postpartum (Small et al, 2000) and serially by Hagan et al. (1999) at two, six and 12 months postpartum.

The outcomes of the two largest trials suggest that participating in a single structured debriefing session in the early postpartum period, prior to discharge from hospital, does not reduce the prevalence of depression or show improvements in health as measured by the EPDS, the BDI, the GHQ or the SF-36 sub-scales (Hagan et al, 1999; Small et al, 2000). One study showed that women in the debriefing arm of the trial fared worse in terms of role functioning-emotional on the SF 36 sub-scale (Small et al, 2000). The trial by Lavender and Walkinshaw (1998) showed reduced levels of anxiety and depression in the group of women who participated in a nonstructured interactive interview.

All of the trials had some limitations making it difficult to draw firm conclusions about the effectiveness of debriefing or non-directive counselling in the early postpartum period. In the study by Lavender and Walkinshaw (1998), the sample size was small (n=114) and determined on the basis of detecting a reduction in the proportion of women scoring above seven on the HAD scale. As the analysis was based on women who scored above ten on the HAD scale, the study may have had insufficient power to detect a true difference between the groups. Furthermore, the HAD scale has not been validated for use with postpartum women, and the levels of depression and anxiety in the control group were well above the norms for this population. Lavender and Walkinshaw (1998) referred to the intervention as 'debriefing' but explained that the intervention did not include in-depth questioning. However, the women participated in an 'interactive interview in which they spent as much time as necessary discussing their labour, asking questions, and exploring their feelings' (p216). Although the intervention was described as an interactive interview the intent of responses by the midwife conducting the intervention were not detailed.

The trials by Hagan et al. (1999) and Small et al. (2000) also failed to clearly explain the intervention used. For example, Henderson et al. (1998) report on the debriefing intervention used in the Hagan et al. (1999) study as the Maternal Individual Debriefing Schedule (MIDS). It is described as a structured discussion which 'allows the woman to tell her birth story in a supportive environment and includes an opportunity to explore her feelings about the experience, normalisation of those feelings and a brief educational component' (Henderson et al, 1998, p38). The exact nature of the educational component is not provided. Small et al. (2000) refer to the debriefing intervention saying women were provided with an 'opportunity to discuss their labour, birth, and post-delivery events and experiences' (p1045) and that the 'content of the discussion was determined by each woman's experiences and concerns' (p1045). In a later response by the authors to a letter commenting on the Small et al. (2000) study the intervention is described as 'active listening; reflection; encouraging the expression of women's experiences; accepting distress, anger and pain; being able to name and normalise the experience; and being able to avoid offering solutions' (Lumley & Small, 2000, p1470). Although these interventions contain some strategies identified in the debriefing protocol detailed above, there are also some steps missing and an overall different emphasis.

It is unclear exactly how the debriefing interventions in these two studies differ from CISD or any other form of debriefing or even how the interventions differ from each other. All three studies reviewed sought the participants' assessment of the intervention with women reporting that they found the intervention helpful, they were satisfied with the information they received and they felt better prepared for returning home (Henderson et al, 1998; Lavender & Walkinshaw, 1998; Small et al, 2000).

Discussion

The available evidence suggests that a single counselling session (referred to as debriefing in the studies) is ineffective in reducing symptoms of depression or improving general health as measured by standardised research tools. The findings of these randomised-controlled trials should be regarded with caution for several reasons. First, an exact description of the intervention has not been documented in any of the studies under review making it diffcult to know precisely what intervention worked or did not work. Secondly, the outcome measures do not match the intention of a debriefing intervention. Debriefing was originally designed to reduce trauma symptoms and prevent PTSD (Mitchell, 1983) yet in the three studies reviewed the outcome measures relate primarily to depression and not trauma (Lavender & Walkinshaw, 1998; Hagan et al, 1999; Small et al, 2000). Although there is a high prevalence of comorbidity of depression and PTSD it may not be accurate to assume that debriefing does not reduce trauma symptoms just because it does not reduce depression.

In light of the high proportion of participants who found debriefing helpful, it is possible that even though debriefing does not reduce postpartum morbidity using 'caseness' criteria of research tools, it does go some way to reducing emotional distress. Other studies support the idea that it is important for the new mother to be able to talk with a supportive listener (Reynolds, 1997). Experts seem to promote postpartum debriefing or 'listening' (Berg & Dahlberg, 1998) and see construction of the birth story as a useful postpartum activity (Affonso, 1977; Eden, 1989; Hillan, 1992; Creasy, 1997; Hammett, 1997).

Despite the problem of no specific documentation of the intervention, the two largest randomised controlled trials indicate that a single session in the early postpartum period does not prevent or reduce psychological morbidity and may increase problems. This finding cannot be ignored as it is consistent with the broader literature on post-traumatic stress debriefing (Wessely et al, 1999; Friedman, 2000a). However, there has also been criticism that these reviews included studies where the reliability and validity of the debriefing intervention had been loosely defined and methodological flaws were evident.

Several factors may explain the possible ineffectiveness of debriefing in reducing psychological morbidity. Women after psychologically traumatic births may be both shocked and numb (Kitzinger S, 1992). They may feel relief that they have survived and 'long to get back to normal'. Post birth, if the baby is well, the mother may feel that a complaint is unjustified or that she should feel grateful for the safe birth of her baby. Some women feel that they should be coping better or that is was their fault that the birth experience left them feeling traumatised (Kitzinger S, 1992; Allott, 1996). All these factors may prevent acknowledgement that there was anything amiss with their birth experience. The emotional numbness and social pressure to accept the birth experience with equanimity may render any attempts to debrief the experience within the first couple of days of the birth useless. In addition, the physical demands of labour and birth and the demands of caring for a baby may result in the woman feeling exhausted and unprepared to fully engage in a review of the birth experience within the first few postpartum days.

Other researchers have suggested that the process of psychological debriefing may not work because it does not allow sufficient acknowledgement of other factors integral to dealing with trauma such as social context, previous stressors, or coping processes (Raphael et al, 1995). Importantly, it may not facilitate a genuinely caring relationship between the woman and the counsellor. By trying to provide a one-off session the counsellor may in some way diminish the importance of this traumatic experience in the woman's life. A single session does not provide for on-going support and may reduce the perception by the woman that the counsellor is truly present and available for them (Kitzinger J 1992).

Future research

Future research should use a large representative sample of birthing women and clearly document the type of intervention used in sufficient detail for another professional to implement. It seems inappropriate to try and review the birth experience whilst women are still in hospital as they tend to be reluctant to criticise their care providers in the early postpartum period (Lumley, 1985). If they have had a difficult birth they may still feel overwhelmed and bewildered and Creasy (1997) suggests women need at least three weeks before they are in a position to formulate a 'birth narrative'.

To date, outcome measures have related to general health and depression. Women who may benefit from talking about their birth may be experiencing trauma symptoms and this should be a measured maternal outcome in studies investigating the use of debriefing. In addition it may be useful to measure anxiety and adjustment to the parenting role. Outcomes should be assessed at various points in time but the final outcome measure should not be earlier than three months postpartum, in line with DSM-IV criteria for chronic PTSD.

In the early postpartum period women are still vulnerable to distressing experiences, such as perineal pain, infections, and breast feeding problems. The additional problems may contribute to the development of a trauma response. Future intervention should reflect a more holistic view of birth-related psychological trauma. This should be reflected in the criteria for inclusion into the study and seek women's perception of the childbearing experience not just the labour and delivery facts.

Kendall-Tackett and Kaufman-Kantor (1993) suggest that there are four main dynamics of birth trauma: physical damage, stigmatisation, betrayal, and powerlessness. From this perspective, future research should test alternative counselling interventions aimed at assisting participants to critically review their childbearing experiences for the purpose of developing insights about what happened and why.

Other factors to take into consideration when designing future research into debriefing or counselling are the venue (home, hospital or clinic), whether it should be provided to the woman alone or include her partner (or significant other) or be conducted with groups of women (Alexander, 1998). If more than one session is to be provided the time interval between sessions needs to be explored. Research should continue into the effectiveness and acceptability of different types of practitioners providing debriefing.

The importance of preventing or reducing postpartum psychological morbidity is well established, however, the strategies for achieving this are uncertain. Whilst postpartum women respond positively about the opportunity to talk to an empathetic midwife about their labour and birth, there is insufficient evidence about the effectiveness of a single structured debriefing session.

REFERENCES

Affonso DD 1977 'Missing Pieces' - a study of postpartum feelings. Birth and the Family Journal 4: 159-164

Alexander J 1998 Confusing debriefing and defusing postnatally: the need for clarity of terms, purpose and value. Midwifery 13: 122-124

Allott H 1996 Picking up the pieces: the post-delivery stress clinic. British Journal of Midwifery 4: 534-536

American Psychiatric Association 1994 Diagnosis and statistical manual of mental disorders. Washington D.C.

Armstrong K, O'Callahan W, Marmar CR 1991 Debriefing Red Cross disaster personnel: the multiple stressor debriefing model. Journal of Traumatic Stress 4: 581-593

Astbury J, Brown S, Lumley J et al. 1994 Birth events, birth experiences and social differences in postnatal depression. Australian Journal of Public Health 18: 176-184

Ballard CG, Stanley AK, Brockington IF 1995 Posttraumatic stress disorder after childbirth. British Journal of Psychiatry 166: 525-528

Berg M, Dahlberg K 1998 A phenomenological study of women's experience of complicated childbirth. Midwifery 14: 23-29

Boyce PM, Stubbs JM 1994 The importance of postnatal depression [editorial]. The Medical Journal of Australia 161: 471-472

Brown S, Lumley J 1998 Maternal health after childbirth: results of an Australian population based survey. British Journal of Obstetrics and Gynaecology 105: 156-161

Campbell S, Cohn J, Flanagan C et al. 1992 Course and correlates of postpartum depression during the transition to parenthood. Development and Psychopathology 4: 29-47

Charles J, Curtis L 1994 Birth afterthoughts: a listening and information service. British Journal of Midwifery 2: 331-334

Creasy J 1997 Women's experience of transfer from community-based to consultant-based maternity care. Midwifery 13: 32-39

Creedy DK, Shochet IM, Horsfall J 2000 Childbirth and the development of acute trauma symptoms: incidence and contributing factors. Birth 27: 104-111

Dalton K 1980 Depression after childbirth. Oxford University Press, Oxford.

Eden C 1989 Midwives knowledge & the management of PND. The Australian Journal of Advanced Nursing 7: 35-42

Everly GS, Jnr., Mitchell JT 1997 Critical incident stress management (CISM): a new era and standard of care in crisis intervention. Chevron Publishing, Ellicott City, MD

Dyregrov A 1989 Caring for helpers in disaster situations: psychological debriefing. Disaster Management 2: 25-30

Field T 1992 Infants of depressed mothers. Developmental Psychopathology 4: 49-66

Fisher J, Astbury J, Smith A 1997 Adverse psychological impact of operative obstetric interventions: a prospective longitudinal study. Australian and New Zealand Journal of Psychiatry 31: 728-738

Friedman MJ 2000a Post-traumatic stress disorder: the latest assessment and treatment strategies. Compact Clinicals, Kansas City

Friedman MJ 2000b PTSD diagnosis and treatment for mental health clinicians. Cassell, London

Green JM, Coupland VA, Kitzinger JV 1990 Expectations, experiences, and psychological outcomes of childbirth: a prospective study of 825 women. Birth 17: 15-24

Hagan R, Pope S, Evans S et al. 1996 Maternal depression following very preterm birth. Paediatric Research 39:1584

Hagan R, Priest S, Evans S et al. 1999 Stress debriefng after childbirth: maternal outcomes [abstract A 84]. Third annual congress of the Perinatal Society of Australia and New Zealand. 95

Hammett PL 1997 Midwives and debriefing. In: Kirkham MJ, Perkins ER (eds) Reflections on midwifery. Baillière Tindall, London

Henderson J, Sharp J, Priest S et al. 1998 Postnatal debriefing: what do women feel about it? Second annual conference of the Perinatal Society of Australia and New Zealand 38 www.medrwh.unimelb.edu.au/PSANZ?Melbourne/program.htm

Hillan EM 1992 Issues in the delivery of midwifery care. Journal of Advanced Nursing 17: 274 - 278

Hobbs M, Mayou R, Harrison B et al. 1996 A randomised controlled trial of psychological debriefng for victims of road traffic accidents. British Medical Journal 313: 1438-1439

Holden JM 1991 Postnatal depression: its nature, effects, and identification using the Edinburgh Depression Scale. Birth 18: 211-221

Holden JM, Sagovsky R, Cox J 1989 Counselling in a general practice setting: controlled study of health visitor intervention in treatment of postnatal depression. British Medical Journal 298: 223-226

Horowitz MJ 1999 Introduction. In: Horowitz MJ (ed) Essential papers on post traumatic stress disorder. New York University Press, New York

Kendall-Tackett KA, Kaufman-Kantor G 1993 Postpartum depression: a comprehensive approach for nurses. Sage, Newbury Park

Kitzinger J 1992 Counteracting not reenacting, the violation of women's bodies: the challenge for perinatal caregivers. Birth 19: 219-220

Kitzinger S 1992 Birth and violence against women. In: Roberts H (ed) Women's health matters. Routledge, London

Lavender T, Walkinshaw SA 1998 Can midwives reduce postpartum psychological morbidity? A randomized trial. Birth 25: 215-219

Lee C, Slade P, Lygo V 1996 The influence of psychological debriefing on emotional adaptation in women following early miscarriage: a preliminary study. British Journal of Medical Psychology 69: 47-58

Littlewood J, McHugh N1997 Maternal distress and postnatal depression: the myth of Madonna. MacMillan Press, London

Lumley J 1985 Assessing satisfaction with childbirth. Birth 12: 141-145

Lumley J, Small R 2000 Authors' reply. British Medical Journal 321: 1470

Mauthner NS 1997 postnatal depression: how can midwives help? Midwifery 13: 163-171

Menage J 1993 Post-traumatic stress disorder in women who have undergone obstetric and/or gynaecological procedures. Journal of Reproductive and Infant Psychology 11: 221-228

Mitchell J 1983 When disaster strikes: the critical incident stress debriefing process. Journal of Emergency Medical Services 8: 36-39

Mitchell J, Dyregrov A 1993 Traumatic stress in disaster workers and emergency personnel. Prevention and intervention. In: Wilson JP, Raphael B (eds) International handbook of traumatic stress syndromes. Plenum Press, New York

Murray L 1992 The impact of postnatal depression on infant development. Journal of Child Psychology and Psychiatry 33: 543-561

Oakley A, Rajan L, Grant A 1990 Social support and pregnancy outcome. British Journal of Obstetrics and Gynaecology 97: 155-162

Raphael B 1986 When disaster strikes. Hutchinson, London

Raphael B, Meldrum L, McFarlane AC 1995 Does debriefing after psychological trauma work? British Medical Journal 310: 1479-1480

Reynolds JL 1997 Post-traumatic stress disorder after childbirth: the phenomenon of traumatic birth. Canadian Medical Association Journal 156: 831-835

Robinson RC, Mitchell JT 1993 Evaluation of psychological debriefings.

Journal of Traumatic Stress 6: 367-382

Rothbaum BO, Foa EB 1993 Subtypes of posttraumatic stress disorder and duration of symptoms. In: Davidson JRT, Foa EB (eds) Post traumatic stress disorder: DSM-IV and Beyond. American Psychiatric Press, Washington

Sinclair A, Murray L 1998 Effects of postnatal depression on children's adjustment to school. British Journal of Psychiatry 172: 58-63

Small R, Astbury J, Brown S et al. 1994 Depression after childbirth: does social context matter? The Medical Journal of Australia 161: 473-477

Small R, Lumley J, Donohue L et al. 2000 Randomised controlled trial of midwife led debriefing to reduce maternal depression after operative childbirth. British Medical Journal 321: 1043-1047

Smith J, Mitchell S 1996 Debriefing after childbirth: a tool for effective risk management. British Journal of Midwifery 4: 581-586

Webster J, Linnome JW, Dibley LM et al. 2000 Improving antenatal recognition of women at risk for postnatal depression. Australia and New Zealand Journal of Obstetrics and Gynaecology 40: 409-412

Wessely S, Rose S, Bisson J 1999 A systematic review of brief psychological interventions ('debriefing') for the treatment of immediate trauma related symptoms and the prevention of post traumatic stress disorder. In: The Cochrane Library. Update Software, Oxford.

Westley W 1997 Time to talk. Midwives 110: 630-631

Wijma K, Soderquist MA, Wijma B 1997 Post traumatic stress disorder after childbirth: a cross sectional study. Journal of Anxiety Disorders 11: 587-597

Midwifery 2002; 18: 72-79

The neonatal examination

A chance to provide health education and influence public health

Mary Mitchell

Within the first 24 hours after birth, every baby receives a detailed physical examination. The aim of this examination is to identify congenital abnormalities, to give reassurance and to provide health education advice to parents. This role had traditionally been carried out by junior medical doctors and GPs (Dunn, 2001). The provision and quality of this service has been much criticised in recent years (Rose, 1994; Walker,1999). Many aspects of the neonatal examination are controversial, not least the issue of who is the most appropriate professional to undertake it. Research studies have evaluated the screening component of the neonatal examination leading to a debate of whether the aims of the neonatal examination are met in reality (Hall, 1999). Indeed Walker (1999) suggests that midwives are in a better position to fulfil the aims of the examination. Hall (1999) argues that research should now concentrate on exploring issues of maternal satisfaction with the conduct of the neonatal examination.

In 1996, Michaelides first introduced the course to prepare midwives to undertake the neonatal examination. Now there are seven centres in the UK offering this course and the impetus for midwives to undertake this course continues. However, the controversies also continue. There is certainly a lack of empirical evidence that supports midwives undertaking this task, but the scene is changing and two research studies will shortly be published that have addressed this issue. The first is a randomised controlled trial of midwives and senior house officers conducting the neonatal examination (Dave, 2001). Preliminary findings have been reported at the Research and the Midwife Conference in April 2001. The second is a study which explored midwives' experiences of conducting the neonatal examination (Mitchell, 2001). In this study, midwives reported spending much time with women, providing information and advice during and after they had conducted the neonatal examination. The mothers gave very positive feedback to the midwives. They appreciated the time midwives spent meeting their needs, addressing practical issues and answering their questions. It is recognised that midwives are in a unique position to provide health information and promote health education. The findings of these two studies, as well as the government agenda to promote health (DoH, 1999; DOH, 1999a) have prompted this article. Midwives conducting the neonatal examination need to be aware of these findings and identify ways in which they can exploit the opportunity provided by conducting the neonatal examination to promote health. However, the message is not just for midwives who have obtained the ENB N96 course, but for all midwives involved in caring for the neonate, as this is a crucial time to influence events.

Crafter (1997) suggests that the time around birth is an ideal opportunity to provide health education for the improvement of health. She eloquently states

'The perinatal period presents a window of opportunity, a sensitive time when the mother and family, with the good of the baby at heart, and feeling the need to review their own way of life, are generally committed to improving their own health and that of their child.'

A variety of definitions of health promotion have led to many different interpretations of the processes involved. For the purposes of this article the term 'health promotion' is used to describe all those activities which are used to enhance positive health and reduce the risk of illness (Dunkley, 2000). Health promotion includes health education, which focuses on individuals and aims to improve healthy behaviour through sharing of knowledge and changing of attitudes (Ewles & Simnet, 1999).

Using the 5 stage model proposed by Ewles and Simnet (1999) it is possible to identify and clarify ways in which the midwife can promote health when undertaking the neonatal examination. However, there is no single right way to provide health education. It is important to recognise that women make health choices in the context of their social and family lives. Midwives must therefore acknowledge the influences on an individual's health behaviour, and modify their approach and advice accordingly. Knowledge of peer pressure, cultural norms and social inequalities will all affect how a midwife approaches this role.

Medical interventions

The aim of this approach is to prevent and rid people of medically defined disease and disability. Much of the neonatal examination is concerned with this medical screening. However, recent studies have highlighted failings in the screening tests employed during the neonatal examination. Failures to detect cataracts, undescended testes, congenital heart abnormalities and developmental dysplasia of the hip have all been reported (Abu-Harb et al, 1994; Jones, 1998; Rahi & Dezateux, 1999; Sarmah 1992). Midwives are in a position to enhance this aspect of the neonatal examination. Midwives place considerable importance on identifying congenital abnormalities whilst conducting the neonatal examination (Mitchell, 2001). They adopted a different approach to that of the GP or paediatrician in that they carried out the neonatal examination often over a period of time. For example, if the baby would not open its eyes they would return later to view the red reflex, or if the baby was fractious they would leave the hip examination until the baby was relaxed and quiet. This is viewed as good practice by Jones (1998) but it would be difficult for paediatricians or GPs to adopt this approach. Their lack of continual presence and workload would make this practice impossible. Midwives also reported auscultating the heart sounds on a number of occasions if there was any suspicion the infant was unwell. Although the NEST Trial (Glazener et al, 1999) failed to show any difference in a two staged check it would be reasonable to assume that auscultation over a period of time and in the event of worrying signs may contribute to identification of cardiac murmurs. On a number of occasions midwives detected abnormalities that had previously been missed by a doctor.

It is recognised that details of relevant history are often missing from records (Tappero & Honeyfield, 1996). Most of the women were known to the midwives and they were aware of their histories and pregnancy details. They supplemented the history in the notes by asking pertinent questions. This adds to creating a complete picture, which contributes to effective detection of abnormalities. Midwives were very aware of their responsibility in undertaking the neonatal examination and thus devoted considerable time and attention to completing this task in a way that maximised the opportunity to detect abnormality.

The behavioural change model

Using this approach, the health promoter seeks to change attitudes and behaviour. It is acknowledged that the change of behaviour is more easily achieved, but changing attitudes is very difficult to achieve (Scriven & Orme, 2001) although individual behaviour at this stage could be influenced. This approach would include giving parents information through the examination, which may lead to a change in behaviour in order to improve the health of their baby and themselves. For example, giving women advice on practices that reduce the risk of cot death, such as putting the baby to sleep on its back, has been shown to reduce the incidence of cot deaths (DoH, 1993). However, recent research highlights a need for improvements in this area. Roberts and Upton (2000) found that few women could remember all five of the preventative factors known to reduce the risk of cot death. Twenty-five per cent of women stated that they placed their infant to sleep on its back. Midwives need to ensure that women understand the full implications of the recommendations and help them develop strategies to implement them with their own baby. One of the most worrying aspects of this study was the high number (29%) of women who stated they smoked and the lack of advice they had been given on the subject. The midwife could expand on this advice and explain the importance of reducing the baby's exposure to other known risks of cot death such as passive smoking, and of the positive factors preventing cot death such as breastfeeding. Midwives should reinforce the smoking advice given in the antenatal period and give actively encourage mothers to stop smoking for the health of their baby. Power et al (1989) found that simple interventions such as this could help women to stop smoking.

The provision of breastfeeding advice that is appropriate and relevant to the individual will support the woman in her choice to breastfeed and assist in its continuation (WHO, 1998). When midwives conduct the neonatal examination they often utilise this as an opportunity to provide breastfeeding advice and support (Mitchell, 2001).

Education approach

There is much overlap with the approach already discussed. Midwives can also use the newborn examination to give the parents factual information about the neonate. Ewles and Simnet (1999) suggest that true educationalists will give the facts and information, laden with as few personal views as possible.

It is not appropriate to try and convince women that our health beliefs and values are the right ones. The midwife will need to be self-aware and have knowledge of how her own beliefs and values may affect the information she is giving. Burnard (1997) believes that self-awareness is important in learning to use ourselves as therapeutic agents. He suggests it helps to avoid stereotyping and making assumptions about others' beliefs and ways of life. Most parents want to do what is best for their babies but some may not adequately understand the baby's needs (Force, 2000). To promote the development of positive parenting the midwife can give information and demonstrate the abilities of the neonate. Parents are often unaware that their newborn can see, smell and recognise their voices. By becoming more aware of this, parents may learn to respond more positively to their infants, have a greater understanding of them and develop the potential to communicate better with their newborn.

Some midwives viewed themselves as role models, believing the way in which they handled the baby and adopted such practices as hand washing gave important messages to the women regarding parenting skills (Mitchell, 2001).

The empowerment model fits well here, where the primary aim is to develop the individual's ability to understand, cope with and influence factors affecting their and their baby's health (Piper, 1998). The midwife can give practical advice to assist mothers in adapting to their new role and assist them to draw on their personal strengths and resources to help with the transition to parenthood.

The client-centred approach

Parents often raise concerns during the neonatal examination. Midwives reported that mothers preferred to discuss their worries about such things as the umbilical stump, skin rashes and subconjunctival haemorrhages with the midwife, as they perceived that the doctors would not have the time to talk (Mitchell, 2001). They allowed the mothers to take the lead in asking questions and then used the questions as an opening to discuss health education issues such as the prevention of infection.

This approach could also be described as one of empowerment. Dave (2001) also reported that one of the significant factors related to higher maternal satisfaction was when healthcare issues were discussed. In this study, healthcare issues were discussed in 61% of cases when the examination was carried out by a midwife and in only 31% of cases when carried out by the SHO.

Midwives should be guided by the questions parents ask to provide information and in this way maximise the opportunity to address client needs. Michaelides (1997) argues that the newborn examination is a time for giving concentrated attention to the newborn in a holistic way: although it is a time when the midwife needs to concentrate fully on what she is doing, it is still also possible to communicate fully at this time with the parents.

The societal change approach

Midwives undertaking the neonatal examination may also contribute to wider public health issues. Midwives' contribution to increasing breastfeeding rates, supporting women in their decision to stop smoking, giving advice that reduces the risk of cot death and encouraging positive parenting will all have an impact on the wider society and influence public health for the better. Midwives who undertake the neonatal examination will be working as part of the multidisciplinary team and as such may be involved in developing policies and protocols and the provision of advice to primary care groups and trusts. Midwives who have undertaken the N96 course report that their skills in all aspects of caring for the neonate have improved and that they are often viewed as 'the experts' in neonatal care by their colleagues (Mitchell, 2001). The midwives also felt that the mothers viewed midwives as the experts in neonatal care.

Midwives can support the development of self-help activities and peer support groups, both of which have shown to be of value in sustaining behaviour change after a specific health intervention (Scriven & Orme, 2001). To help meet the government agenda to improve midwives' role in public health and to improve maternal satisfaction with the neonatal examination, midwives need to maximise the opportunity provided by the neonatal examination to provide health education. A variety of approaches can be utilised to this effect. Although in reality there is considerable overlap between the approaches, it is a useful starting point to illustrate the areas in which midwives can use their expertise and exploit the potential to provide health education and influence the health of the nation. Midwives are in an ideal position to influence health, as Dunkley (2001) suggests that health promotion is more effective at a level that is within the context of people's everyday lives. The evidence is emerging that midwives are the most appropriate professional group to undertake the neonatal examination and to fulfil all three of its aims.

REFERENCES

Abu-Harb M, Hey E, Wren C. 1994. Deaths in infancy from unrecognised congenital heart disease. Archives of Disease in Childhood, 71, 3-7

Burnard P. 1997. Know yourself: self-awareness activities for nurses and other health professionals. London: Whirr Publishers Ltd

Crafter H. 1997. Health promotion in midwifery: principles and practice. London: Arnold

Dave S. 2001. Maternal satisfaction with routine examination of the newborn: Preliminary results. National Conference on Research in Midwifery Paper. Birmingham, April 2001

Department of Health. 1993. The sleeping position of infants and cot death. London: HMSO

Department of Health. 1999. Making a difference: Strengthening the nursing and midwifery and health visiting contribution to public health. London: HMSO

Department of Health. 1999a. Saving lives: Our healthier nation. London: HMSO

Dunkley J. 2000. Health promotion in midwifery. London: Balliere Tindall

Dunn P. 2001. Examination of the newborn in the UK: a personal viewpoint. Journal of Neonatal Nursing, 7(2), 55-7

Ewles L, Simnet I. 1999. Promoting health, a practical guide. Fourth edition. London: Balliere Tindall

Force S. 2000. Establishing effective parenting: The midwife's role. MIDIRS Midwifery Digest, 10(2), 232-4

Glazener C, Ramsey CR, Campbell MK et al. 1999. NEST: a randomised controlled switchback trial of alternative policies for low risk infants. BMJ, 318(7184), 627-32

Hall DBM. 1999. The role of the routine neonatal examination (Editorial). BMJ, 318(7184), 618-20

Jones DA. 1998. Hip screening in the neonate: A practical guide. Oxford: Butterworth-Heineman

Michaelides S. 1996. A deeper knowledge. MIDIRS Midwifery Digest, 6(2), 197-9

Michaelides S. 1997. Midwifery examination of the newborn. MIDIRS Midwifery Digest, 7(3), 359-61

Mitchell M. 2001. Midwives undertaking the neonatal examination: an exploratory study. University of the West of England

Power FL, Gillies PA, Madely RJ et al. 1989. Research in an antenatal clinic: The experience of the Nottingham mothers stop smoking programme project. Midwifery, 5(3), 106-12

Piper S. 1998. The theory and practice of health education applied to nursing: A bipolar approach. Journal of Advanced Nursing, 27(2), 383-9

Rahi J, Dezateux C. 1999. National cross sectional study of detection of congenital and infantile cataract in the United Kingdom: Role of childhood screening and surveillance. BMJ, 318(7180), 362-5

Roberts H, Upton D. 2000. New mothers' knowledge of sudden infant death syndrome. BJM, 8(3), 147-50

Rose S. 1994. Physical examination of the full term baby. BJM, 2(5), 209-13

Sarmah A. 1992. Late diagnosis of cryptochidism: A failure of medical screening. Archives of Disease in Childhood, 67, 728-30

Scriven A, Orme J. 2001. Health promotion: Professional perspectives. Second edition. Basingstoke: Palgrave Publishers

Tappero EP, Honeyfield ME. 1996. Physical examination of the neonate. California: NICU

Walker D. 1999. Role of the routine neonatal examination. BJM, 318, 1766

World Health Organisation. 1998. Evidence for the 10 steps to successful breastfeeding. Family and Reproductive Health Division. Geneva: WHO

The Practising Midwife 2002; 5(5): 32-34

Breastfed babies

To supplement or not to supplement?

Sarah Hunt

Step Six of the WHO Ten Steps to Successful Breastfeeding (Gorab, 2000) states 'Give newborn infants no food or drink other than breastmilk, unless medically indicated'. To support this in the community setting, the Seven Point Plan directs that 'all providers of community health care should: have a written breastfeeding policy', and 'should: train all staff involved in the care of mothers and babies in the skills necessary to implement the policy'.

However, there seems to be a dearth of research-based information in the area of what to do when potentially breastfed babies need to be fed for clinical reasons, particularly when quantities of expressed colostrum are very small – a situation which is familiar to many midwives working on busy postnatal wards.

The reasons for breastfeeding failure in many cases may be partly caused by the increasing medicalisation of childbirth which often means that mothers request and receive pain relieving drugs in labour, and that skin-to-skin contact and the first breastfeed are delayed, thus missing the optimum time for initiating and teaching about breastfeeding. Women who have experienced long and difficult labours and births may not receive sufficient extra support from over-stretched midwives and healthcare workers to enable them to make up for the lost first feed, and the knock-on effect to breastfeeding failure is sadly an all-too-familiar scenario.

In addition, midwives and other health professionals may lack the skills and experience needed to effectively support breastfeeding mothers who are experiencing problems.

The effects on the initiation of breastfeeding of pain-relieving drugs given to women in labour are well documented. Rajan's (1994) summary of the research in this area in the 1970s and 1980s highlights the potential difficulties with initiating and sustaining breastfeeding that mothers who have received pain-relieving drugs or epidurals in labour may encounter. Rajan's own study on the impact of obstetric procedures and analgesia and or anaesthesia during labour and delivery on breastfeeding, further stresses the need for particular support to these mothers as they are more likely to encounter breastfeeding difficulties.

Similarly, Weetman (2000) highlights the particular breastfeeding difficulties often experienced in babies born to mothers who have received pethidine in labour. These babies may have skin-to-skin contact immediately after birth, and may be given every opportunity to breastfeed within the first hour after birth, but due to the depression of the suckling reflex do not feed successfully either at birth or for many hours afterwards.

Both Rajan and Weetman identify potential breastfeeding problems, and both recommend that mothers are advised antenatally about the possible effects of pethidine on breastfeeding. However, neither offer any very practical solutions, other than for midwives to identify these babies and to be particularly proactive in their breastfeeding support, teaching women to recognise when their babies may be receptive to feeding, helping women to position their babies in the best possible way and teaching hand expression of colostrum which may be offered to the baby by syringe, cup or bottle and teat.

And this is where the gap in the link to breastfeeding success may lie. There is no doubt that there will always be times when despite the best efforts of midwives and mothers, the baby needs to be fed and there is simply not enough milk. As Samuels (1999) reminds us, 'The mother is asking you to do something and that something is usually to give the baby a bottle'.

Not enough milk

For Samuels, cup feeding hand expressed colostrum or formula milk provides a stop-gap answer which has the advantage over feeding by bottle and teat that the baby will usually take a smaller quantity of milk.

We have all seen the case where a baby has been cup fed the 4mls of colostrum that her mother has painstakingly hand expressed, and then either because the baby remains unsettled or because we cannot believe that such a small volume can be sufficient, proceeds to wolf down 40 mls of formula milk from a bottle and teat. Not surprisingly, the baby then sleeps for a considerable period of time, and is then not satisfied at the breast when it is next offered, as the baby's stomach is expecting a considerably larger volume. For the mother, seeing her lovingly-produced colostrum does not satisfy her baby, and then watching it fall asleep for 4 or 5 hours afters 40 mls of formula, does very little for her breastfeeding confidence and can sound the death knell for breastfeeding.

Johanna Gorab, a lactation consultant, has also observed this phenomenon and suggests that a baby's stomach naturally expands as the milk supply increases, so that giving an unnaturally large volume at an early stage confuses the stomach and the baby will not feel satisfied with subsequent physiologically small volume feeds (Journal of Human Lactation, 2000).

Inch and Fisher (2000) recognise the physiologically small volumes of colostrum and breastmilk that are normal for the first few days after birth and suggest that in cases where there is a need for either additional or alternative fluids for a breastfeeding baby, banked expressed milk or 10% dextrose could be offered. Both these alternatives avoid the possibility of sensitising the baby's immature gut with cows milk proteins, but banked breast milk is extremely hard to come by, and there appears to be very little information on the giving of 10% dextrose to healthy term infants who require fluids where breastmilk is not available.

Inch and Fisher do not specify what quantity they suggest giving to babies or whether a baby is encouraged to take as much as it requires either by cup or syringe rather than bottle and teat.

So what quantity of alternative fluids should we offer to breastfeeding babies if there is a need to do so?

Available statistics indicate that an average breast feed in the first 24 hours after birth will produce between 7 and 7.5 mls of colostrum, with an average total intake over the first 24 hours of 37mls. These volumes increase to 14mls, 38mls, 58mls and 70mls per feed over the subsequent 24 hour periods, although this very much depends on the number of breastfeeds given.

While the quantity of colostrum in the first few days appears quite small, the stomach volume of a baby at 3 hours old is 30mls and at 4 weeks 70mls which explains why such large volumes can be tolerated by even very young babies (Henschel and Inch, 1996; Inch and Fisher, 2000; Minchin, 1998; RCM, 2002).

We should also be asking ourselves whether giving very large quantities of formula milk to any baby could be in any way implicated in the current epidemic of obese children and young adults and the corresponding rise in childhood diabetes.

It seems reasonable to suggest therefore, that if we are to offer fluids other than colostrum and breastmilk to babies, that we should be offering quantities which are similar to those that a baby would receive at the breast and that there should be clear guidelines for midwives to follow and clear explanations given to women.

More research needed

The new 3rd edition of Successful Breastfeeding produced by the Royal College of Midwives states 'There is no evidence that healthy term infants need fluid in any greater quantity than is made available physiologically', (RCM, 2002), but gives no further hint of where this evidence is gathered from.

More research is also needed into giving small volume feeds of water or 10% dextrose to babies who are temporarily not fully breastfeeding, to supplement the available small amounts of expressed colostrum, thus avoiding the giving of formula milk with its problems of possible sensitisation and its undermining psychological effect on potential breastfeeding mothers.

If we are to increase breastfeeding rates and duration, clear guidelines on how to deal with common problems in the early days of feeding are needed. There is research which clearly shows the benefits of early skin-to-skin contact and many babies are now routinely laid on the mother's abdomen immediately after birth (Renfrew, Woolridge and McGill, 2000). We are becoming better educated about how to recognise a good latch, and how to help mothers to position their babies to achieve the best possible latch.

However, we still struggle with babies who do not feed in the first few hours after birth, those who, for whatever reason, do not successfully latch on, and babies who do not settle after being at the breast. Instead of giving a bottle feeding answer to a breastfeeding problem by giving a large volume feed of formula milk, we should work towards a breastfeeding solution based on a physiological rationale for a breastfeeding problem.

REFERENCES

Gorab J. 2000. Supplementation in the Hospital Setting. J Human Lactation, 16(4), 294-5

Henschel D and Inch S. 1996. Breastfeeding: A Guide for Midwives. Oxford: Books for Midwives

Inch S and Fisher C. 2000. Breastfeeding: early problems. The Practising Midwife, 3(1), 12-15

Minchin M. 1998. Breastfeeding Matters. Australia: Alma Publications

Rajan L. 1994. The impact of obstetric procedures and analgesia/anaesthesia during labour and delivery on breastfeeding. Midwifery, 10, 87-103

RCM. 2002. Successful Breastfeeding. Edinburgh: Churchill Livingstone

Renfrew M, Woolridge M, McGill HR. 2000. Enabling Women to Breastfeed. London: HMSO

Samuels P. 1999. Cup feeding: How and when to use it with term babies. MIDIRS Midwifery Digest, 9(2), 215-17

UNICEF. The UNICEF UK Baby Friendly Initiative: a brief guide for health professionals.

Weetman J. 2000. Pethidine, difficult births and breastfeeding. Are these babies at risk? The Practising Midwife, 3(10), 18-19

The Practising Midwife 2002; 5(6): 20-21

Promoting successful preterm breastfeeding
Part 1

Liz Jones, Andy Spencer

Breast milk is species-specific and has been adapted throughout human evolution to meet the nutritional requirements of the human infant to enable growth, development and survival. Breastfeeding helps an infant to make the adaptation to an extra-uterine environment by providing protection against pathogenic organisms, for which active immunity will only be developed later in life. The immaturity of the immune system is profound in preterm infants, since the placental transfer of IgG to the fetus is shortened by early delivery. The autoproduction of many immune factors is also delayed, leaving the vulnerable neonate at risk of opportunistic infections. Although optimal nutrition for preterm infants remains controversial, many neonatologists prefer human milk as it is better tolerated and carries a lower risk for infection than formula feeds.

Protection against infection

Specific factors in human milk, such as secretory lgA., lactoferrin, lysozyme, oligosaccharides and growth factors may reduce the incidence of sepsis in preterm infants who are fed mother's own expressed milk (Goldman, Garza, Nichols et al, 1982; Mathur, Dwarkadas, Sharma et al, 1990; Goldman, Goldblum & Hanson, 1990). There is evidence that human milk may stimulate the functional maturation of the gastrointestinal tract and may stimulate the baby's own immune system. Enzymes, hormones and growth factors appear to play an important protective role in both gut growth and immunity. A large non-randomised study of hospitalised preterm infants reported that the incidence of necrotising enterocolitis (NEC) was significantly lower in infants fed at least some human milk, compared with infants fed formula (Yu, Jamieson & Bajuk, 1981). This study documented suspected cases as well as confirmed incidences, and in both circumstances the incidence was significantly greater in premature infants solely fed formula.

In another study, NEC when acquired appeared to be less severe and there was a lower incidence of gut perforation in preterm infants who had received human milk compared with formula (Covert, Barman & Domanico, 1995). Although these results provide some evidence that human milk may enhance the premature infant's host defences through local and systemic actions, the reasons for the protective role of human milk in NEC remain unclear.

Early postnatal nutritional influences on the growth and development of the human brain are observed through childhood. There is a maternal-fetal transfer of long-chain polyunsaturated fatty acids (LCPs) across the placenta in the third trimester. Eighty per cent of the LCPs present at term accumulate during this crucial period (Clandinin, Wong & Hacker, 1985). LCPs are essential components of cell membranes and are important in the developing brain and retina. Therefore, preterm infants are at a greater risk of deficiency. Human milk is a rich source of LCPs, and enzymes found in breast milk such as lipases facilitate lipid absorption. Therefore, LCPs are absorbed better from human milk than from preterm formula (Carlson, Rhodes & Ferguson, 1985).

Recent studies suggest that human milk may confer some neurodevelopmental advantage (Scott, Janowsky, Carroll et al, 1998) and ensure more normal retinal development (Hylander, Strobino & Dhanireddy, 1995) than formula, although it is difficult to exclude social factors in making this assessment. Preterm mothers' own expressed milk contains a higher concentration of direct-acting antimicrobial agents (secretory IgA, lactoferrin and lysozyme) than milk from mothers who deliver at term (Michaelsen, Skafte & Badsberg, 1990). In addition, preterm milk has higher concentrations of lipids, protein, sodium and calcium than term milk, which may help to meet the extra nutritional requirements of a preterm infant (Stein, Cohen & Herman, 1996).

Handling and storage

Preterm infants derive the most benefit from mother's milk, which has been freshly expressed with a minimum of handling and storage. This is because many immunological components become inactive after refrigeration and freezing and some nutrients are lost on exposure to light (Bates, Liiu, Fuller et al, 1985). Although the use of pasteurised donor, drip and unfortified term expressed human milks may be useful in initiating gastric feeds, they are nutritionally inadequate to support long-term growth in the very low birth weight infant (VLBW). Other detrimental effects of pasteurisation include the destruction of heat labile vitamins, the denaturation of bile salt stimulated lipase, and the reduction of some of the immunological components.

The composition of expressed breast milk is extremely variable. Lipids in human milk provide 40% to 50% of the energy requirements and are vehicles for fat-soluble vitamins. Lipids in human milk vary more than other components, showing both diurnal variation and increase during a single feeding from foremilk to hind milk. In addition there is a significant inter-individual variation (Hall, 1979). It is important to estimate the fat content of expressed breast milk through the creamatocrit method (Lucas, Gibbs & Luster, 1978) to ensure that both fore and hindmilk have been expressed in order to deliver a feed that is nutritionally adequate. It is also prudent to remember that lipids are poorly miscible, and separate from the milk, adhering to feeding tubes and collection containers. This may result in milk that is sub-optimal for infant nutrition. Bottles of expressed breast milk must be gently shaken before use to ensure the homogeneity of milk. When human milk is administered continuously or via slow infusion the syringe must be positioned to allow delivery of the fat portion first, as there is a risk of large fat loss.

Nutritional composition

When the nutritional composition of mother's milk approaches that of term mature milk the preterm infant is at increased risk of growth failure. Although well infants (>1500 g) may tolerate greater volumes, precluding the need for fortification, many preterm infants are restricted in fluid intake for various reasons.

If an increase in feeds is not feasible, another solution to overcome poor weight gain is to utilise high-energy hind milk in order to deliver a higher percentage of calories (Valentine, Hurst & Schanler, 1994). Hind milk can be obtained from a single expression by the collection of fore and hind milk in two separate containers. Fore milk can be defined as the milk collected for 2-3 minutes after milk begins to flow. Hind milk is the remainder of the milk collected by complete breast emptying. However, this will not remedy protein insufficiency and may not always improve weight gain (Spencer, Hendrickse, Roberton et al, 1982). Furthermore, if the mother is already producing milk with a high fat content, there is a danger of delivering too much fat, so the use of hind milk should always be monitored. The use of a breast milk fortifier may be necessary to ensure adequate growth.

A major concern with human milk fortificaton is whether the added nutrients cause either a reduction or a complete loss of some of the immunological components in expressed milk, leading to a reduced protection against infection. In a review of prospectively collected data on morbidity and diet in premature infants in Houston, Texas, infants fed exclusively on fortified human milk had significantly lower incidence of NEC and sepsis, and fewer positive blood cultures, than infants fed preterm formula, or a mixture of fortified human milk and preterm formula (Schanler & Oh, 1996). The infants in the exclusively fortified human milk group had more episodes of skin-to-skin contact with their mothers than those fed preterm formula.

Since one of the important protective effects of human milk on the recipient infant operates via the enteromammary immune system, skin-to-skin contact may be particularly important since mothers can be induced to make specific antibodies against the nosocomial pathogens in the neonatal environment. The researchers argue that the lower incidence of infection in the exclusively human milk group suggests strongly that skin-to-skin contact may be a means of providing species-specific antimicrobial protection for both term and premature infants. However, there is a need for a randomised controlled trial to assist in the development of a proper evidence base to test this assumption.

Effect of mother's diet

A mother's diet can affect both the quality and quantity of breast milk. Although it can be argued that in the United Kingdom it is unlikely that a mother's dietary intake in respect to energy and protein will be insufficient to adversely affect the quality of breast milk, inadequate vitamin intake is possible. The vitamin content of human milk is directly influenced by a mother's vitamin status, particularly in the case of water-soluble vitamins (Atkinson, 1992). Mothers on a strict vegan diet should be referred to a dietician to ensure their diet is adequate in respect to vitamin B12. During the last trimester of pregnancy there is a massive accretion of minerals. Unfortunately, even if a mother has an optimal nutritional intake, human milk may not provide an adequate source of some vitamins and minerals when an infant is born preterm.

In conclusion, human milk contains immunologic and host defence cells, which help to prevent the proliferation of pathogenic bacteria, reducing the incidence of sepsis in preterm infants. Enzymes, hormones and growth factors also play an important role in gastrointestinal growth and maturity. Since human milk may be inadequate on its own to promote optimal growth in infants born extremely preterm, it is common practice to supplement expressed breast milk with a commercial fortifier. Studies need to be performed to determine if the addition of fortification alters both the function and composition of milk constituents. When compared to preterm formula there is some evidence that the administration of fortified breast milk may provide substantial protection from infection for an infant born preterm. The potential stimulation of an enteromammary pathway through skin-to-skin contact also appears to be feasible as a means ot providing species-specific protection for preterm neonates. However, human milk can only be used to support the nutritional requirements of preterm babies if adequate volumes are produced.

REFERENCES

Atkinson SA. 1992. Feeding the normal term infant: human milk and formula. In: Sinclair and Bracknell (eds). Effective Care of the Newborn Infant. Oxford: OUP

Bates CJ, Liiu DS, Fuller NJ et al. 1985. Susceptibility of riboflavin and vitamin A in breast milk to photodegradation and its implications for the use of banked breast milk in infant feeding. Acta Paediatr Scand, 74, 40-4

Carlson SE, Rhodes PG, Ferguson MG. 1985. Docosahexaenoic acid status of preterm infants at birth and following feeding with human milk or formula. Am J Clin 44, 798-804

Clandinin MT, Wong K, Hacker RR. 1985. Synthesis of chain elongation-desaturisation products of linoleic acid by liver and brain microsomes during development of the pig. Biochem J, 226, 305-9

Covert RF, Barman N, Domanico RS. 1995. Prior enteral nutrition with human milk protects against intestinal perforation in infants who develop necrotizing enterocolitis. Pediatr Res, 37, 305A

Goldman AS, Garza C, Nichols B et al. 1982. Immunologic factors in human milk during the first year of lactation. J Pediatr, 100, 563-7

Goldman AS, Goldblum RM, Hanson LA. 1990. Anti-inflammatory systems in human milk. In: Bendich A, Phillips M, Tengerdy RP (eds). Antioxidant Nutrients and Immune Functions. New York: Plenum Press

Hall B. 1979. Uniformity of human milk. Am J Clin Nutr 32,304-12

Hylander M, Strobino D, Dhanireddy R. 1995. Human milk feedings and retinopathy of prematurity among very low birth weight infants. Pediatr Res, 37, 2114A

Lucas A, Gibbs JA, Luster RL. 1978. Creamatocrit: simple clinical technique for estimating fat concentration and energy value of human milk. BMJ, 1, 1018

Mathur NB, Dwarkadas AM, Sharma VK el al. 1990. Anti-infective factors in preterm human colostrums. Acta Paediatr Scand, 79, 1039-44

Michaelsen KF, Skafte I, Badsberg HH. 1990. Variations in micronutrients in human milk: Influencing factors and implications for human milk banking. J Pediatr Gastroenterol Nutr, 11, 229

Schanler RJ, Oh W. 1996. Fortified human milk improves the health of the premature infant. Pediatr Res, 40, 551A

Scott DT, Janowsky JS, Carroll RE et al. 1998. Formula supplementation with long-chain polyunsaturated fatty acids: are there developmental benefits? Pediatr, 102, E59

Spencer SA, Hendrickse W, Roberton D et al. 1982. Energy intake and weight gain of very low birth weight babies fed raw expressed breast milk. BMJ, 285, 924-6

Stein H, Cohen D, Herman A. 1996. Pooled pasteurized breast milk and untreated own mother's milk in the feeding of very low birth weight babies: a randomised controlled trial. Pediatr Gastroenterol Nutr, 5, 241-7

Valentine C, Hurst N, Schanler R. 1994. Hindmilk and weight gain in LBW infants. J Pediatr Gastroenterol Nutr 18, 4

Yu VY, Jamieson J, Bajuk B. 1981. Breast milk feeding in very low birthweight infants. Aust Paediatr J 186-90

The Practising Midwife 2002; 5(4): 18-20

Promoting successful preterm breastfeeding
Part 2

Liz Jones, Andy Spencer

The mother who chooses to breastfeed her acutely ill premature baby experiences many needs and problems that clearly distinguish her from the mother who breastfeeds a healthy term infant (Meier & Brown, 1996).

The immediate period following preterm birth is a time of extreme anxiety and stress for parents. The initiation of lactation may be delayed, since many mothers have experienced Caesarean deliveries or may be very ill in the immediate postpartum period due to obstetric complications. In addition, the initiation of an expression schedule may be difficult to achieve since it may necessitate a strong commitment to the future that is impossible to make.

Furthermore, prolactin bioactivity is significantly less in mothers who deliver prematurely, suggesting deficiencies in the initial stimulus for milk production (Ellis & Picciano, 1993). Poor initial milk production which then declines is common in these women (Hopkinson, Schanler & Garza, 1988). Despite desperately wishing to provide breast milk for their ill baby, many women face mammary involution within several weeks of preterm delivery. Mothers of preterm infants experience both physiological and emotional challenges that are beyond the scope of a term breastfeeding programme. The provision of uniform, research-based information and specialist advice should be the 'standard of care' for all mothers who wish to breastfeed their preterm infant (Neifert & Seacat, 1988).

Manual expression

Mothers dependent on the manual expression of milk to sustain lactation should express as soon as possible following delivery and continue to do so regularly throughout the day. Initially, milk volume is hormonally driven, and mothers should express frequently in order to ensure the sensitisation of prolactin receptors. However, 30-60 hours following delivery, maternal milk volume is directly related to the frequency and quality of milk removal (Prentice & Wilde, 1989).

The advice given to mothers on the frequency of expression must be based on the stage of lactation and the storage capacity of the breast. It is extremely important that the initial milk expression sessions are supervised, to ensure that mothers understand the principles of milk expression and that pump assembly and expression technique is quickly understood and mastered.

Breast pumps

It is important to understand that a breast pump does not suck or pull milk out of the breast. When oxytocin is released, the myoepithelial cells contract, and as milk fills the available space into the alveoli, intra-mammary pressure rises. Oxytocin then reduces resistance to the outflow of milk from the alveoli, by shortening and widening the ducts, thus allowing the internal pressure of the breast to push milk out.

At first, the milk ejection reflex is unconditioned, but it quickly becomes conditioned and as such can become inhibited by stress, sore nipples and other worries. Unless the oxytocin response is elicited, milk flow will be compromised and mothers will be tempted to use excess suction to try to tease more milk out. This will lead to sore nipples, and a declining milk supply.

Breast massage

Massage should be used to elicit the milk ejection reflex before milk expression is performed. Both oxytocin and prolactin respond favourably to tactile stimulation. It is also apparent that prolactin is complementary to oxytocin release, with levels rising sharply, coinciding with milk ejection. Prolactin is not inhibited by maternal stress, although the mechanisms underlying prolactin release are poorly understood. When mothers on our

Neonatal Unit were asked about techniques to improve milk flow, the two most frequently mentioned were nipple and breast massage. The technique of breast massage involves gentle tactile stimulation of mammary and nipple tissue using a hand action that rolls the knuckles downward over the breast, beginning at the ribs and working towards the areola. This technique does not involve manual expression of milk (Lang, 1997).

Expression technique

The technique of milk expression is also very important. Women should be advised to sit comfortably with a straight back. Before positioning the milk collection set, it may help to support the breast from underneath, with fingers flat on the ribs and the index finger at the junction of the breast and ribs. This will support the breast tissue forward into the funnel, which should be placed with the nipple central. The funnel should be held close enough to mammary tissue to obtain a patent seal, but not so firmly to the breast that the milk flow is inhibited.

Milk collection sets should be measured to the size and shape of individual mothers, since women with large or wide nipples may have difficulty with a set that has a small opening or narrow slope. Unless a collection set is used which fits the anatomical configuration of the breast, milk drainage will be compromised, leading to maternal engorgment and a decrease in milk production. Mothers will also complain of sore nipples and there will be an increase in the incidence of mastitis.

In a randomised controlled trial performed by the authors to compare methods of milk expression following preterm birth (Jones, Dimmock & Spencer, 2001) there was disparity between breast and collection set sizes in ten cases. Large glass funnels can be purchased in the UK from Central Medical Supplies, Leek, Staffordshire.

Obstetric complications

Although premature birth does not appear to inhibit the initiation of lactation, several factors arising from obstetric complications do – prolonged bed rest, low maternal haemoglobin, postpartum haemorrhage, fatigue, stress, low prolactin bioactivity and irregular milk expression.

All available literature supports the practice of early milk removal to promote the development of prolactin receptors (DeCarvalho, 1983).

Studies suggest that there may be a 'critical period' early in lactation during which the breasts must be emptied to assure a sufficient volume (Zuppa, 1988). A faltering milk supply in the following weeks may be attributed to the lack of sufficient prolactin receptors and infrequent breast stimulation while lactation is being established. The relationship between prolactin release and quantitative milk yield is unclear.

The prevention of secondary engorgement is also crucial to lactation success. As alveolar pressure rises, with subsequent milk stasis, lactation suppression begins. When milk production begins in the absence of a baby, pumping frequency may need to be temporarily increased to prevent involution of the alveoli caused by the back-up pressure of milk on the build up of suppressor peptides, which down-regulate milk volume. Although the breast is under hormonal control initially, the regulation of milk volume switches to autocrine control with the arrival of transitional milk 30-60 hours following birth (Daly & Hartmann, 1995).

Advice given to mothers regarding milk expression should address the fact that volume is directly related to the frequency of removal, the degree of breast emptying and the storage capacity of the breast. Advice must be individually tailored.

Ejection triggers

The key to a sustainable milk supply can be found in triggering milk ejection. Simultaneous milk expression is the most efficient way to capitalise on the rapid transfer of milk following milk ejection, by removing milk as soon as it flows from the alveolar spaces into the ducts. In this way, the breast and the pump work together, facilitating breast emptying.

In a randomised-controlled trial performed by the authors on the Neonatal Unit at North Staffordshire

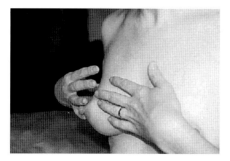
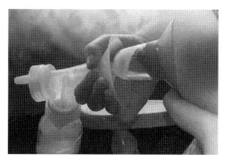
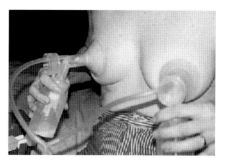

Hospital, milk weight in grams was compared between non-breastfeeding mothers of preterm infants, who used either sequential or simultaneous pumping for 4 days (Jones, Dimmock & Spencer, 2001). The fat content of expressed milk was also evaluated.

The effect of breast massage and non-massage on milk weight and energy yield was also compared, using each mother as her own control. Mothers who used simultaneous pumping produced significantly higher milk yields than those who used sequential pumping (P = <0.01) on all four days of the trial. Breast massage versus non-massage was also significant at the P = <0.01 level.

Fat concentration was similar between all groups. The time taken to express was less in the simultaneous group. In cases of prolonged milk expression the difference in time commitment may have an influence on a mother's willingness to continue to express her milk.

Decreasing volume

The phenomenon of a deceasing milk volume, especially during the second month of milk expression, has not been examined. Recent studies examining milk volume in term lactation have suggested that milk volume is limited by infant demand rather than by a finite capacity of a mother to produce milk (Hurst, Valentine & Renfro, 1997).

The increased difficulties that mothers of preterm infants experience regarding prolonged milk expression appear to point to the fact that a breast pump cannot mimic an infant's responsiveness, which might be a prerequisite for the optimal long-term regulation of milk volume. Therefore, encouraging skin-to-skin contact may represent the only realistic intervention available in preventing insufficient milk volume.

Conclusion

In conclusion, time must be spent with mothers in the immediate post-partum period to ensure that they understand both the principles and the technique of milk expression. The creamatocrit technique (Lucas et al, 1978) is extremely helpful in terms of milk quality surveillance. The healthcare professional and the mother need to evaluate both the quantity and quality of mother's milk at no later than one week postpartum to determine if intervention is needed to ensure an adequate supply of milk to feed the preterm infant at discharge is available.

Frequent and complete removal of milk will enhance milk production, although advice on the frequency of expression should also be tempered with knowledge of mammary storage capacity.

The use of simultaneous pumping and breast massage will also maximise lactation success, ensuring that the breast and the pump work together and that the time needed to express is substantially reduced.

Skin-to-skin contact between mother and baby should also be encouraged on a daily basis until breastfeeding is fully established. The transition from naso-gastric feeding to preterm breastfeeding is a complex process and requires highly skilled support.

In our next article (page 215), we will be discussing positive ways to manage and support the establishment of successful preterm breastfeeding.

REFERENCES

Daly SEJ, Hartmann PE. 1995. Infant demand and milk supply (1): Infant demand and milk production in lactating women. J Hum Lact, 11, 21-6

DeCarvalho MD. 1983. Effect of frequent breastfeeding on early milk production and infant weight gain. Pediatr, 72, 307-11

Ellis L, Picciano M. 1993. Prolactin variants in term and preterm human milk: Altered structural characteristics, biological activity and immunoreactivity. Endocrine Reg, 27, 181-92

Hopkinson J, Schanler R, Garza C. 1988. Milk production by mothers of premature infants. Pediatr, 81, 315-20

Hurst N, Valentine C, Renfro L. 1997. Skin-to-skin holding in the neonatal intensive care influences maternal milk volume. J Perinataol, 17, 213-7

Jones E, Dimmock PW, Spencer SA. 2001. A randomised controlled trial to compare methods of milk expression after preterm delivery. Arch Dis Child, 85, F91-5

Lang S. 1997. Breastfeeding Special Care Babies. London: Balliere Tindall

Lucas A, Gibbs JA, Luste RL. 1978. Creamatocrit: simple clinical technique for estimating fat concentration and energy value of human milk. BMJ, 1, 1018

Meier P, Brown L. 1996. State of the science: breastfeeding for mothers and low birth weight infants. Nurs Clin North Am, 31, 351-65

Neifert MM, Seacat J. 1988. Practical aspects of breastfeeding the premature infant. Perin Neonatol, 12, 24-30

Prentice A, Wilde J. 1989. Evidence for local feedback control of human milk secretion. Biochem Soc Trans, 17, 489-92

Zuppa A. 1988. Relationship between maternal parity, basal prolactin levels and neonatal breast milk intake. Biol Neonate, 53, 14-47

Establishing successful preterm breastfeeding
Part 3

Liz Jones, Andy Spencer

Following neonatal admission to the Neonatal Intensive Care Unit, we encourage parents of preterm infants to touch and caress their tiny babies as soon as possible. When an infant's physical condition is stable, skin-to-skin contact 'kangaroo fashion' is facilitated. Skin-to-skin contact can be achieved even with a ventilated infant. This helps a mother to gain confidence in handling her tiny infant and provides an opportunity via the enteromammary pathway for mothers to make specific antibodies against the nosocomial pathogens in the neonatal environment (Hurst, Valentine & Renfro, 1997). When an infant no longer requires ventilation or continuous positive airway pressure (CPAP) and is haemodynamically stable, breastfeeding can commence.

Mothers must be supported and guided by neonatal staff during early breastfeeds. An under-arm breastfeeding position works very well, since the baby's body can be coaxed into a position of flexion; an attitude that for the preterm baby will help to promote a coordinated oral response. Hyperextension of the neck during feeding should also be corrected, since it reduces jaw stability, increases cheek retraction and reduces the seal between baby's lips and his mother's breast (Vanderberg, 1996). Since the preterm head is heavy in relation to the weak musculature of the neck, a neonate's head and neck must be supported with gentle pressure. The position adopted must provide neck stability because undirected head movements can easily collapse the airway, causing apnoea and bradycardia (Neifert & Seacat, 1988).

By using hand expression a stream of milk can be produced to provide olfactory and sensory stimuli. Preterm babies often exhibit considerable excitement by nuzzling closer and licking the milk with their tongues. Occasionally they simply open their mouths and swallow the milk, which drips directly into their mouth. Most early breastfeeding problems are related to immaturity and inconsistency (Kavanaugh, Mead &

Table 7.7.1 Monitoring preterm breastfeeding in the community

Ensure correct attachment and positioning
Ascertain that that the baby is capable of nutritive suckling patterns
Ensure baby is able to receive hindmilk (patterns of breast use/maternal milk supply)
Ensure that parents understand that that initially the maximum interval that should elapse between feeds is 3 hours, with no fewer than 8 feeds daily.
Advise parents to supplement poor feeds when necessary
Monitor whether or not hospital-based stooling patterns are maintained
Ensure that the baby is maintaining his/her temperature
Weigh twice weekly
Plot weight, length and head circumference on centile chart weekly
Reassure parents that the ability to feed well consistently is related to maturity.

Meier, 1995). Preterm infants are unable initially to co-ordinate a suck/swallow/breath response and are often incapable of rhythmic suckling. Sucks are irregular and the pauses between sucks are prolonged which may inhibit milk ejection and fluid intake. When the nervous stimulation becomes overwhelming, they abruptly go to sleep and the remainder of the feed will need to be given through a feeding tube. A preterm baby's ability to breastfeed is maturationally dependent. The desire to sleep may over-ride feelings of hunger and ability to feed for weeks, and mothers have to be very patient during the transition from feeding tube to full preterm breastfeeding.

It is very helpful for a mother to stimulate her milk flow by manual expression before putting her baby to her breast. In this way, the infant quickly receives post-ejection milk and so conserves his energy. If a breast pump is used (briefly) before putting the baby to the breast the nipple will be elongated helping the small infant to latch onto the breast. This is especially useful when an infant has demonstrated suction pressures too weak to retain the nipple in his mouth during feeding. Occasionally a preterm nipple shield is a useful tool, especially for mothers with both large and flat nipples. The use of the shield will help to facilitate the transition from non-nutritive to functional suckling. When the baby becomes larger and stronger, mothers should be encouraged wean off the device to promote more effective mammary stimulation and to provide swifter milk transfer. At no time should the shield be trimmed or modified. The soft moulded edges will become sharp and could tear or cut delicate oral tissue.

If a mother has stimulated her milk supply so that it is in excess of infant requirement, she may need to suppress volume by a reduction in the frequency of expression to ensure that a baby will receive hindmilk when put to the breast before breastfeeding can be successfully established. Mothers feel very vulnerable during the transition from tube feeds to breastfeeding. Mothers are very concerned about infant milk intake and indeed many infants although apparently adequately hydrated do not take in a sufficient volume of milk to achieve growth. Although a modified cue-based feeding is feasible during this period, mothers should wake their babies if they do not demand to feed within 3 hours. If a mother feels that a baby has taken insufficient milk at a feed, she should be encouraged to top up a poor breastfeed with a supplement of expressed milk by cup. Many infants are not capable of self-regulation until they are between 36-38 weeks gestation.

Some mothers become conditioned to manual expression. Even when a preterm infant's suckling pattern matures and becomes functional, mothers experience a delay in milk ejection when an infant is put to the breast. It is not uncommon for a tiny baby to become frustrated by a period of ineffectual suckling and simply to go to sleep before milk flow begins. Using a breast pump or hand expression to elicit flow is helpful, but will not always remedy the situation. Sometimes it is necessary to place an infant on one breast and the breast pump at the other to provide more intense stimulation. Often the infants respond by suckling eagerly and for a sustained period of time and consume adequate amounts of milk. Gradually as the effectiveness of suckling increases extra mammary stimulation becomes unnecessary and milk ejection becomes conditioned to infant demand.

In the immediate discharge period, support must be available from healthcare professionals who are skilled in preterm breastfeeding. There is no longer a weight criterion for discharge from many units and occasionally neonates are sent home with a naso-gastric tube in situ to establish breastfeeding in the community. Indices used to evaluate breastfeeding for term babies such as wet and dirty nappies and the pattern of feeds are not always appropriate for an infant born preterm. Members of voluntary support groups do not always have this knowledge, although it is important to keep them involved and informed regarding local preterm breastfeeding guidelines and protocols. The concerns that mothers have about the adequacy of breastfeeds are realistic and not just the result of their experience in hospital. The risk of under consumption is a very real concern, necessitating skilled advice and support. A discharge plan should be made in conjunction with parents to ensure continuity of care and to provide anticipatory advice. Access to hospital breastfeeding co-ordinators can also make an enormous difference in emergency situations such as the baby refusing to feed or significant weight loss. Planning well in advance will help to alleviate parental anxiety by providing a raft of practical breastfeeding support.

REFERENCES

Hurst N, Valentine C, Renfro L. 1997. Skin-to-skin holding in neonatal intensive care influences maternal milk volume. J Perinatol, 17, 213-17

Kavanaugh K, Mead L, Meier P. 1995. Getting enough: Mothers' concerns about breastfeeding a premature infant after discharge. J Obstet, Gynecol and Neonatal Nurs, 24, 23-32

Neifert M, Seacat J. 1988. Practical aspects of breastfeeding the premature infant. Perin Neonatol, 12, 24-30

Vanderberg K. 1996. Nippling management of the sick neonate in the ITU: the disorganised feeder. Neonatal Network, 9(1), 9-15

The Practising Midwife 2002; 5(6): 18-19

Thrush and breastfeeding

Jancis Shepherd

This article discusses a breastfeeding case history of a mother who presented with sore nipples and a positioning problem, who subsequently developed breast thrush. The literature about thrush in the breast will be drawn upon to illustrate the difficulties the condition raises.

Jane (a pseudonym) presented in the breastfeeding clinic when her baby Tom was five days old. Jane stated that she was breastfeeding Tom and that he was an unsettled baby. This is not unusual when positioning is sub-optimal and breast milk stimulation may be diminished.

When mothers attend the breastfeeding clinic, an informal history is taken about the birth of their baby, their feeding experiences and what they perceive to be the difficulty. Jane had a normal labour and vaginal delivery of Tom who weighed 10lbs 10oz. He was offered the opportunity to breastfeed in the labour ward soon after delivery, but did not feed well. During the next 24 hours Tom was reluctant to feed and Jane said he had received top-ups of formula. When Tom started to breastfeed, Jane was transferred to the care of her community midwife. Over the next few days Jane continued to breastfeed, Tom but her nipples became sore and painful.

In discussion with Jane we learned that she had breastfed her previous baby for 12+ weeks before weaning him onto formula milk. She expressed a strong desire to be able to breastfeed Tom for a similar length of time but was at the point of discontinuing because of the pain. Jane had a normal pregnancy but received three courses of antibiotics, two of these in late pregnancy, for a severe chest infection.

As Jane was quite distressed and said her nipples were very painful, Tom was examined to eliminate any other possible reasons for her sore nipples before attempting to put him to the breast. He appeared a healthy baby, his mouth and palate were a normal shape, he had no tongue tie or evidence of thrush on his tongue, cheeks or palate. He demonstrated a rooting and gape reflex and was willing to feed.

Jane was asked to show us how she held Tom to position and latch him onto the breast. Difficulties were noted with her latching technique. Although both nipples were sore with abrasions, the right nipple was the more painful and Jane found positioning on this side more difficult. The principles of achieving pain-free positioning were discussed and demonstrated. The positioning was improved by holding Tom closer in a 'tummy to tummy' position, bringing his bottom in closer to Jane's abdomen and teaching her to wait to elicit a wide gape. When Tom opened his mouth wide, with his tongue down, he was brought to the breast and latched well. Due to Jane's understandable anxiety about nipple pain she was asked to breastfeed on the less painful side first.

A pain score was used to evaluate how sore her nipples had been during the preceding breastfeed, 10 being the most pain imaginable and 0 no pain at all. Jane said the pain had been '8-9' and was now a '5-6'. Advice was given that the key to reducing the nipple pain was to continue to optimally position Tom, and as she became more adept the pain score should subside. In 24 hours a marked improvement in pain scores and in her ability to optimally position Tom was expected. Written information with a pictorial guide to positioning was given to reinforce optimal positioning. The relevant documentation was completed for her to communicate with her midwife. An invitation was given to revisit the clinic if she wished.

When Jane revisited the clinic 5 days later, her skills at positioning had progressed and the nipple trauma had improved. The right side still caused her some difficulty but she felt this would resolve given time. The importance of optimal positioning was reiterated.

Two days later Jane contacted us to say that she could

successfully latch on the right side. However she had a 'searing pain' particularly in the right breast that continued during and after the feed had finished. Tom was unsettled and did not stay well latched to the breast during the feed. Jane's previous nipple trauma and typical history led us to suspect thrush in the breast (see Table 7.8.1). When Tom was examined he had visible white plaques in his mouth and a sore bottom, indicative of thrush (see Table 7.8.2). Jane was advised to visit her General Practitioner for treatment for herself and Tom, as it was thought she had thrush in her breasts. General advice on diet, hygiene, and how to cope with thrush was given.

Candida albicans is a single celled yeast commensal. Infections have been reported in almost all organs of the human body (Odds, 1988) but are commonly found in warm moist environments (e.g. the gastrointestinal system or the mucosal surfaces of the mouth or vagina) where it may be referred to as thrush. When conditions are right for its growth it is an opportunistic pathogen which proliferates, giving symptoms. It may affect the nipple and thrive on milk secretions or within the lactating breast ducts.

Unlike vaginal thrush, which is recognised and treated, breast thrush may be the unrecognised cause of unresolved breast pain in lactating women. This may lead to early cessation of breastfeeding. The incidence, risk factors and most effective management of mammary thrush are still relatively unevaluated. Heinig et al (1999) suggest that some healthcare practitioners are sceptical of its existence. There are some case histories reported in the literature (Hoover, 1999; Bodley and Powers, 1999) but no overall incidence is given. Anecdotally the condition seems to be common: Broadfoot et al (1999) report that 12% of callers to the Breastfeeding Network Supporterline had a possible problem with thrush but the actual number who went on to have a diagnosis made is not given. Within the breastfeeding clinic our audit and diaries identified 12 women with a diagnosis of thrush in 1998, rising to 44 women out of 679 in 2001. This gives an incidence in the population that visited the clinic of 6.4%. The reason for this rise in cases is unclear. It may represent an increased awareness on the part of the staff, or be the nature of a specialist clinic where women with a diverse range of difficulties are seen. It is also possible that other changes in practice such as the introduction of prophylactic antibiotic therapy at Caesarean section may have influenced the numbers.

The condition may be under- or over-diagnosed. As the incidence is low and health professionals may not have seen the condition or be unaware of the significant clinical signs, the condition may not be considered. Difficulties of under-diagnosis may mean some women having unresolved breastfeeding pain leading to

Table 7.8.1 Symptoms of thrush – mother

Nipple pain that is not improved with optimal positioning
Unhealed nipple trauma
Onset of nipple or breast pain days/weeks after pain-free feeding
Nipples – painful, pink, shiny, purple, itchy or flaky, very sensitive
Severe deep breast pain during and/or after a feed, described as shooting, stabbing, burning

Table 7.8.2 Symptoms of thrush – baby

Pulls off the breast and does not remain well latched when feeding as mouth is sore
May make a clicking sound
Unsettled, fretful, anxious, difficult to settle
Visible white patches in the baby's mouth, gums or palate that do not rub off easily
Tissues may be inflamed or bleed if plaques removed
Redness, rashes, soreness and broken skin on bottom

discontinuation of breastfeeding. Alternatively practitioners may be tempted to diagnose thrush before excluding other more likely causes of nipple and breast pain such as poor positioning or mastitis. Deep breast pain attributable to Staphlyococcus aureus has been reported in breastfeeding clinics (Livingstone et al, 1996) and care should be taken to differentiate this from thrush. Thrush should be considered only after other possible causes of nipple or breast pain are excluded. Over-diagnosis, especially if the diagnosis is incorrect, may lead to women being treated inappropriately for a condition they do not have, whilst the original problem remains unresolved. It will also lead to a loss of confidence of the skills of the breastfeeding advisor by other colleagues, further diminishing the difficulties associated with thrush.

Odds (1988) suggests four classifications of factors that may predispose to thrush: natural, dietary, mechanical and iatrogenic. Although this is not specific to breast thrush, these factors can play a part in the diagnosis and management. Natural factors are biological, physiological, infections, congenital disease and age that make the individual more susceptible to thrush. Pregnancy is a physiological state where vaginal yeast infections are a common occurrence, affecting up to one third of women by the end of pregnancy (Blashke-Hellmessen, 1998, cited by Heinig et al, 1999), the majority being caused by Candida albicans. Symptoms are usually recognised by the mother and treatment sought. Pregnant women benefit from longer courses of treatment than non-pregnant women: a four-day course of imidazoles has been shown to effect a cure in just over half of the infections and a seven-day course cures over 90% (Young and Jewell 2000). Between 22% and 24% of babies may acquire infection during delivery (Blashke-Helmessen, 1998, cited by Heinig et al, 1999). The infection may then be transmitted from the baby's mouth to the nipple and breast. The increasing number of babies who are colonised as they get older suggests other factors: care giver practices, hygiene and use of dummies may play a role (Darwazeh et al, 1995). Dietary factors such as excess or deficient nutrients that alter the normal gut microbiological flora, or excess sugar or yeast in the diet may have a bearing: Horowitz et al (1984) suggest a relationship between sugar intake and microflora. Diabetes is associated with yeast infections, possibly related to glucose saturation of tissues (Odds, 1988), therefore women who are diabetic during pregnancy may be predisposed to breast thrush.

Mechanical factors such as nipple trauma, poor positioning, or prolonged damp nipples from wet breast pads may predispose to yeast proliferation. Intact skin should provide a barrier to Candida albicans but when trauma is present this may allow entry of Candida albicans from the baby's mouth when it latches to the breast. Odds (1988) suggests iatrogenic factors that predispose to thrush are drug treatments including antibiotic exposure during surgical procedures, steroid use and oral contraceptives. Amir (1996) also considers that nipple damage and postpartum antibiotic use may predispose to thrush. Whether prophylactic antibiotics given intravenously at Caesarean section affect the incidence is currently unknown.

Where thrush is on the surface of the nipple, visually the appearance of the nipple can range from slightly pink and shiny in a Caucasian woman or, as Tanguay (1994) reports, a red or purple colour. This may not be so evident on a dark skinned woman. Amir et al (1995) suggest a white growth may be present. Mothers may describe their nipples as sore, flaky, itchy or burning. A rash with tiny blisters may be noted (Mohrbacher and Stock, 1997).

Where the infection has spread within the breast to the ducts, a deeper breast pain may be present. This may be described as shooting, stabbing or razor pains, within the breast during and after a feed. The pain may radiate to the back/arm/shoulder and may be present for a considerable time after the feed (Heinig et al, 1999).

When attempting to breastfeed, the baby can appear hungry but not stay well latched. A clicking sound is sometimes heard as he does not form a strong seal with his mouth (Mohrbacher and Stock, 1997). The baby may come off the breast frequently, as the mouth is sore, or appear to pull at the nipple. Examination of the baby may reveal the characteristic white plaques or spots in the mouth, on the tongue, within the folds of the cheeks or far back on or behind the palate. A torch may be needed to visualise the mouth adequately. The plaques do not rub off easily and if removed the underlying tissues may be inflamed and bleed. As the baby has difficulty in staying well attached to the breast he/she may be unsettled and unhappy, sometimes appearing windy, anxious and hungry. The nappy area may be pink/red and sore or the skin broken. For the health professional, visible signs of thrush in the baby confirms the diagnosis. However, the baby may be asymptomatic (Heinig et al, 1999). If so, a careful diagnosis based on the history and clinical symptoms of the mother is required.

Management of thrush

Mother and baby need treating simultaneously to prevent re-infection. Thrush on the nipple may respond to topical application of miconazole cream four times a day. This should be continued for at least 48 hours after the symptoms have resolved. This can sometimes prevent spread of the infection into the deeper breast tissues. Even if asymptomatic, the baby should have miconazole oral gel or nystatin drops four times a day after feeds to prevent re-infection of the mother. With miconazole gel, ensure all surfaces of the mouth are treated: application via a clean finger may be a practical solution. The hands should be thoroughly washed afterwards. If nysatin is given the medication dropper should not reintroduced into the bottle if contaminated. Nystatin given via a medicine spoon that can be boiled/sterilised, or applied by a cotton bud, is a viable alternative. Hoppe (1996) in a randomised controlled comparison trial of two nystatin oral gels with miconazole oral gel found that miconazole was significantly more effective than nystatin.

Where deep breast pain continuing after a breastfeed is unresolved with optimal positioning, thrush may be deep in the breast ducts. Treatment for this is either with nystatin or fluconazole.

Nysatin 500,000 units six hourly is a well-known treatment for thrush and is licensed for use with breastfeeding mothers. Oral absorption is poor and the breast pain may continue for around 10 days, therefore it should be continued for at least 48 hours after symptoms subside. Treatment may need continuing for 14 days or more.

Fluconazole capsules are currently unlicensed for use by breastfeeding mothers. However the drug is licensed for neonatal use at doses significantly higher than is found in breastmilk. The amount secreted in breast milk is around 1% of the maternal dose and less than 5% of the recommended paediatric dose (Hale, 1998), therefore the amount in breastmilk is unlikely to effectively treat the neonate. A loading dose of half the daily dose (up to 400mg) is suggested by Hale (1998) depending upon the severity of symptoms. The Breastfeeding Network (1999) suggest a loading dose of 150mg followed by 50mg twice a day. Heinig et al (1999) suggest 200mg, followed by 100-200mg per day in divided doses morning and evening for a minimum of 10 days. Where fluconazole is prescribed it would seem prudent to commence with the smallest dose that will effectively treat the condition.

As fluconazole is unlicensed for use with breastfeeding mothers this creates a dilemma for health professionals. They may feel this is in the best interests of the mother but are asking another professional to prescribe an unlicensed medicine. On the one hand nystatin will treat breast thrush given time, up to 10 days elapsing before pain subsides. However the practitioner may be faced with a mother who is in extreme pain and on the point of reluctantly discontinuing breastfeeding. If treatment with fluconazole is commenced the pain is likely to resolve within the first few days, perhaps enabling the mother to continue breastfeeding. A doctor may be willing to prescribe fluconazole on his own responsibility, however any untoward consequences resulting in an action for damages being sought would lie with the doctor rather than the manufacturer (UKCC, 2000). As this is an unlicensed treatment the doctor should gain the informed consent of the mother, having explained any likely effects. The most common complications reported are vomiting, diarrhoea, abdominal pain and skin rashes. Experience has shown that nystatin is the more frequently prescribed medication.

These issues were discussed with Jane, who made an appointment to see her GP. A week later Jane revisited the breastfeeding clinic. She now seemed able to latch Tom well on most occasions but continued to have a searing pain in her breast after a breastfeed, lasting up to 20 minutes. Jane had been prescribed fluconazole 50mg once a day and miconazole gel on her nipples, Tom was having nysatin oral suspension and miconazole cream on his extremely sore bottom twice a day.

As the dose of fluconazole seemed small and she had not had a loading dose, her medications and the advisability of a loading dose of fluconazole 150mg was discussed with a pharmacist. It was suggested that she discuss with her GP having a loading dose of 150mg of fluconazole followed by 50mg twice a day. Miconazole cream rather than gel on her nipples should be increased to at least 4 times a day after feeds. Tom's bottom was being treated 4 times a day with miconazole cream and remained sore. The importance of hand hygiene, and other measures to reduce the risk of re-infection were reiterated. It was suggested that towels, flannels, underwear and baby clothes should be laundered daily on a very hot wash. Breast pumps, bottles and teats should be sterilised, as should dummies or plastic toys

Table 7.8.3 Self help
Careful hand washing after nappy changing and before touching breasts
Laundering of clothes (preferably cotton) on a hot wash daily
Separate towels for each family member, laundered on a hot wash
Thorough cleaning of baby's changing mat
Sterilisation of breast pumps, bottles, teats and dummies by chemical or heat methods – careful washing with hot soapy water to remove milk deposits is essential
Sterilisation of plastic toys that have come into contact with the baby's mouth
Discard breast milk frozen when thrush present
Simultaneous treatment of mother, her sexual partner, baby and other siblings may be required
Change breast pads after each feed

Factors that may help but are unevaluated include:
  – Acidophylus tablets may help to restore the normal gastro-intestinal flora and reduce reoccurrence
  – Low yeast diet
  – Eating of live yoghurt

that come into contact with the baby's mouth. Care should be taken to remove any milk deposits on feeding equipment by washing in hot soapy water and using a bottle brush. The manufacturer's instructions for length of time to sterilise bottles should be adhered to. Any expressed breastmilk that was frozen while suffering from thrush should be discarded. Partners of women with thrush may also require treatment to prevent re-infection.

Jane's GP changed her treatments and Jane took the loading dose of fluconazole 150mg followed by 50mg twice a day. Within 24 hours of changing the dose the pain in her breast had dramatically subsided. This emphasised the importance of having a loading dose of fluconazole rather than a possibly sub-therapeutic dose. Tom's sore bottom rapidly responded to treatment with miconazole and hyrocortisone cream applied 4 times a day.

It is essential to follow up the mother and baby to evaluate effectiveness of the treatment. Chetwynd et al (2002) report a case where the mother received fluconazole for 11 weeks and the baby was treated with oral nystatin for 13 weeks before it was realised that the nystatin was ineffective. On changing the baby to oral treatment with fluconazole both mother's and baby's symptoms resolved. With this in mind we are currently developing an audit tool to evaluate the treatments the mothers receive, the effectiveness and the outcomes.

The following week Jane, her husband and older son became unwell with 'flu. Jane contacted us to seek advice for a blocked breast duct. This suggests that perhaps positioning still may have not been optimal or possibly the obstruction was from a poorly fitting brassiere. In view of her history and her 'flu-like symptoms, the possibility of mastitis was explored. Foxmann et al (2002) suggest that the application of anti-fungal creams is associated with a three-fold increase in the risk of mastitis in their study. The authors conclude that further research is required and question if the underlying presence of a fungal nipple infection, a change in nipple flora as a result of the treatment or if the exposure to pathogens from fingers to nipples are the predisposing factors.

Advice was given on how to apply warmth to the breast and to hand express to relieve the blocked milk duct. At this point Jane felt she and her family were so unwell that she could no longer continue to breastfeed. It was suggested that her breasts may be more comfortable if she waited until the breast duct was cleared and then gradually discontinued breastfeeding. Neither did she have to change to exclusive formula feeding. Jane was supported in her decision and no value judgements were made. Despite her difficulties she valued the time she had breastfed Tom. Jane is similar to the 90% of women in the Infant Feeding Survey, (Hamlyn et al, 2000), who would have liked to have breastfed for longer if she had not been deterred by other problems. All credit is given to Jane who persevered for as long as she could despite more than the usual number of difficulties experienced by a breastfeeding mother.

REFERENCES

Amir LH, Garland SM, Dinnerstein L et al. 1996. Candida albicans: Is it associated with nipple pain in lactating women? Gynecologic and Obstetric Investigation 41(1): 30-34

Bodley V, Powers D. 1997. Long term treatment of a breastfeeding mother with fluconazole resolved nipple pain caused by a yeast: a case study. Journal of Human Lactation 13 (4): 307-311

Broadfoot M, Britten J, Sachs M. 1999. The Breastfeeding Network Supporterline. British Journal of Midwifery 7 (5): 320-322

Blashke-Hellmessen R. 1998. Subpartial transmission of Candida and its consequences. Mycoses 41 (Suppl 2): 12-36 [in German]

Chetwynd E, Ives T, Payne P et al. 2002. Fluconazole for postpartum candidal mastitis and infant thrush. Journal of Human Lactation 18 (2): 168-170

Darwazeh AMG, Al-Bashir A. 1995. Oral candidal flora in healthy infants. J Oral Pathol Med 24: 361-364

Foxmann B, D'Arcy H, Gillespie B et al. 2002. Lactation mastitis: occurrence and medical management among 946 women in the United States. Am J Epidemiol 155: 103-114

Hamlyn B, Brooker S, Oleinikova K. 2000. Infant Feeding. London: The Stationary Office

Hale T. 1998. Medications and mothers milk. 7th edition. Texas: Pharmasoft Medical Publishing

Heinig J, Francis M, Pappgianis D. 1999. Mammary candidosis in lactating Women. Journal of Human Lactation 15(4): 281-288

Hoppe JE, Hahn H. 1996. Randomized comparison of two nystatin oral gels with miconazole oral gel for treatment of oral thrush in infants. Antimycotics study group. Infection 24 (2): 136-139

Horowitz BJ, Edelstein S, Lippman L. 1984. Sugar chromatography studies in recurrent Candida vulvovaginitis. Jnl Reprod Med 29: 44-43

Hoover K. 1999. Breast pain during lactation that resolved with Fluconazole: Two case studies. J Hum Lact 15 (2): 98-99

Livingstone VH, Willis CE, Berkowitz J. 1996. Can Fam Physician 42: 654-9

Mohrbacher N, Stock J. 1997. The Breastfeeding Answer Book. Revised Edn. Schaumburg, Illinois: La Leche International

Odds FC. 1988. Candida and Candidosis. London: Baillière Tindall

The Breastfeeding Network. 1999. Thrush and Breastfeeding. London: The Breastfeeding Network

Young G, Jewell D. 2000. Topical treatment of vaginal candidiasis in pregnancy. The Cochrane Library Issue 2, The Cochrane Collaboration.

UKCC. 2000. Guidelines for the administration of medicines. London: UKCC

The Practising Midwife 2002; 5(11): 24-27

Reflecting on life after birth

• Whether you have formal or informal systems set up for 'debriefing' where you work, what do you feel about the value of this practice? Does the term 'debriefing' accurately describe the experience that is offered to women, or can you think of a better word or phrase?

• How do you feel about the role you play in examining new babies, whether you undertake the brief neonatal check that all midwives perform after a baby is born or the extended examination of the newborn? Which of the area(s) of health promotion that Mary Mitchell discusses do you feel most reflects your practice in this area?

• Whether or not a particular midwife practises in an area where she looks after preterm babies, most midwives have contact with their mothers, during birth or on postnatal wards. How good are communication systems between neonatal units and maternity wards when it comes to supporting breastfeeding women? Do you feel equipped to support and advise women who are breastfeeding preterm babies?

If you feel like writing...

• Have you worked with a woman and baby recently where you have gone out and researched an area to gain more understanding? Could you write a case history, like Jancis Shepherd's, to share your experiences and what you have found out with other midwives?

If you feel like taking action...

• What are the policies in your area on supplementing breastfed babies? When does this happen, and what quantity of milk is usually given? Could you take the ideas in Sarah Hunt's article forward as a topic for discussion among midwives and other relevant people?

Focus on:
Alternative Therapies

SECTION CONTENTS

Chiropractic for midwives

An Introduction

Christine Andrew

If Chiropractic means 'treating bad backs' to you, then read on. It is so much more. Chiropractors diagnose and treat myriad conditions, including but not limited to musculoskeletal disorders.

I find it helpful to think of chiropractic as promoting the restoration of normal function through its influence on the neurological system. After all, it is the neurological system that controls all aspects of function within the human frame.

The World Federation of Chiropractic (1999) defines chiropractic as a health profession concerned with the diagnosis, treatment and prevention of mechanical disorders of the musculoskeletal system and the effects of these disorders on the function of the nervous system and general health. There is an emphasis on manual treatments including spinal manipulation or adjustment.

Chiropractic may appear to be a relatively new science, taking its modern principles from the work of Daniel D Palmer, an American student of anatomy and physiology, who in 1895 devised the specific spinal adjustment that is used today. There are, however, early historical records to show that in 2700 BC the ancient Chinese used spinal manipulation. Hippocrates, the Greek physician writing in the fourth century BC, was a proponent of spinal manipulation and said 'Get knowledge of the spine, for this is the requisite for many diseases'. Modern chiropractic has developed from these early roots to establish itself as the third largest health profession, following allopathic medicine and dentistry, in the world. It is a drug-free healthcare system that is delivered by hand.

For those concerned with the health and wellbeing of the pregnant woman, chiropractic care may not immediately be considered to be a part of antenatal care. As a midwife for many years, chiropractic did not feature in my repertoire of recommendations to those in my care. However an experience at a birth made me re-consider.

Case study 1

Trudy was well established in labour when I was called as her community midwife to attend her birth at home. In this, her first uncomplicated pregnancy, she had reached full term before spontaneously starting labour. Progress was good, with excellent support from her partner in the quiet, calm environment that a home setting provides.

I spent most of the night there and as dawn approached Trudy reached full dilatation and began bearing down to birth her baby. Despite wonderful contractions and continued effort from Trudy the baby did not arrive. All the old midwifery skills were called into action, change of position, resting, walking, up and down the stairs, you name it, we tried it. The baby was in an occipito-anterior position, resting at the level of the spines, but nothing could persuade it to come out. As I was considering a hospital transfer, Trudy and her partner suggested calling her cranial-osteopath. He duly arrived, listened to the story, then gently examined Trudy and performed what seemed like magic to me (a pelvic adjustment). Within minutes there was rapid descent with the contractions and the baby was born, to much joy all around! The baby arrived, healthy and breathing, but within a few minutes was softly 'grunting' The cranial-osteopath cradled the baby's head and slowly, gently used cranial technique to ease the baby's distress. Before long she was breathing easily and ready to breastfeed, where she stayed for nearly an hour, alert and sucking. It was an amazing experience. How I wanted to have those skills!

Seven years later I am now a chiropractor. Why chiropractic and not osteopathy? Well, I pondered for a few years on the difference between osteopathy, chiropractic and cranio-sacral therapy. Osteopathy and chiropractic both offer a registered qualification following four years full time degree level study and

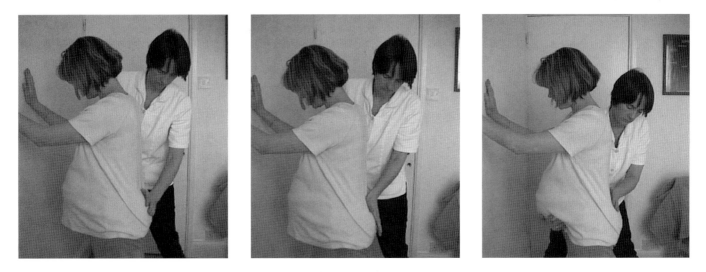

entry into a statutory regulated profession. Both provide a thorough training in manual medicine, with the main difference being the application of technique. The course I undertook in chiropractic was the right one for me. Additionally, I knew that whichever training I did, I would then pursue postgraduate training in craniopathy, like the cranial-osteopath at the birth I witnessed.

The outcome of that birth made me think more deeply about pelvic alignment and its influence over the birthing process. Since then I have been involved in the care of many women with pelvic dysfunction in pregnancy, which often brings very disabling pain. Sometimes classified as symphysis pubis dysfunction, this peripartum pelvic pain affects not only the symphysis pubis, but also the whole ring structure of the pelvis and the spine, and often has considerable knock-on consequences. This may involve compensatory dysfunction in other parts of the spine and cranium that has a bearing on the woman herself, and also on the position of the uterus and therefore on fetal positioning. The pioneering work of Jean Sutton (1997) has highlighted the significance of the pelvis in her publications on Optimal Fetal Positioning. I have found in my work that when pelvic dysfunction is treated and normal alignment restored there is often a positive effect on fetal positioning.

Case study 2

Claire sought chiropractic care in the 30th week of her second pregnancy as she had begun to experience low back and pelvic pain. She had previously suffered with low back pain during her last pregnancy, which considerably worsened immediately following the birth of her baby. She found that she had difficulty walking due to the pain in her back and pubis, which made caring for herself and her new baby almost impossible. She was keen to avoid this happening with her second birth. The chiropractic assessment diagnosed a pelvic dysfunction due to instability of the pelvic ring structure affecting both the sacro iliac joints and the symphysis pubis. The chiropractic treatments were focused on improving pelvic and spinal stability and included soft tissue work on the associated muscles and ligaments. Claire had felt that her baby was lying in an uncomfortable position for her and examination revealed that her baby was lying in a right lateral position with its bottom pushed up into her liver. This was uncomfortable for her and her baby. Further examination revealed that Claire's sacrum was tilted to one side (a left posterior sacrum) with a corresponding taut round ligament of the uterus on the opposite side. (The round ligaments act as 'guy' ropes to the uterus and have their attachments in to the pelvic fascia; if taut, they can rotate the uterus to an extent that the fetus has less available space and may adopt a less than optimum position). Treatment comprised a gentle sacral adjustment followed by a myofascial release technique to the round ligament (see Webster in utero constraint technique, below). At the next visit Claire was feeling more comfortable and her abdomen had visibly changed shape allowing the baby to use all the space available. Interestingly, this baby engaged early and was lying very well down in the pelvis several weeks before the birth. Claire continued to have chiropractic care on a weekly then fortnightly basis as her back and pelvic pain resolved. Her uterus continued to stay in good shape, and apart from feeling as though she was going to give birth any minute because of the deep engagement of her baby's head, she did not experience further back or pelvic pain. The birth was swift and straightforward, with no repeat of the back pain and disability that she experienced first time around. Claire continued with her chiropractic sessions postpartum for three weeks. She now returns, on an occasional basis, when she feels that

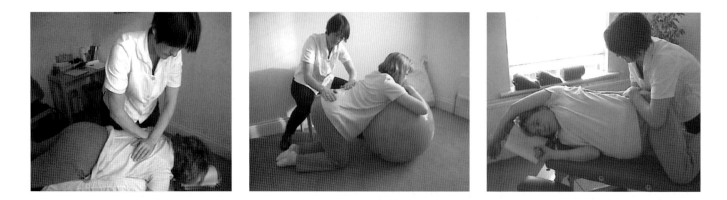

she is not in perfect alignment as she is able to detect the subtle changes in her body that indicate to her that she needs 'adjusting'.

In utero constraint

The Webster in utero constraint technique was pioneered by the American chiropractor, Larry Webster DC. He noticed the errect of a rotated sacrum and corresponding taut round ligament had upon the uterus and fetal position. By adjusting the sacrum and releasing the round ligament he noted the often immediate alteration of uterine position, freeing the fetus to change position. During his lifetime he used the technique widely. He used the technique to encourage the breech fetus to turn to cephalic with very good success rates. For a detailed explanation of this technique I recommend reading Kunau (1998), who also documents case studies based on her work with the Amish community.

Chiropractic approach in pregnancy is based upon the assessment and correction of spinal and pelvic alignment, maximising the neurological function to the viscera and muscles, optimising the space in utero and thus reducing in utero constraint and possible malposition/ presentation, facilitating normal birth and recovery postpartum. Maternal uterine contractions are reliant on good neurological function, as are all the structures involved in labour. The aim of chiropractic care is to provide optimal neurological function to all these structures.

Chiropractic care in pregnancy requires knowledge of the physiological adaptations of pregnancy, labour and the puerperium. It requires the ability to assess the structure and function of the body in relation to the changes that occur in pregnancy i.e. hormonal changes, musculoskeletal adaptations, changes in the centre of gravity and the consequences of postural adaptations. We know that pregnancy places additional biomechanical stresses on the musculoskeletal system and that these changes are believed to originate from postural alterations and ligamentous laxity. These changes are of a dynamic nature as the body is continuously changing in response to the demands of the growing fetus and uterus. Physical assessment and treatment promote good spinal health.

When treating pregnant women I aim to:

- Improve the body's functional ability
- Maintain the body's ability to function at its optimal level
- Promote prevention of pelvic instability
- Facilitate optimal fetal positioning; maximising the room in utero
- Prevent malposition/ presentation
- Improve the general wellbeing of the mother and fetus.

A pregnant woman experiencing chiropractic care during pregnancy can expect a detailed initial consultation where a full case history will be taken followed by a physical examination. History taking is of paramount importance as it enables the chiropractor to establish a differential diagnosis and to exclude other disorders that can mimic spinal/ pelvic pain. Once a diagnosis has been established a treatment plan will be discussed together. Treatment during pregnancy will need to be adapted to accommodate the changing shape of the pregnant woman, and to respect the presence of the fetus in utero. Many chiropractic treatment benches are able to be adapted for the pregnant woman to lie comfortably. Alternalively a 'doughnut' pillow can be used to enable the pregnant woman to lie in a comfortable prone position.

Treatment may involve gentle chiropractic adjustment to the spine, pelvis and extremities, as required. These adjustments, in which a specific hand contact is applied to a particular part of the involved joint, are fast and light and usually painless. Due to the ligamentous laxity in pregnancy very gentle treatment will produce the required result. Treatment will also concentrate on any muscular and ligamentous imbalance in order to restore normal function. Many chiropractors also use cranial techniques to achieve the subtle changes that will correct dysfunction occurring within the neuromusculoskeletal system.

Chiropractors will also provide education on posture, activities of daily living and ergonomic advice for home and work. The demands of other children can often be a factor in exacerbating spinal and pelvic dysfunction as mothers lift and carry other children and cope with the less than ergonomic designs of equipment, such as infant car seats. Exercise that provides strength and stability to the core stabilisers of the spine, such as yoga or Pilates, has been found to be beneficial to some women with pelvic dysfunction in pregnancy (Andrew, 2001).

A range of conditions can be treated during pregnancy. These include low back pain, sacroiliac and symphysis pubis dysfunction, myofascial syndromes, thoracic spinal joint problems, postural strain and imbalance, tension headaches, headaches of a cervicogenic origin, neck pain, arm pain with paraesthesia and carpal tunnel syndrome, to name a few.

Chiropractic technique is safe in pregnancy with few side effects or contraindications to treatment. The main side effect may be a feeling of tiredness as the body responds to the changes that have been made.

Contraindications to treatment may include:

- threatened miscarriage
- active pathology
- active inflammatory conditions.

Chiropractic offers care complementary to other healthcare providers such as the woman's midwife. It is my belief that chiropractic helps the pregnant woman to feel a sense of strength and vitality while she is pregnant, and to feel confident in her preparation for labour. Chiropractors can be part of a team chosen by the pregnant woman, offering support both to the woman and family and linking with other healthcare providers to offer holistic care. It is important for the chiropractor to be aware of both their own and others' professional boundaries and responsibilities. Like midwives and doctors, chiropractors are bound by their own standards of proficiency and code of practice, and are subject to statutory regulation for the protection of the public.

As a chiropractor I feel privileged to work on two spines, the woman's and that of her unborn baby. By facilitating good neurological function to the mother, and enabling her to approach labour with a well-aligned pelvis and a fetus in its optimal position, the likelihood of in utero constraint will, I hope, be lessened. There is work to be done now on auditing practice and compiling data.

For a more comprehensive account of treatment in pregnancy and a review of the research related to chiropractic in pregnancy I would recommend the chapter by chiropractor Tone Tellefsen in Complementary Therapies for Pregnancy and Childbirth, edited by Denise Tiran and Sue Mack.

Education

Four year BSc courses arc offered at the following universities:

- University of Glamorgan
- University of Surrey
- Anglo-European College of Chiropractic, Bournemouth.

Graduates of these institutes will be fully educated in anatomy, physiology, biochemistry, pathology and differential diagnosis, with an emphasis on musculoskeletal and neurological physiology. Students are also educated in radiology to nationally accepted standards.

A final vocational year occurs post-graduation during the first year in practice to obtain the professional qualification of DC (Diploma in Chiropractic).

Chiropractic has a professional register maintained by the General Chiropractic Council (GCC). It is illegal for anyone in the UK to use the title 'chiropractor' or to imply that they are a chiropractor unless they have applied for registration with the GCC. The GCC is the statutory body that regulates chiropractic in the UK.

To find a chiropractor, all registered chiropractors are listed on www.gcc-uk.org in alphabetical and geographical order, or phone the General Chiropractic Council on 0845 601 1796 (local rates apply).

REFERENCES

Andrew C. 2001. A study into the effectiveness of chiropractic treatment for pre and postpartum women with symphysis pubis dysfunction. University of Surrey. Unpublished MSc Thesis.

Kunau PL. 1998.Webster Technique. Journal of Clinical Chiropractic Pediatrics 3(1), 212-6

Sutton J, Scott P. 1997. Understanding and teaching optimal foetal positioning. Tauranga, New Zealand: Birth Concepts

Tellefsen T, 2000. The Chiropractic Approach to Health Care During Pregnancy. In: Tiran D, Mack S (eds). 2000. Complementary Therapies for Pregnancy and Childbirth. 2nd edtion. Edinburgh: Ballière Tindall

World Federation of Chiropractic 1999. In: General Chiropractic Council. 2001. What can I expect when I see a chiropractor. ISBN 1-903559-12-X

Massage for childbirth and pregnancy

8 years on

Linda Kimber

Initially my aims in implementing massage within my practice as a community midwife were to support labouring women with a coping strategy and give the birthing partner an active role. It was also a way of empowering the couple by equipping them with a pleasurable skill.

In 1993-94 I taught 50 couples some massage techniques for them to use during childbirth (Kimher, 1998a) and observed 22 of them using it. From the observation and the women's feedback it became very apparent that for this to work effectively the massage had to be used in combination with the woman's breathing and needed to be performed with each contraction. Random massage was not as useful. (Kimber, 1998b; Kimber/Talking Pictures). With the frequent feedback given by the couples and midwives over the years this programme continues to evolve and is now considerably broader in its concept, content and use than I had first envisaged.

Current trends

The interventionist and medicalised approach appears to be commonplace, with the widespread use of epidural anaesthesia and the rate of Caesarean sections increasing in many areas (Thomas &: Paranjothy, 2001). It appears that many women seem to have lost or do not know how to find their own strengths and resources and also how to feel confident working with other disciplines to achieve a drug free and natural birth. They feel that they are not able to approach childbirth without the certainty that they will have an epidural or Caesarean section. They possibly do not believe in the concept of natural childbirth, or, for that matter, that they could be able to manage it.

I feel there is a need for each practising midwife to reflect on why epidural anaesthesia and Caesarean sections have become so frequently requested and used

(Castro, 1999). Maternity units have become busier and we read that there is a midwife shortage and in some areas a problem with the retention of staff (RCM, 2001). Have our attitudes as midwives changed because of the increased technology and stress? (MIDIRS, 1999)

Professor Lesley Page comments:

'The modern management of labour is highly aggressive. Induction of labour and active management of labour are commonplace; the increased epidural rate and routine use of electronic fetal monitoring have resulted in a very high rate of instrumental and Caesarean birth.'

I was later struck by the following comment by Professor Page:

'Unless we change, I foresee a time when it will be considered to be quaint and old-fashioned to labour and give birth vaginally.'(Page,2000)

Supporting women/couples during a natural childbirth is undoubtedly hard work emotionally for midwives, and possibly the use of epidural anaesthesia is perceived to be an easier option for some. If the necessary support is not available when the couple needs reinforcement and encouragement then anxieties and heightened pain perceptions may occur.

The immediate issues of the shortage of midwives and therefore the stresses involved within already stretched midwifery units cannot be changed immediately, but I believe that there are certain coping strategies that can be put into place for midwives and couples.

The use of this massage programme is an example of this, and can, I believe, not only empower the couples but also extend the range of support offered by the midwife.

The development of the programme

At present I am working at the Horton Maternity Hospital in Banbury and due to the enormous support and encouragement from my managers I am teaching this massage programme to interested couples and midwives. Ideally the couples are taught antenatally and come to a one-off session with me. There are also organised workshops that I run for the midwives.

Due to the fact that breathing control and massage are used simultaneously I had envisaged that both would be used at all times. The information I am getting is very interesting and reinforces the effectiveness of this programme by the use of its different components together or separately.

Women are reporting that from time to time massage is not possible. For example, when the partners are driving them to the hospital. At such times visualisation of the massage may be used to maintain the breathing pattern and relaxation.

The women are able to adapt to different situations by drawing on the various components. I have also been witness to couples using the principles of this massage programme while immersed in water.

The following enumerates the evolving benefits of this massage programme in different stages of childbirth.

Antenatally

- Ideally this massage programme starts between 35 and 36 weeks, and encourages couples to spend more time together.
- Reduction in backache and help with insomnia have been reported.
- Couples are reporting an increased sense of confidence for the forthcoming labour and a reduction of anxiety. (The fact that the birthing partner is equipped with a practical skill tends to influence their decision to spend longer at home before coming into hospital)
- A stronger belief that the woman and her partner can and want to manage childbirth normally with the support of their partner and midwife.
- It encourares women to get into optimum positions at the end of their pregnancies. (Sutton, 1994)

Labour

- This programme can be used effectively even if an interventionist approach has to be taken such as induction of labour.
- It makes the couples more self reliant, so they are not so dependent on the midwife.
- It encourages the woman to stay upright and mobile during childbirth.
- It helps the woman achieve and maintain her breathing pattern.
- It creates a hypnotic effect, and the use of visualisation plays an important and positive role.

- It helps women work with the pain experienced during childbirth.
- It can be used when women are in the birthing pool.
- For some women it helps them not to start with active pushing as second stage commences (because of the rhythmic pattern of breathing for some there is a gentler transition into second stage.) (Sutton, 1999)
- It promotes skin-to-skin care. (With calm non-interventionist labours and normal deliveries the initiation of skin-to-skin following delivery is more likely.)(Sheridan, 1999)
- It increases a sense of wellbeing and creates better outcomes.

Postnatally

- Many women are reporting a feeling of extreme happiness and sometimes surprise to have managed the labour without analgesia.
- Their baby appears calm and placid.
- Possible positive Iinks with successful breastfeeding (Chen, Nommsen-Rivers, Dewey et al, 1998).

In Turner's study (Turner, Altemus, Enos et al, 1999) the levels of plasma oxytocin in normal cycling women were measured and it was found that there tended to be an increase in these levels following relaxation massage.

The benefits of this massage programme have not been formally researched as yet, but it would appear that there is some evidence for a possible physiological mechanism for its observed effects.

Through animal and human experiments it is thought that endogenous oxytocin is released in response to some sensory stimuli such as touch and massage. Also activation of the sensory nerves by touch significantly increases plasma levels of oxytocin in several animal species.

There has also been research on the possible relationship between raised state and trait anxiety scores in pregnancy and lengths of labour, the need for synthetic oxytocin and pharmacological pain relief (Haddad, Morris, Spielberg, 1985; Haddad, 1989.)

Massage will not always be a viable option for everyone and the wishes of the individual to opt out of massage need to be respected. This not only applies to the couples but also to the midwives.

Midwives and massage

However, because the actual massage is not randomly performed and the focus is always on the partner or friend as the primary provider of the massage, not the midwife, some midwives who would normally not want to be involved are happy to do so. The very fact that the programme also involves working with breathing and visualisation may encourage the midwife who would not instinctively want to support solely a massage care option.

Midwives are offered a workshop to teach them how to support the use of this programme. Initially I wanted all my colleagues to share my passion and believe in the powerful effects of using massage, breathing and visualisation together throughout childbirth. This, of course, did not happen and still does not happen. What did happen, however, was that I embarked on an extremely valuable learning experience, one where I had to realise that I could not hand my passion over to someone else – they had to develop their own type of passion. My passion, of course, is being fuelled by seeing the sense of wellbeing and satisfaction coming from the couples.

The workshops I run for midwives are intended to encourage them:

- To reflect on why they think the epidural and Caesarean section rates are rising.
- To reflect on how they look after women/couples in labour and particularly their thoughts on pain relief.
- To teach them the concepts and hands-on use of this massage programme so that they can support women and their birthing partners throughout labour.
- To encourage the midwives to introduce various coping strategies like this massage programme first, before resorting to pharmacological forms of analgesia.
- To encourage them to try it out, if it makes sense to them, assess it and see if a passion for it develops in them.

Many interesting issues are arising as I run the workshops and receive feedback from midwives.

In Banbury, if a couple using this programme comes into the hospital, a midwife who has been to the workshop, if possible, is allocated to that particular couple.

There have been a number of women that have arrived in the labour ward who have not learnt this programme antenatally and some of the midwives have taught them in early labour showing some very good results. For example, women do not need analgesia or only use small amounts of entonox, have normal deliveries and the couples report high levels of satisfaction. Midwives also experience high levels of satisfaction.

We are using the massage programme for women who are being induced and find that as long as we can safely monitor them, as they remain upright, the massage and principles of this programme can be implemented very successfully.

There seem to be only a few situations where this programme cannot be used:

- Women with severe PET that may need increased support and help in the form of drugs and epidural anaesthesia
- Women having elective LSCS
- Premature labours.

Primigravid women who have been induced or augmented with large amounts of syntocinon have used this programme and managed well with the use of massage (visualisation/breathing) and sometimes with small amounts of entonox as they approach second stage.

Likewise, women who have had a previous Caesarean section have used this programme, managing very well with none or small amounts of entonox as they approach second stage.

The massage programme encourages the women to remain upright and mobile throughout labour, as long as they can be monitored safely.

Some of the reports from the midwives using this programme are extremely positive and are shown in Box 8.2.1.

The midwives that are using this programme and witnessing couples using it report that:

- It helps the couples to feel in control, calm and confident in their ability to progress through childbirth naturally.
- Its use also encourages and supports midwives to use their basic midwifery skills rather than relying on high tech equipment.
- Instead of giving the midwife more work to do, midwives are reporting that it helps them when it is busy, as they know the couple have a coping strategy and are managing well with their labour even if the midwife is unable to be with them all the time.
- For women who are being induced its use helps couples to still feel in control, calm and confident in achieving a natural birth without the addition of analgesia/anaesthesia.

Women's views

The feedback I receive from couples also highlights various important issues:

- Many couples report that they need encouragement and support from the midwife for this programme to show its full potential.
- As mentioned I had expected the three disciplines to work throughout labour. Certainly because the breathing control and massage are used simultaneously I had envisaged that both would be used at all times. This is not always the case as some

Table 8.2.1 Reports of Midwives using the massage programme

From the onset of incorporating this massage programme into their experience she was focused and calm... They were united on emotional, physical and spiritual levels with apparent ultimate focus on the birth of their child. It was wonderful as a midwife to be able to support them using my basic midwifery skills, to ensure safety and not have high tech equipment in the room. The lights were low, there was minimal interruption and she was mobile. I was able to work within non-intrusive but safe parameters and was available whenever they required my assistance. The massage programme enabled them to feel empowered and positive, which in turn resulted in a magical birth experience for them and a truly satisfying one for me.' (Midwife A)

'By helping couples to help themselves I feel we hand back some of the "control" modern obstetrics has robbed them of. By helping them explore ways of coping without interfering with the flow and rhythm of labour, I believe we can improve the number of uncomplicated deliveries by avoiding the so-called "cascade of intervention"... I have used this programme with several first time parents. On each occasion I have been struck by the tremendous strength couples appear to draw on as labour unfolds in a beautifully untampered with way... There does not appear to be a stereotype who chooses to try it...' (Midwife B)

'We were extremely busy as there were 6 women in and only 2 midwives. I felt much happier being able to equip the couple with this coping strategy as I could not be with them totally. A few occasions have arisen where I have not been able to spend a great deal of time with the couple due to all the demands of the day. Knowing that the couple have a coping strategy makes me feel much happier.' (Midwife C)

'Using it on a woman having an induction certainly opened my eyes. I didn't feel as if the massage would enable her to have a drug free labour. The results were incredible.' (Midwife D)

of the women report that when massage is not possible then they visualise the massaging partner's hands and this keeps their breathing rhythm steady.

- Some women report very quick labours and for that reason do not have a chance to start the massage component of the programme.
- The couples' reports of wellbeing are not confined to labour but extend to the postnatal period as well.

All this information leads me to reflect on what I hope for, and I have come to the conclusion that if couples find using this programme of any value to them at all antenatally, during childbirth or postnatally then something positive has been put in place.

Conclusion

I feel it is important for midwives to put in place something that reinforces a belief that childbirth is essentially a normal phenomenon and that, to a point, we all create our own realities through our positive or negative thoughts.

We also need to equip the women and their birthing partners with those thoughts, by helping them to use their own inward strengths and/or adopt whichever coping strategies they feel appropriate for them.

Empowering couples very often means we need to stand back as midwives and observe couples making choices that are right, safe and that work for them.

At the same time, for this programme to work effectively, it needs the support and encouragement of the midwife, as the birthing partner may have been massaging for some hours prior to admission to hospital. This support is also necessary if the woman is having a home confinement.

With the increasing rate of analgesia/anaesthesia use, if some midwives find that it supports them in keeping childbirth as normal as possible without resorting to medical intervention and drugs, then it has a very important place.

It is an extremely exciting time as this massage programme continues to evolve and new interesting issues unfold. Massage can convey a message of support and reassurance, and possibly an increase in plasma oxytocin levels: something we can all help to achieve with touch.

REFERENCES

Castro A. 1999. Increase in Caesarean sections may reflect medical control, not women's choice. BMJ 319(7222), 1401-2

Chen DC, Nommsen-Rivers L. Dewey KG et al. 1998. Stress during labor and delivery and early lactation performance. American Journal of Clinical Nutrition 68(2), 335-44

Haddad F. 1989. Effect of anxiety in pregnancy. Contemporary Reviews Obstetrics & Gynaecology, 1, 123-32

Kimber L. 1998 (a). Effective techniques for massage in labour. The Practising Midwife, 1(4), 36-9

Kimber L. 1998 (b). How did it feel? The Practising Midwife, 1(12), 38-41

Kimber L. A practical guide to childbirth massage techniques. The video. Talking Pictures

Page L. 2000. MIDIRS Midwifery Digest, 10(4)

RCM Midwives Journal. 2001. Numbers of practising midwives continue to fall. February 2001.

Sheridan V. 1999. Skin-to-skin contact immediately after birth. The Practising Midwife 2(9), 23-8

Stock S, Uvnas-Moberh K. 1988. Increased plasma levels of oxytocin in response to afferent electrical stimulation of the sciatic and vagal nerves and in response to pinch and touch in anaesthetised rats. Acta Physiologica Scanda, 132, 29-34

Sutton J. 1994. Optimal fetal positioning: a midwifery approach to increasing the number of normal births. MIDIRS Midwifery Digest, 4(3), 283-6

Sutton J. 2000. Birth without active pushing. The Practising Midwife, 3(4), 32-4

The art of midwifery: lost to technology? 1999. MIDIRS Midwifery Digest, 9(1)

Thomas J, Paranjothy S. 2001. RCOG Clinical Effectiveness Support Unit. The National Sentinel Caesarean Section Audit Report. London: RCOG Press

Turner RA, Altemus M, Enos T et al. 1999. Preliminary research on plasma oxytocin in normal cycling women: investigating emotion and interpersonal distress. Psychiatry

Self-hypnosis in midwifery

Joyce Reid

When Gillian went into labour with her first child, the pain was so intense she was sure she would not be able to go through with the birth. After telephoning the hospital to say she was on her way, her next phone call was to Agnes Steven, her hypnotherapist.

'I can remember vividly the contractions coming,' says Gillian. 'My Mum was really worried about me, but when I spoke to Agnes she told me to close my eyes. She put me into hypnosis and the pain was gone.' To her mother's astonishment, Gillian walked out of the door calmly, telling her she was going to be fine.

Using techniques which have been around since the 1700s, Agnes teaches mothers-to-be how to relax and get in touch with their unborn child during pregnancy. She can also show them how to anaesthetise parts of their body, taking control of, and reducing, pain.

'The hardest part about having a baby is trying to get your breathing slow,' said Agnes. 'The next thing is getting your mouth moist. The saliva dries up when you are panicky and the breathing speeds up. I can teach women psychological anaesthesia to numb different parts of the body. I can also teach them the tap method – they can turn the taps off, which in effect turns off the nerves.'

Dr Sam Prigg, consultant obstetrician and gynaecologist with Ayrshire and Arran Acute Trust, has been very impressed with Agnes' work and now refers patients to her. 'I was very sceptical to be honest,' explained Dr Prigg. 'But I have seen with my own eyes the difference that Agnes makes. Her great strength is that she gives women confidence to deal with whatever is happening.'

Dr Prigg has described seeing Agnes' work with people as 'staggering'. 'One patient delivered under hypnosis and I have never seen anyone so relaxed in labour,' he said. The midwives working in the trust were all equally sceptical to begin with, but are now very convinced that hypnosis works.

Dr Prigg feels that a lot antenatal care is about telling women what is going to happen, and that can frighten some of them. Agnes makes them feel in control, which takes away their fear. He often refers women in early pregnancy to Agnes. Women who are suffering from hyperemesis or who simply need shelter them from what is happening at home – other children to look after, perhaps – do not need to be hospitalised. That is an expensive way of doing things. When Agnes becomes involved, she can say to women 'OK, you feel sick – here's what we can do about it. We can make sure it doesn't get you down.' In other words, she does not solve their problems, she shows women how to deal with them effectively.

'What Agnes does is not evidence-based medicine, but I think she really has got something to offer,' said Dr Prigg. 'She gives women confidence and that counts for so much. Community midwives now know of her work and will often ask me to refer patients to her. They are responding to the results they have seen.'

As is her way, when Agnes first spoke to Dr Prigg about her work, she did not simply give him the theory. She showed him what she could do. 'She picked up a fold of skin from my forearm, put a hypodermic needle right through it and it didn't hurt at all,' he recalled, still with a degree of astonishment in his voice. 'It is very convincing stuff, and proves that the brain is very important in the control of pain.'

This is the technique Agnes uses for those with a needle phobia, which is very common and can become a real nightmare during pregnancy. It can be very beneficial to women who know they will be having an epidural.

Agnes' work also takes in infertile couples. She can help where there is no physical reason why a woman cannot get pregnant. Lest there be any confusion, she is quick to point out that she only works with those who have been medically checked, and does not work in isolation. 'I always work with the patient, the doctor, the occupational health nurse or consultant,' she said. 'We need to work together. I always work on the referral of a medical person.' She often sees men because if they are stressed their sperm count will be low. When working with men and women, the most important thing is that they talk things through, and look at why stress could be causing the problem.

When it comes to teaching self-hypnosis, Agnes wants her patients to get the mind and body back into balance. She asks them to close their eyes and talk into themselves (not out loud) counting from forty back to zero. Each time the patient breathes out she should count down another number. It doesn't matter if the mind wanders or someone forgets which number they are at, they simply bring the mind back to another number and carry on from there. When they reach zero, they go back to forty and start counting down again. Agnes advises, 'Do this as often as you like. It will enable the body to heave a sigh of relief and slide itself down into a state of hypnosis. You will feel wonderfully at ease.'

Now Agnes can concentrate on any problems from the past. Is there anything there that needs to be removed? She stresses that you cannot change your past, only how you look at it, how you feel about it. 'The subconscious mind protects you, so if there is a block it thinks it is looking after you,' she explained.

In her book 'How to rush slowly…and avoid panic attacks', Agnes recounts working with a woman whose subconscious mind was 'protecting' her by not allowing her to become pregnant.

'When Joyce was three years old she overheard a part of a conversation between her mother and her aunt who had just undergone surgery for cervical cancer. What Joyce heard was her mother ask her aunt if she thought that having children had contributed to her having contracted the disease. Joyce's three year old mind had stored its own particular adaptation of the information and now years later her subconscious mind was equating cervical cancer with having a child.

'I asked Joyce's subconscious mind to allow her to remember and hear the rest of that conversation. Joyce saw and heard her aunt reply "having children has been the best thing that could have happened. The cancer was spotted during a routine antenatal. I was able to have the treatment straight away and because of the quick diagnosis the surgery has been successful. I have been given the all-clear. I was very lucky."

'Joyce was shocked that she couldn't remember the incident at a conscious level, yet it appeared to be having such a profound effect on her own life. The fertility part of her subconscious mind was trying to protect her by not allowing her to become pregnant.'

After a few sessions with Agnes, Joyce became a much more relaxed person and did indeed become pregnant – with twins!

Once Agnes feels that the patient is ready she goes onto the next stage. They must begin by imagining that they can look down, or go into, the womb and must tell Agnes what they see – she is not looking for medical terms and gets a great variety of answers. Some women see their womb as being black; black indicates depression. It may well be the woman is depressed about not getting pregnant. Agnes will then introduce self-hypnosis, during which everything will come into balance; the depression will be brought to the surface and can be dealt with.

If a woman is depressed because she has had a miscarriage or termination, she may be experiencing guilt or loss. Sometimes she may not have come to terms with it because she does not know where her baby is. In that case, Agnes will talk the woman into self-hypnosis and take them to the other side to be with their baby. We are not talking about heaven here, just where they imagine their baby could be. The woman can then lift the baby into her arms, cuddle the baby and talk to the baby. Agnes then tells the woman she can see someone walking towards them – the woman always sees it as a Gran or a Mum – and tells them that that person is going to look after the baby. You cannot over-estimate how relived many women feel when they know their unborn baby has someone to look after it.

Having dealt with blocks, Agnes goes on to ask women to imagine they are building a nursery in the womb; she is aware that in the cold light of day, this can seem slightly ridiculous, but there is no doubt that it does work. She wants them to imagine putting up the curtains, the wallpaper, putting down the flooring and putting in the furniture. They must then imagine a cot or a crib.

The next step is for the woman to go to the door and hear all the little blackcurrant men from the Ribena advert. They are all roaring with laughter and chattering. They come rolling into the room, from the top of the door to the bottom. They jump into the cot and they are all carrying on, boxing each other, making a racket.

All of a sudden everything goes silent, all the little Ribena men put their fingers to their lips and say "Shhhhh", and then "Awwww." They move back to reveal a little baby in the crib. All the little men tip toe out of the room, whispering to themselves. The woman goes and shuts the door and then she goes up and cuddles her baby, telling the baby 'I am your Mum'. Psychologically, she has closed the door, so will not have a miscarriage.

Is this giving couples false hope? Agnes answers: 'The one thing people in this situation are saying to themselves is "I will never be pregnant". The mind goes by pictures and they always imagine an empty womb. The mind also works on feelings, so if you have built a nursery in the womb for the baby, you will have moved on from emptiness.' She cannot give a success rate for infertile couples, but she can say that even if the woman does not become pregnant, the couple will have had the chance to look at other parts of their lives and sort themselves out.

Gillian first saw Agnes when she was trying to become pregnant and built the little nursery in her womb. She remembers it clearly. 'At one stage, Agnes asked me if the door was open or closed and I said it was closed. She told me to open it but it kept closing. She told me to put it on a big hook so it couldn't close. I visualised myself doing that. We often went back to see if the door was open.

'Each time I went into my nursery, there were more and more things in it, it was becoming more homely. There was a rocking chair and I could see myself sitting in it. I got all the feelings. It was amazing.'

Another patient, Barbara, came to see Agnes after suffering several miscarriages. She feels that the hypnotherapy enabled her to accept what had happened and that was a really big step forwards. Agnes accompanied her when she went for a laparoscopy and did hypnotherapy with her prior to Barbara going into the theatre. 'It was a phenomenal experience,' said Barbara. 'I was not scared at all, I was so relaxed and felt no pain afterwards. It was a very positive experience.'

Unfortunately, Barbara went on to have an ectopic pregnancy. Once again Agnes accompanied her to the hospital and did deep relaxation and hypnotherapy before the operation. 'Obviously this could never be described as a positive experience, but it did help,' said Barbara. 'I am convinced it did made a big difference and if I ever need another operation I will definitely consult a hypnotherapist again.'

Agnes believes that many women experience fertility problems because they are terrified of giving birth. 'The romantic picture of childbirth soon goes away when we realise that the baby has to be delivered,' she says. 'These women come along and talk about their fears and begin to see them in a much more manageable way. I can then teach them childbirth hypnosis and it can make them feel more relaxed than they have done in a long time. I am not saying they won't be worried; it's just that the worry isn't so important to them.

Gillian used childbirth hypnosis during her 16-hour labour. Agnes stayed with her throughout. Gillian was aware of people talking and at one time heard someone say that she needed painkillers. 'I panicked and came out of the hypnosis,' she said. 'Agnes took me back under and asked me if I needed painkillers, but I said no and became quite calm again.'

Gillian used the taps method of pain relief. She recalled, 'I ended up with 46 taps in my tummy, which I kept switching off when I felt pain. It took away a lot of the pain, though it did not go completely.'

Two hours before Gillian's daughter was born, Agnes brought her out of the hypnosis as the baby was too relaxed. Gillian is happy, however, that she felt herself give birth. She is sure that she would do the very same again if she was ever having another baby.

Another aspect of Agnes' work is helping women to relax during their pregnancy. 'I can take the woman down into the womb so that she can see her baby, hold the baby and tell it how much she is looking forward to its arrival.' While the mother does this, the baby often moves, confirming that all is well. Agnes suggests that if a mother ever becomes worried because she can't feel any movement, she can go down into the womb in her imagination and lift the baby up, cuddle it, tickle it under the chin or count its toes.

This can obviously lead to a greater bonding between mother and baby. It has also been said that self-hypnosis during pregnancy and childbirth can help to shield the baby from stress and give relief from morning sickness. It can keep down blood pressure and help the woman to sleep. Certainly, a baby whose mother has performed childbirth hypnosis is often much more relaxed at birth.

During the labour, mothers can use the same self-hypnosis they used to talk to their baby during pregnancy to check on both the baby and the cervix. 'If the cervix is not opening up enough, the mother can tell her mind to do it,' said Agnes. She stresses that the subconscious mind will not do anything that is dangerous to the mother or the baby, so women should not worry that they might do any harm. She knows of no adverse effects caused by childbirth hypnosis and has found that it can calm clown the situation, bringing benefits also to fathers who often find it distressing to see their wife or partner in trauma. Midwives have been stunned to see mothers smiling through contractions. However, Agnes does not want mothers to be under the illusion that there will be no pain and that they will be lying back smiling throughout the birth. When she is talking a woman through relaxation, she never takes her right to the point of delivery, as she is convinced the woman needs to feel she has actually given birth.

Frances is expecting triplets, who will be born at around 32 weeks by Caesarean section. She is worried about not having a pre-med before the epidural, but Agnes will be with her, doing relaxation for about an hour beforehand. 'Agnes has assured me I will not feel the needle going in,' said Frances.

It was a midwife who suggested that Frances go to Agnes as she, Frances, was extremely worried about the triplets, having suffered two previous miscarriages. 'I realise now that I did not deal properly with the miscarriages, particularly the one at 18 weeks when I had to go through a stillbirth and a funeral. I thought I was fine, but I wasn't,' she said. Talking things through with Agnes has been enormously helpful, and Frances now admits that where before she was tired because she was not sleeping and was constantly tearful, she is now quite calm and optimistic.

Although her husband will also he present at the birth, Frances feels that having 17 people in the theatre when she gives birth will be quite daunting, and she will be very glad to have Agnes on hand, to support her.

In her quest to pass on her knowledge, Agnes spends some of her time teaching psychological anaesthesia to GPs at Glasgow University, and lectures on stress for both trainee midwives and those who are studying for their BSc. 'Nurses and doctors are here to look after patients, but first of all they must know how to look after themselves,' said Agnes. 'We need positive stress, but I work with them to give them some tools to take away in order that they can deal with stress effectively.'

In every aspect other work, this is Agnes' message. 'I help people to help themselves and that is a wonderful thing,' she beamed.

Postscript: Frances' triplets were safely delivered at the beginning of December (2001). She had two girls and one boy, and all are doing well.

The Practising Midwife 2002; 5(3): 14-16

Working with babies

Enhancing the future through resolving the past

Graham Kennedy

Working with babies provides a unique opportunity to resolve many of the difficulties that can become imprinted early in life and can go on to affect our full development and potential as we mature.

One of the most formative experiences that we all undergo is the experience of birth. It is becoming increasingly recognised that the quality of our prenatal life and the nature of our arrival into the world is fundamental to, and may have significant impact upon, our future development.

In the United Kingdom in the middle part of the twentieth century, as the hospitalisation of birth was encouraged, birthing women were organised from the viewpoint of obstetricians and other medical practitioners. This led to the development of birthing practices that favoured the medical professionals but actually made the birth more difficult for both mother and baby.

Later on, the active birth movement lead the way for the de-medicalisation of birth and focussed on how the mother could empower herself during her pregnancy and while she gave birth.

In recent years, health professionals in various fields of research have been considering the birth process from the baby's point of view. This has been very challenging, especially since, as recently as 1995, most parents and healthcare professionals believed babies to be too small and undeveloped to be affected by their prenatal life or birth.

A number of pioneers in this field have developed unique approaches to working with babies, children and their families in order to help resolve those issues that have their origins in prenatal life and the birth process. These issues within a baby can, over time, affect the dynamic of the whole family. It is therefore important to work with the baby within the context of their family system.

In developing these approaches, practitioners and teachers have drawn from a wide range of modalities including craniosacral therapy, polarity therapy, psychotherapy, trauma resolution work, and birth simulation work. Combining this with a detailed study of midwifery and obstetrical practices, embryology and neurology, a powerful method of working with babies and their families has emerged.

These revolutionary approaches look at the effect upon the baby of its prenatal life, the birth process and current birthing practices and how these effects may be resolved to ensure good health and optimum potential.

One of the challenges that is often faced in working with babies is what I call the 'inside-outside' dilemma. The baby is on the inside and has its own unique experiences of its life in the womb and the nature of its arrival into the world. The baby's parents, other family, doctors, midwives and everybody else are on the outside, and they also will have their own experience of these times. In many cases, the experiences of the baby and the parents are not the same.

I have worked with a number of mothers who have stated that, to them, the birth was wonderful. However, when we start working with babies it becomes clear that they may still be holding some left-over issues around their arrival into the world.

Case history: Emily

Sally brought her baby Emily to see me for a check-up following the birth. Sally was a week overdue and the doctors informed her that she had two options regarding the delivery of her baby. One of these choices was induction, the other was elective Caesarean section. After weighing up the pros and cons of each option, Sally chose to have a section, in the belief that it would be the safest alternative of the two.

When she brought Emily to see me, she stated that she was completely satisfied with the way the birth had gone, although she did have a little regret about it not starting 'on time'.

As I began to work with Emily, she started to express a lot of anger and upset that was directed towards her mother. At the same time, she initiated pushing movements with her legs, in the same way that a birthing baby would push against the back of its mother's womb.

As we worked over a number of sessions, it became clear that Emily (although only 3 months old) blamed her mother for not allowing her to have a 'normal' birth.

As we made clear to Emily that mum made what she thought was the best choice in the circumstances, and we supported her to express her strong feelings, she eventually began to soften and settle.

After this course of treatment, Sally reported that the degree of bonding between her and Emily was greatly improved and she was a much more content baby.

Our early life

Every parent must surely be aware that the conception, gestation and birth of a child are miraculous events. One needs only to look into the eyes of a newborn baby to be wonder-struck by the miracle of life.

Today, many prospective parents are deliberately taking the time prior to conceiving their child to take steps to resolve any issues in their physical and emotional wellbeing as well as in their relationship with each other. They are consciously taking this time in the understanding that the more of these issues they resolve, the healthier will be their sperm and egg and the new life that results from their union.

It is becoming clear that this type of conscious conception, as well as active parental responsibility during gestation, can contribute to easier birthing and bonding.

Impaired bonding of the infant to its parents has been shown to be one of the major factors in the development of aggressive and violent behaviour as well as relationship difficulties later in life (Chamberlain, 1995; Prescott, 1996). Contrary to many beliefs, bonding can, and ideally should, take place while the child is still in the womb.

In contrast to the ideal scenario, most parents do not undertake any preconceptual healthcare, nor do they consciously conceive their child. The effects of this may adversely impact on the baby while it is developing in the womb.

Table 8.4.1 lists a number of potentially disturbing events that may imprint the prenate while it is still in the womb. This, and the information in Table 8.4.2, is derived from the work of Dr William Emerson.

Table 8.4.1 Potentially disturbing events for the prenate

Unwanted pregnancy
Conception by force, manipulation or rape
Conception under the influence of alcohol, cigarettes or drugs (recreational/pharmaceutical)
Thinking about, planning or attempting abortion
Intrauterine toxicity (from alcohol, cigarettes, drugs, medications, strong negative emotions)
Prenatal twin loss – research has shown that up to 70% of all pregnancies begin as multiple conceptions (Keith et al, 1995)
Fetal surgery, invasive antenatal testing and ART
Planned adoption
Accident, illness or injury during pregnancy
Divorce or separation of parents
Death of a loved one

The birth process

For the first nine months of its life, a baby has been growing and developing within the relative safety of its mother's womb. As this time draws to a close, both mother and baby release certain hormones that initiate the contractions of labour. The baby, therefore, possesses an inherent wisdom as to when it is ready to birth itself.

During a normal delivery, the baby descends head first, through the mother's pelvis and down the birth canal. In order for the baby to pass through its mother's pelvis, certain physiological changes need to occur. The widest part of the baby is its head. Fortunately, for both mother and baby, the head is able to mould in order to facilitate its passage through the pelvis. This moulding is able to take place because the bones of the skull have not yet 'fused' together. They are like large plates that are floating on the membranous surface of a water-filled balloon.

As the baby begins its passage through the pelvis, the various bones of the skull naturally move and distort in particular ways, in order to facilitate the descent. This may include one or more bones overlapping each other. The overall effect of the birth process upon the baby, and particularly upon its head, is one of compression.

New parents are often alarmed by the degree of moulding that is present in their baby's head. Medical professionals often state that this is nothing to worry about as moulding is a natural process that will fully resolve itself in a matter of days.

It is true that moulding is a natural process and that a certain degree of resolution occurs quite quickly. However, it is often the case that due to the strong compressive forces that the baby experiences during its birth, the bones of the skull may not fully release and return to their natural position. If these bones remain locked together they can interfere with the natural growth and development of the skull and the brain.

The compressive forces of the birth process are often fed into the spine and pelvis resulting in a greater degree of tension and less freedom of movement in certain joints and in particular areas of the body. These effects may have body-wide repercussions and potential long-term consequences on the child's health and wellbeing.

Many conditions described as 'normal' during infancy may have their origins in the rigours of the birth process. In fact, it would be more appropriate to describe these conditions as common, reflecting the commonality of the experience that we have all gone through, rather than normal. To suggest that something is normal implies that it is something necessary for the baby to experience and is indicative of good health.

Common conditions related to unresolved cranial moulding are difficulties with feeding and sleeping, constant crying, colic, ear problems, squint and other visual disturbances. Other conditions, that may not manifest until later in life, include asthma, autism, behavioural and emotional problems, dyslexia, epilepsy, hyperactivity etc.

Case study: Sarah

Sarah, a 4-week-old baby, was brought to see me suffering with severe colic. Her parents were concerned by the fact that she would scream inconsolably for several hours in the evenings, pulling her legs up into her body as she did so. Although she was breastfeeding, Sarah was unable to digest the milk when her mother ate fruit, vegetables and other foods, and was also suffering from smelly green stools. Consequently, her mother was living on a diet of dairy products and chocolate, as these seemed to provide the least distress to Sarah.

Sarah's mother stated that her labour was very quick and had been induced for the convenience of the consulting obstetricians. Consequently, she felt very angry at what she considered to be the mismanagement of her labour. Inductions generally have the result of creating more intense uterine contractions and have the potential to produce more pronounced shock and cranial moulding patterns.

This was certainly the case with Sarah. Just looking at her, I was struck by the strong asymmetry that was present, particularly in her face. By taking a light contact onto the back of her head I became aware of the strong degree of compression that was present throughout her body. Some of her cranial bones were compressed and misaligned in relation to their neighbours.

From just the very first session, I could feel some of the tension in her body begin to relax. Her occiput softened and there was a lengthening throughout her body as the tight soft tissues released their tension.

Sarah's parents noted that the day after the treatment she had continuous bowel movements that gradually became less green and smelly. By the next time I saw her, Sarah was obviously a different baby. She seemed much more at ease and relaxed, and the powerful screaming, that was the initial cause for concern, had stopped. These improvements continued over the few more sessions that Sarah and I had together.

Assisted delivery

In many cases, interventions are used that are intended to make the birth process easier for both mother and doctor. Often, such interventions are necessary for the safety of both the mother and baby. However, such interventions can potentially have long-term side-effects. The use of such tools as forceps and ventouse, for example, can often create more extreme moulding patterns, body tension and shock in the baby. In these cases, it can often take longer to get a resolution of the underlying problem.

The use of pain-relief medication can also create long-term side-effects. Dr Lennart Righard, of the University of Lund, Sweden, produced a study showing that babies born from a medicated birth were often unable to attach to their mother's breasts and begin feeding (Righard, 1990). This may then set up an early pattern for bonding and relationship difficulties. More recent studies, from the University of Gothenberg, have linked high doses of opiates and barbiturates, used as painkillers in labour, with increased likelihood of substance abuse later in life.

Caesarean sections

It has often been reported that babies born by Caesarean section have an easier time and suffer less as a consequence than those born vaginally, primarily because they don't experience the cranial moulding from the birth canal. Indeed, many parents (especially in the USA, and increasingly so in the UK) are now opting for elective Caesareans as a way of avoiding the pain and discomfort of the birth process. Research has estimated that a Caesarean section rate of only 6-8% is medically justified. This is in comparison to the UK national rate of upto 20% (up to 50% in some parts of the USA)(Sakala, 1993).

Caesarean-born babies have a different experience to vaginally-born babies. They undergo many physiological and psychological changes, over a very short space of time, as they make the transition from life in the womb to the outside world. They also experience a sudden pressure change as the uterus is surgically opened.

These factors can actually imprint a significant amount of distress into the baby's system albeit, in certain circumstances, without any cranial moulding.

Case study: Hayley

Michael and Amanda had been trying to conceive a child for 11 years. Having given up hope of having a child of their own, they decided to adopt a little boy, Simon. As the adoption process reached its final, critical stage, Amanda fell pregnant.

This was a very stressful time for everyone. Amanda was very sick for the whole 9 months of her pregnancy. The stress of the adoption process, the stress of wondering whether the adoption agency would take Simon away and finally the stress of finding out that the baby was in a breech position, with her head wedged under Amanda's ribcage, and she would need to have a Caesarean section.

Amanda brought Hayley to see me when she was 22 months old because she had been very sick as a baby and now had extreme temper tantrums.

As I started working with Hayley, she always seemed to settle into her Mum's lap in exactly the position she had been stuck in the womb, with her head tightly pressed into Amanda's ribs.

Over time, by allowing Hayley to express the feelings she had about being stuck and having to be born surgically, she was able to move from her stuck place, turn around, and go through a symbolic birth process, head first. By empowering Hayley to move from her stuck place she was able to re-pattern the shock that had become imprinted at the time of her birth. She was also able to let go of the emotional charge that had built up as well. Today, Hayley is a much happier little girl and no longer has the violent temper tantrums that plagued her early life.

Table 8.4.2 gives a list of interventions and other conditions that can potentially give rise to shock and trauma during the birth process. However, it must be reiterated that many of these interventions are often necessary and can even be life-saving.

Shock

It has been estimated that approximately 95% of all babies experience some degree of shock, whether mild or severe, at some stage during their prenatal life or their birth process (Castellino, 1995). In my experience, a significant number of parents also suffer some shock during this time, and often have unresolved emotions concerning the management of their labour.

If the shock naturally works its way out of our system, then no lasting damage is done. However, oftentimes the complete discharge of this shock is hindered by external pressures and social 'norms'.

Unresolved shock and trauma accounts for a great deal of physical, psycho-emotional and social problems.

Table 8.4.2 Potentially traumatic birth events

Obstetrical interventions i.e. forceps, ventouse, labour induction, premature rupturing of membranes
Obstetrical anaesthesia/analgesia e.g. gas and air, pethidine, epidurals, general anaesthesia
Caesarean section
Birth complications e.g. placenta praevia, cord compaction and oxygen deprivation, nuchal cord, fetal distress, cephalo-pelvic disproportion, breech presentation
Prematurity
Separation from mother for cleaning, weighing, suctioning etc.
Post-natal testing
Early cutting of umbilical cord

To a birthing baby, the physical rigours of the birth process may be a direct contrast to its time in the womb. It may feel threatened by the whole process, and so it is not uncommon for newborn babies to have their muscles clenched, as if to protect themselves.

At the same time, the baby may enter a state of hyperarousal, even panic. It is, therefore, also common for newborn babies to be incredibly angry, frustrated or even frightened following their birth.

Another effect of shock imprinting at the time of birth, is for the baby to go into a state of hypoarousal. In this case, the baby would withdraw into itself and appear to sleep a lot. Many parents have commented that they have really good babies who seem to sleep all the time, when actually they are suffering the effects of shock.

Later on in life, as the child grows and matures, these stress responses may become habitual. This may mean that the child habitually responds to difficult and stressful situations with the same degree of overwhelm as they did at birth. In other words, stressful situations can take us back to responses that had their origins in prenatal and birth-related trauma. Whilst these responses were appropriate at the time, today they may cause us to react out of proportion to the situation at hand. At the same time, they may cause further agitation to the tissues of the body and a possible entrenching of the original trauma.

Hence, many physical and psycho-emotional disorders that we suffer from as both children and adults may have their origin in prenatal life or the rigours of the birth process. It is therefore a primary responsibility for the therapist to help the baby to negotiate safely the complete release of any imprinted shock from its early experience.

Treatment process

Fortunately, these imprinted shocks are not locked away, never to be accessed. If we can learn to observe babies and children in a new way, we will see that they are constantly showing us how it was for them in their early life.

Obviously, babies and children are not telling us a verbal story of their history but express themselves through their body and eye movements, their expressions as well as through their play. The practitioner works by monitoring the subtle energetic and physical cues that the baby presents, and responds appropriately. With older children, some of the work may involve play with toys or some re-enactment of the birth process using balls, tunnels or other games.

It is also important that the parents recognise these cues and learn how to modulate their responses to the newborn at home, thus providing self-help and care directly within the family environment.

I truly believe that through helping babies and children to resolve some, or all, of their early patterning we can help to create a more positive future for them, where they can begin to realise their full human potential and sow the seeds for a more loving and caring generation.

REFERENCES

Castellino R. 1995. The Polarity Therapy Paradigm regarding Pre-conception, Prenatal and Birth Imprinting. Santa Barbara.

Chamberlain DB. 1995. What Babies are Teaching us about Violence. Pre- and Perinatal Psychology Journal, 10(2), 57-74

Emerson W. Shock – a Universal Malady. Prenatal and Perinatal Origins of Suffering. Emerson Training Seminars. Petaluma CA

Keith L et al. 1995. Multiple Pregnancy: Epidemiology, Gestation and Perinatal Outcome. New York: The Parthenon Publishing Group

Prescott JW. 1996. The Origins of Human Love and Violence. Pre- and Perinatal Psychology Journal, 10(3), 143-188

Righard L. 1990. Delivery Self-attachment. Lancet, 336, 1105-7

Sakala C. 1993. Medically Unnecessary Caesarean Section Births: Introduction to a Symposium. Social Science & Medicine, 37(10), 1177-98

The Practising Midwife 2002; 5(6): 14-17

Reflecting on holism

Ishvar Sheran

We live in a society where most people have been brought up to view health and healing as the domain of doctors and technology (Robbins 1996). However there is a growing dissatisfaction with 'conventional' forms of health care as evidenced by the increased use of complementary and alternative medicine (CAM) (Long et al 2001)[1]. The field of CAM, and healthcare in general, contains many competing ideologies and opinions about what causes disease and how to restore health (Hay 1996, Robbins 1996). Although pregnancy and birth are not diseases in any sense of the word, this area is relevant to those caring for childbearing women for two reasons. Firstly because, whether we like it or not, Western maternity care is offered within the same healthcare systems that diagnose and treat sick people, which means that childbearing women who receive care within these systems or from those people educated within this framework may be subject to similar tools and procedures of diagnosis and treatment. Secondly, even where patterns and styles of care for those women whose childbirth experiences are 'normal' have become more holistic, some pregnant and birthing women do experience pathology, which seems to lead to an immediate movement into what has become known as 'the medical model'.

Medical doctors within the Western tradition spend vast amounts of time learning about the mechanics of the body with much training focused on pathology, disease states and interventions rather than prevention, a problematic issue that has been raised many times in debates on birth (Davis-Floyd and St John 1998). One of the primary criticisms of conventional healthcare is the view of the body as a machine that must be 'fixed' when things go wrong, using symptoms to indicate what needs repairing (Weed 1989). This attitude has kept the reins of power firmly in the hands of the medical elite who alone are trained to diagnose and advise on disease states using their medical technology. This preoccupation with pathophysiology has also meant that what constitutes health is far less well understood in conventional medicine than what constitutes disease (Achterberg 1991, Weed 1989). For health is not merely the absence of disease; it is a state of well being that allows an individual to realise their full potential to enjoy life (Newman Turner 1990).

The original goals of medicine have become increasingly clouded amidst a morass of technological gadgets (Robbins 1996), and the normality of birth as a social event has provided it no immunity from this aspect of Western culture. Of course, much of the improvement in the health of society is not due to advances in Western medicine but due to improvements in nutrition and hygiene. (Achterburg 1991). The inventions of the flush toilet, steam pumps and damp-proofing have, according to Robbins (1996), done more for the health of humanity than all surgeons put together.

However, this is not to say that advances in medical technology are not valuable. Robbins (1996) describes conventional medicine as 'crisis medicine', which is unrivalled where trauma is concerned. There is little doubt that the Caesarean section has saved the lives of many women. Yet, in paraphrasing Hippocrates, Robbins (1996: 227) reminds us that:

'The natural healing force in each one of us is the greatest force in getting well.'

It is this natural healing force that practitioners of CAM seek to support and enhance, decreasing drug reliance, and contributing to a greater sense of wellbeing. They believe that health is our natural state of being, which involves maintaining harmony with ourselves and the natural world (Weed 1989, Robbins 1996). The art of healing is seen as bringing the body, mind and spirit into greater balance and wholeness (Robbins 1996).

Of course to over 80 per cent of the world's population, so called 'alternative' medicine is the basis of the healthcare system (Larsen 1999)

As midwives will know, the practitioner of CAM is less concerned with the external physical symptoms and seeks to find the underlying cause for the disease. Conventional medicine seeks to follow a precise formula of treatment for defined pathologies, often leading to a 'one size fits all' approach. Recent cultural shifts towards the notion of evidence-based medicine have only served to enhance this, where Government-funded bodies have been set up to appraise literature and clinical trials in specific areas in order to discover the 'best' approach for any given condition or state. There is an inherent danger that 'best' is taken to mean 'universal'.

In contrast to this approach, practitioners of alternative medicine seek to do what, in their opinion, is best for the individual rather than follow prescriptive treatments based on symptoms (Larsen 1999). For this reason practitioners of CAM see their approach to healing as fundamentally different from that of conventional physicians.

However, it could be argued that many CAM therapists are merely treating symptoms of dysfunction that occur in the more subtle emotional or mental bodies to restore health in the physical body. Surely this is the same approach adopted by conventional doctors, albeit a more in-depth method of fixing problems on more subtle levels? Both systems view the patient as an individual who needs 'fixing'. Something has gone wrong and whether your view is that it requires drugs, surgery, a new diet or lifestyle, acupuncture or spinal manipulation to restore that balance does not alter the attitude behind this point of view (Weed 1989). For example, a woman might choose to see an acupuncturist at 42 weeks of pregnancy to attempt a more 'natural' induction of their labour than to go immediately to a hospital for a medical induction. Yet, while the former approach is often a pragmatic decision taken within a framework of complex social and professional pressures, the same outcome is being sought in both cases. Is this holistic?

A holistic midwife who I interviewed recently placed a lot of emphasis on informed choice, and said she would not make any decisions for women, except in an emergency situation where the women was unconscious or unable to express a choice. She sees her role as facilitating women's decisions, and provides information but tries 'not to influence their choices on their journey'. In my experience as a naturopath people sometimes perceive that they will be treated in the much the same way that they would be treated by a doctor in the Western model. When illness occurs many people still seek a 'magic bullet' that will effect a cure, albeit with an emphasis on using natural remedies to achieve this over drugs. I have found some people prefer this even to simple lifestyle changes, and I know from talking to midwives that they sometimes face the same kind of situation, particularly when working within 'the system'.

So what does it really mean to be a holistic practitioner? According to Shealy and Myss (1988) 'holistic' is not a technique; it is a way of approaching healing that incorporates different therapies, and to be truly holistic conventional approaches must be included in this paradigm. As an illustration of this, Robbins (1996) states that, when truly needed, he gratefully uses Western medicines, but does so with awareness of adverse effects while doing everything possible to heal the underlying problem.

However, if a holistic or integrative practitioner is one who selects the best treatment from all traditions, then surely no one can be a holistic practitioner? For to be truly holistic you would need to be trained in so many different systems of healing that there is just too much to know (Wilber and Schlitz 2003). As experts of normal childbirth, midwives can hardly be expected to have also undertaken study in all of the different holistic therapies that women may want to use. Some of the midwives I know who attend home births are very honest about the fact that this has become their expertise to the detriment of skills they may have once held in assisting in surgery, or supporting women who are severely ill and needing intensive care. Conversely, midwives who support women in these high-tech situations may not have the range of skills needed in an out-of-hospital setting. With such a wide range of differing approaches to diagnosis and treatment a single practitioner may, in any case, be hard pressed to reach a conclusion on what is 'best'. It could therefore be argued that going to just one therapist for everything is no more holistic than a diet that includes only protein; just as we need a balance of foods, so we also need to care for mind, body and spirit, not just the body.

Yet I see holistic as being greater than the sum of the best conventional and alternative medicine has to offer. My research and reflection has led me to conclude that both conventional (treat the disease) and alternative (treat the whole person) medicine still view disease as something 'bad' that must be 'treated'. The very word 'patient' seems to imply that in some way you become less valid if you become ill (Weed 1989). The treatments, as with the induction example above, simply differ in the extent to which they are perceived as 'natural' or 'medical', which is somewhat paradoxical when we consider that most pharmaceutical drugs originated from plants.

Weed (1989) proposes a different approach that she terms the Wise Woman way. The difference here is that 'disease' is not seen as a problem to be cured, but rather as a transformative doorway to wholeness. This gives the 'patient' a more positive and healthy respect for their body's messages (Wysong 1996). The Wise Woman tradition sees health as flexibility, groundedness and openness to change and transformation. In this paradigm the therapist – or midwife – is the facilitator of change rather than someone who heals or cures (Weed 1989). I see the role of facilitator in the same way as a teacher who, although unable to pass an exam for the student, can help the student develop the tools to succeed. As one of my own teachers says:

'The true healer is within the body and the practitioner only facilitates healing by giving the body the right conditions in which to heal.' (N Sofroniou, personal correspondence, 2004).

As an aside, from my perspective as a male healer, the term 'Wise Woman' appears somewhat exclusive, focusing as it appears to on women. Undoubtedly the Wise Woman way is known by many names in different cultures, but it is a paradox that a holistic approach to health that embraces disease does not, on the surface, appear to embrace men!

Weed (1989) suggests we do not try to avoid pain and problems, which can be paths to greater wholeness and more vital health. According to Nouwen (1994), those who avoid the painful encounter with the unseen live boring and superficial lives! Hindsight may allow us to see the value of suffering what at the time seemed like an unwelcome illness or problem. The problem may have taught us something valuable: it may be we learned to adopt a healthier lifestyle or diet that prevented a more serious complaint arising, or we may have gained an insight into suffering that allows us to empathise with others as a result, and may even lead to a new career in the healing professions (Achterberg 1991).

Laudable and logical as it appears, the 'heroic' approach of CAM that asks us to follow natural laws to achieve health strikes me as quite a controlling vision. It seems to suggest that to be healthy and whole we must follow certain rules or we will be punished with disease (Weed 1989). This is a very patriarchal viewpoint, which led me to realise that conventional Western medicine and CAM are not as different as I once thought. Despite its holistic language, much of CAM adopts the same approach as conventional medicine by seeking the cause of the disease and eradicating it, albeit on more subtle levels with gentler treatments. But if CAM is truly holistic perhaps it should move beyond treating physical, emotional, mental and spiritual 'diseases', however naturally this is accomplished.

I invite midwives to reflect on how this translates into their practice, again acknowledging that their starting point is different from mine. Perhaps the time has come to consider whether the way forward is in presenting alternative, 'natural' therapies to treat discomforts, problems or conditions faced by childbearing women, or to attempt to move from the rhetorical to the real as far as the 'journey' of pregnancy is concerned, and completely re-frame the situations that Western medicine sees as problematic within the Wise Woman or a similar approach. A truly holistic perspective will embrace all experiences be they termed disease or health. By transforming our views of health and disease we can begin to overcome the labels that often pigeon hole our experiences as problems to cure, and start seeing them as a call to embrace a more expansive perspective and a greater vision of who we can become.

REFERENCES

Achterberg J (1991) Woman As Healer. Rider, London

Davis-Floyd R and St John G (1998) From Doctor To Healer; the transformative journey. New Brunswick, NJ; Rutgers University Press

Hay L (1996) You Can Heal Your Life. Enfield, Middlesex; Eden Grove Editions

Long L, Huntley A, Ernst E (2001) Which complementary and alternative therapies benefit which conditions? A survey of the opinions of 223 professional organisations. Complementary Therapies in Medicine 2001; 9: 178-185

Newman Turner R (1990) Naturopathic Medicine; Treating The Whole Person. Wellingborough, Northamptonshire; Thorsons Publishers Ltd

Nouwen HJM (1994) The Wounded Healer. London; Darton, Longman & Todd Ltd

Robbins J (1996) Reclaiming Our Health; Exploding the Medical Myth and embracing the Source of True Healing. Tiburon, CA, USA; HJ Kramer Inc

Shealy CN & Myss CM (1988) The Creation of Health; Merging Traditional Medicine with Intuitive Diagnosis. Walpole, NH, USA; Stillpoint Publishing

Weed S (1989) Healing Wise; Wise Woman Herbal. Woodstock, NY, USA; Ash Tree Publishing

Wysong RL (1996) Wysong Health Letter. Available at http://www.wysong.net/healthletter/hl_mar96.shtml (accessed on 2nd January 2004)

Stories and Reflection

SECTION CONTENTS

Once upon a time, midwives learned from stories told by their elders, many of which have been forgotten in the mists of time. Nowadays, we have the ability to write stories down to share with a wider audience. Happily, despite the prevalence of scientific approaches to being and knowing in our modern culture, midwives still love telling and hearing stories. This final section is a compilation of stories and reflection on other ways of knowing from the different perspectives of midwives and others.

Janice Marsh-Prelesnik, an American midwife who learned her trade by apprenticeship, writes about intuition; how this may manifest for women, and how we can help women tap into their deepest ways of knowing. Helen Eatherton provides another perspective on women's knowledge, and how this may clash with professional knowledge, and examines some of the conflict between the two. Jill Parker and Karen Dunlop both reflect on practice situations that further demonstrate the impact of a medical philosophy on birth and the need for midwives to consider their responses to this.

Artist Xavier Pick offers another perspective on birth, and his paintings depict another way of storytelling, while Charlotte Walker shares her reflections and resources on the use of creative writing as a tool for self-expression and learning. Rosalind Holland then reflects on two births she attended in Kenya. Her story highlights the stark differences experienced by women giving birth in different parts of the world today, and her own experience of hope-based practice. Finally, Jenny Fraser's story not only serves to emphasize the complexity of good midwifery and an optimal environment for birth, but also provides the happy ending that we tend to like at the end of our stories…

How can midwives assist women to trust their intuition?

Janice Marsh-Prelesnik

During the childbearing year, when all of a pregnant woman's senses are heightened, including intuition, how can midwives assist the women they are serving to trust, and access, their intuition? Whether a baby is *in utero*, being born, or in his or her mother's arms, intuitive ways of knowing can be instrumental in the mother's decision-making. Of course, rational, linear thinking is highly valued in Western culture. Many midwives consider it their role to support women in decision-making based on intuition.

So what is intuition? It is a form of intelligence and a fine tuned sense. It is a life force and a way to access deep, inner ways of knowing. Intuitive information is unique to the individual and the experience. Perhaps intuition is a culmination of our entire being. The dictionary defines intuition as, 'an immediate cognition; sharp insight; the act or faculty of knowing without the use of rational process.'

Women need to understand that intuitive knowledge can come to them in many different ways. It may be experienced as a gut feeling, a voice (either their own or another's), a response to move, a peaceful feeling, a flutter or a pain in the heart, while dreaming, an 'aha' experience, or other individual ways. Many people understand intuitive messages as the Higher Spirit (replace with God, Allah, Goddess, as you will) speaking through them. As a midwife, think back on an intuitive thought or feeling that you yourself have experienced. What form did it take? Do you value intuition as a valuable tool for decision-making? Do you honour your own intuition? Share your experiences with the women you assist.

All women have the ability to access, and trust their intuitive ways of knowing:

'It's a new perception. It's as though it allows us to notice what we haven't noticed and acknowledge what we perhaps already know but have forgotten in some way. The interesting thing is that as soon as you start paying attention to intuition,

it does become more available. It's as though it responds to attention, and so it's really not that difficult.' (Vaughn, 1999)

When asking a woman her opinion on a subject, ask her what the deepest part of her being thinks or knows. Assure her that all ways of acquiring knowledge, whether rational or intuitive, are valid. Midwives may be one of the few people in a woman's life that support her ability to make holistic decisions based on the culmination of all of her senses and her whole being. Just as we trust women's bodies to grow and birth their babies, we also can trust a woman's knowledge to know what is right for her.

There are many levels of intuition. In general, it is down to earth and used in practical ways every day. When a pregnant woman just knows not to ride her bike anymore, for fear of hurting her baby, that is intuition speaking to her. Linda, a mother of seven children, said that intuition spoke to her loudly one night by demanding that she eat liver. She says:

'The night before my last baby was born I was craving liver. LIVER! I never eat liver. So I bought some, and ate it up. It was great. I hadn't eaten liver my entire adult life. I had liver, onions and bacon that night. I had a wonderful meal. I just gravitate to the things I need to do. Like food cravings. It's not a voice telling me. It is more of a gut feeling for me.'

During labour, moving and choosing different positions is an intuitive process on the mother's part. Any interventions by the midwife, no matter how small, will alter the intuitive process for the mother and distract her from the rhythm of her birthing energy. Midwives must truly believe that the mother they are with knows what is best for her. Intuition will be her guide during labour and birth.

Larger decisions in life can be enhanced with intuition, leading to women living a more authentic life. Decisions such as place of birth, and choosing a parenting style are more readily accessible when a woman is accustomed to following what her inner most self tells her. Today, this level of intuitive knowledge can often be backed up with research. Finally, science is validating what women have already known throughout the centuries!

Occasionally messages are given that scream 'all is not well' leading to instinctual behaviour to protect. A sense of doom, or lack of health and well being for either the mother herself, or her baby, of course, must at once be acknowledged. Sometimes it can be difficult to differentiate the difference between a deep-seated fear and an intuitive message. Deep fears often are discussed and recognised antenatally. These may be fears surrounding childhood issues, fear of birth, or mothering. Often these kinds of unresolved issues are constrictive and can stop birthing energy from flowing. Intuitive messages, that all is not well, come on suddenly and gnaw at the depths of your being. They are expanding and insist on swift action. It is imperative that both midwives and mothers listen to these messages.

Recently I interviewed mothers on how intuitive knowledge came to them. Here are some of their words.

'I first feel it as a wave: as vibrations running through my body telling me what I am supposed to do. It starts out spiritual and then becomes physical. If I am not paying attention, or I do something against what my intuition tells me, I feel it in my tummy. If I don't listen to that I hear voices in my head.'

'I just feel it in my whole body. I just know what to do.'

'If fear is involved I feel it in my solar plexus. It says, "Run, you are not safe". If information has been processed and intuition is giving me answers, I hear voices in my head. If emotions are being dealt with, I feel it in my heart.'

'An inner drive pushes me forward into behaving in a certain way. Fortunately, this drive, so far, has made right decisions for me. When I first started paying attention to this drive I was worried that it would be wrong. It hasn't been, though, and it has brought me many blessings. I am glad I pay attention to it.'

'I just feel guided along by something much more than myself. I guess this would be a higher power. It is God telling me what to do.'

These words came from seasoned mothers who have learned to follow their intuitive voice. Several of the mothers mentioned that they had to relearn the ability to listen to their intuition. They felt as though they were taught to think in a linear, black and white fashion, where there was one answer for every question. As young children they were encouraged to think as the majority of people did, and not think, or feel, for themselves.

Now as grown women and mothers it has been a challenge for them to listen to information that was intuitively given to them on a deep personal level. Many of the mothers mentioned that it was important for them to find the support of other like-minded women. Midwives can be a wonderful resource for women to find one another. Why not organise a mother's group where women can meet one another?

It can be a great change for women living in modern culture to make decisions based on intuition. The challenge for midwives is to support women and their intuitive decisions when books, family, friends, the 'experts' and mainstream culture, and even midwives themselves, may give information that is counter-intuitive to an individual woman's deep ways of knowing. Lorene, a mother I interviewed, calls this clouding. She says:

'Clouding means that someone says something against what you innately feel is right. Then you start doubting yourself. You start clouding up. It is important to keep yourself in a place where you don't get clouded. My La Leche League friends didn't cloud me.'

A mother needs support for her intuitive ways of knowing. Although intuitive messages may be clear to her, the logistics of how to carry out this intuition may not always be straightforward. Lorene continues:

'Most people who offer advice want to solve a problem the easiest way possible. They want you to feel better as soon as possible. That is not what you want to hear. You want to hear choices for working through a problem until it comes out right. You want to feel encouraged.'

While women gather information from books, health care providers, family and friends, midwives can remind women that they must make decisions based on their individual belief system and life style. In a world where women are encouraged to follow mainstream culture and the collective consciousness, a midwife may be one of the few people in a woman's life that advocates and trusts the woman's ability to make individual decisions.

As Sheila Kitzinger writes in *Rediscovering Birth*: *'Traditionally the midwife is not merely a birth attendant with special expertise. She has a spiritual function in helping the baby to birth, the woman to become a mother, and in creating the setting for birth and the time immediately following it so that it is right for this spiritual transition.'* (Kitzinger, 2000)

So much of this spiritual transition is grounded and rooted with the ability for women to listen deeply to their inner selves. Midwives have the awesome ability to support women in this most elemental time of their lives. In fact, it may be one of the few times in a woman's life where another woman says with all sincerity that she totally trusts and honours her way of knowing how to birth and mother her baby. The supportive words of a midwife can give strength to a new mother for the rest of her life.

Many people think of instinct and intuition as one and the same. Although intuitive thoughts may transpire from an instinctual response they are not the same.

'Intuition is the bridge that connects instinct and all its survival responses with our emotions and their elegant instruction on how to thrive. Intuition is a higher order of embodied response than either instinct or emotion.' (Reeves, 1999) Instincts are consistent within species. Intuition is individual. We all have the same instinct to protect our young, and ourselves, and to react when danger threatens our existence. Instinct causes us to react quickly to the situation. If mothers perceive a danger to their baby or themselves they physically react. Heart and breathing rates increase as adrenaline rushes through the body. Every cell in the body says to protect. The woman experiences the fight or flight phenomenon.

It is so important that mothers and the midwives they work with understand this. Mothers need to know that during labour, if they experience fear, or a feeling that they are unsafe, the oxytocin loop will be disrupted and contractions will stop or slow down. I believe that this needs to be discussed with women antenatally as a means to bring up discussion on unresolved fears, creating the ideal birthing environment, and having support people present who are truly supportive.

So how can midwives teach women to access and develop their deep ways of knowing? First of all, remind mothers that growing a baby is the ultimate creation. The creative process beckons time for internal work, and asks for the sensations of the heightened senses to be celebrated, and honoured. Remind your mothers to allow themselves plenty of time to daydream and relax during pregnancy. Encourage them to have plenty of time each day to quiet their body and mind in order for them to learn to pay attention to the messages of their inner selves.

To attain this, recommend that women spend time alone, without distractions, in nature, whenever possible. Suggest that they just sit, or lie quietly, and feel their emotions and any tension held in the body. Where are the different emotions held in the body? Where does she experience muscle tension? Teach her to breathe deeply, and find the peaceful, quiet place within herself. Intuitive insights often come to women during this relaxed, blissful state. Encourage her to strive to maintain this calm feeling as much as possible throughout the seasons of her pregnancy. This skill will serve her well during labour, and as a new mother.

Intuitive ways of knowing are indeed valid. Especially during the seasons of pregnancy, the ultimate culmination of creative process, a mother's intuition is a gift that leads to true and honest mothering, and womanhood. The beauty of midwifery care is that midwives truly do honour and listen to the authentic, intuitive voice of each mother that we are asked to be with.

REFERENCES

Kitzinger, Sheila. (2000). Rediscovering Birth. New York: Simon & Schuster

Reeves, Paula. (1999). Women's intuition: unlocking the wisdom of the body. Berkeley, California: Conari Press.

Vaughan, Frances (1998). Awakening Intuition. Transcript from Thinking Allowed: Conversations on the Leading Edge of Knowledge and Discovery with Dr. Jeffrey Mishlove. www.intuition.org

Trust in women...

Don't trust the 'patient'

Helen Eatherton

'Well, this is our star patient tonight.' A few clinical details are given followed by, 'She came in pushing, had to have a wheelchair brought to the front door, then when we examined her we found she was only a multips os'. Everyone sniggers. 'I went into her room this evening and said 'Oh, you haven't had it yet then.' (laughter) 'But just to be on the safe side, VE her before you send the boyfriend home, it's his first and there'll be hell to pay if he misses it.'

So went the handover on the antenatal ward; the scene is set which colours the rest of the night. At the time, I did not question this unsympathetic picture. Although I cared for Susan to the best of my ability, I must admit, I did not believe what she was saying. This article explores some of the issues which arise from working in a culture which values medical and technological knowledge over that of women. The italicised comments are from my reflective diary.

At 2230 I did a vaginal examination and found no change in the cervix. The contractions were scarcely palpable but Susan claimed they were getting worse.

Susan was having contractions although the clinical findings did not support this. It is a clear indication of the extent to which medical knowledge is seen as authoritative when a woman's testimony is laughed at. 'What the woman knows and displays... has no status in this setting... Worse, her knowledge is nothing but a problem for her and her staff' (Jordan, 1997). The way in which the midwife had unfavourably described Susan clouded my professional judgement and that of my colleague. Although camaraderie at handover is an indication of caring for colleagues (Hunt & Symonds, 1995) it remains a sad fact of hospital culture that there exist many prejudices and biases. In current practice, it is my personal observation that mistaking the onset of labour is a great sin, second only to that of poor personal hygiene or obesity. As Hunt and Symonds (1995) state, 'the morality of an admission is related to the dilatation of the cervix'. Susan was sneered at because midwives have come to be a part of the medical system and so share the same prejudices. This system is self-perpetuating as midwives are trained in this milieu.

Two hours later, Susan buzzed again. She said the pains were even stronger. I sat with her for a while and palpated and timed her contractions again; clinically, the picture remained unconvincing. I discussed the need for a further vaginal examination with my senior colleague, Theresa. I had been chatting to staff earlier that night about evidence-informed practice, suggesting that vaginal examinations performed by different people were an inaccurate way of assessing progress. *She sneered, 'Oh come on, you know what you were reading, you can't keep doing all these VEs!'* I was relatively inexperienced and this remark perturbed me... consequently I didn't examine Susan again.

Why couldn't she have supported me in working through this situation? Instead, she joked about my interest in 'the literature'. Why do so many colleagues feel threatened by new information? As obstetricians have established their knowledge as authoritative, and policies have been drawn up exclusively around this arrogance, midwives in hospitals often scorn knowledge that is not disseminated hierarchically. Experienced midwives either develop into wise women or remain firmly encased in the medical model, so comfortable in this role that they feel threatened stepping beyond its boundaries. Skills of intuition, common sense and experience have not been fostered, even worse they have been ignored or derided. Theresa could have been in the position of a wise woman, confident, generous with her expertise, supportive. Instead she is a product of a culture in which women have lost out and react defensively in order to preserve the little prestige they have left, and even that has been gained with medical approval.

Susan buzzed again. This time she wanted her mother

in with her. I refused to call her; quoting hospital rules, horrified at the thought of having two demanding women instead of one.

How does the midwife become the focus of care instead of the woman? Midwives in the hospital are often walking a tightrope between hospital policies and the needs of the woman. Versed in clinical judgement and taught to devalue their own, midwives fear reprisals from the hospital hierarchy and often other midwives. By refusing to believe Susan I avoided conflict with labour ward staff who had their own set of clinical rules, but Susan and her mother would have been too much for me to ignore. Childbirth was not meant to be a power contest between midwives and women. If midwives can be taught or shown how to adjust the power base and to allow other evidence to inform their practice, the gap between themselves and women will diminish.

Susan became more and more vociferous about her pains and her need for her mother. I became desperate. I rang labour ward and spoke to the midwife in charge, 'Marion, I don't know what to do!' 'Bring her down here,' she said. I will always be grateful.

This is an example of an experienced midwife fulfilling her role as a wise woman.

She is supporting a less experienced colleague in a crisis, which has repercussions for the entire unit and a new generation of midwife. Marion was drawing on her common sense/intuition/experience or a mixture of all three to make a decision that was both clinically inaccurate and risked incurring the criticism of her colleagues. How we extol that attitude or regard it in our current system is hard but perhaps knowing that she was right was reward enough. This experience has also had a profound effect on me, which is, maybe, the way it is perpetuated. She was prepared to sweep aside medical guidelines showing that this knowledge was not authoritative for her (Davis-Floyd & Davis, 1997). Such small measures can go a long way to empower both women and midwives and to destabilise the power base in childbirth.

I started to take Susan to the labour ward in a wheelchair accompanied by her boyfriend. On the way Susan said that she wanted to go to the toilet. When she was in the toilets she called out to me and said that she felt like pushing. Realising my mistake, I quickly ushered her back into the wheelchair and rushed her downstairs to the labour ward as quickly as I could. 'But Helen, haven't you done another VE?' was what greeted me on labour ward. I felt ridiculous.

Susan was understandably angry and talked of complaining. This anger, albeit hard to deal with, is a healthy sign of women asserting their rights for their knowledge of evidence to be a part of decision-making. During the last century and continuing into this one, the patriarchal medical system has portrayed itself as the owner of authoritative knowledge. Technology has been coupled to science to strengthen this cultural leaning. These two allies form a formidable opponent for women.

Reflecting on the issues

Since this scenario happened, I have reflected on the situation and begun to question my own prejudices and preconceived ideas about different situations. The first question the scenario raises is, 'How have midwives become so divorced from women?' Midwives in the hospital setting have been torn away from their roots gradually but inexorably during the twentieth century and have become 'with doctors' instead of 'with women'. In this role, midwives have learnt to reinforce the culture in which they themselves, as women and professionals are victims, thereby becoming collaborators. As midwives have become 'with doctors' they have accepted medical knowledge as authoritative and thus dismissed other sources of knowledge as unreliable (Jordan, 1997). This has to be perpetuated to be maintained.

Anthropological studies advocate the tenet that birth has always been a spiritual, social, emotional and cultural event (Stuart-Macadam & Dettwyler, 1996). Yet the medical world has attempted to reduce it to a purely physical or pathological one by refusing to view the woman holistically and aided by the fact that science has become our culture's authoritative knowledge. Birth does remain, however, more than just a physical event, which can be seen by the activities which surround it: cards, new clothes, knitting, and excitement as evidenced just a few years ago when the country found out that Cherie Blair was pregnant.

Authority has been wrested from women in the western world throughout history and midwives have often been the focus of attack (Mander, 1998). Christianity viewed pain in labour as a punishment for Eve's sin (Genesis Ch3 v16). Midwives were persecuted by the church for using herbs to relieve pain in labour and were often burnt as witches. Others were thus discouraged from using their skill and power (Mander, 1998). The Age of the Enlightenment saw the rise of science to provide an explanation for our lives and bodies. 'Women were no longer linked to the powerful mysteries of nature but become objects of science'(Carter, 1995).

Throughout their lives women are trained to accept this authoritative knowledge and be obedient. Women are reined in during the antenatal period with hospital visits, long waits, brief séances with a lack of opportunity to ask serious questions (Szurek, 1997), reminding women of their place. The silent participation of many women in these proceedings confirms their position

(Sargent & Bascope, 1997). Midwives, too, are subject to these influences. Most midwives were themselves born in hospitals, in a system which taught their mothers to obey (Szurek, 1997). The role of the GP in women's lives reinforces his or her authority as the arbiter of long-term sickness certificates.

Compounded to all this, most practising midwives today were initially trained as nurses, which helps explain why midwives have not seized the opportunity offered by Changing Childbirth (1993) to change maternity care. This is not only because they lack confidence to expand their role by including a greater degree of autonomy (Hunter, 1998) but also because, for many, midwifery was initially not the job they signed up for. Despite the recent influx of direct entry midwives, the majority of midwives today were originally nurse trained, and view midwifery merely as an extension of that role. This is, of course, a generalisation; there are midwives in the National Health Service (NHS) who are willing to pay more than lip service to woman-focused care. So many, however, find the medical model of childbirth safe and operating within it keeps them within their personal comfort zone.

Despite the depressing aspects of current midwifery practice which this incident highlights, it also serves to illustrate how even within our care system, encumbered by the medical model of childbirth and stifled by the present day authoritative knowledge, midwives can call upon other sources of knowledge to inform their practice. And this incident has been, of course, an invaluable episode in my experiential learning.

REFERENCES

Carter P. 1995. Feminism, Breasts and Breastfeeding. London: MacMillan

Davis-Floyd R, Davis E. 1997. Intuition as authoritative knowledge in midwifery and home birth. In: Davis-Floyd R & Sargent C. Childbirth and Authoritative Knowledge: Cross Cultural Perspectives. California: University of California Press

Department of Health. 1993. Changing Childbirth, Part 1: Report of the Expert Maternity Group. London: HMSO

Genesis, Chapter 3 Verse 16. In: The Holy Bible, New International Version. 1990. London: Hodder and Stoughton

Hunt S, Symonds A. 1995. The Social Meaning of Midwifery. London: Macmillan

Hunter B. 1998. Independent Midwifery – future inspiration or relic of the past? BJM, 6(2)

Jordan B. 1997. Authoritative knowledge and its construction. In: Davis-Floyd R & Sargent E. 1997. Childbirth and Authoritative Knowledge: Cross Cultural Perspectives. California: University of California Press

Mander R. 1988. Pain in Childbearing and its Control. Oxford: Blackwell Science Ltd

Sargent C, Bascope G. 1997. Ways of knowing about birth in three cultures. In: Davis-Floyd R & Sargent E. 1997. Childbirth and Authoritative Knowledge: Cross Cultural Perspectives. California: University of California Press

Stuart-Macadam P, Dettwyler K. 1996. Breastfeeding: Biocultural Perspectives. New York: Walter de Gruyter Inc

Szurek J. 1997. Resistance to technology – Enhanced childbirth in Tuscany. In: Davis-Floyd R & Sargent E. 1997. Childbirth and Authoritative Knowledge: Cross Cultural Perspectives. California: University of California Press

The Practising Midwife 2002; 5(7): 32-33

9.3

Artist in residence
Rochdale Infirmary Maternity Unit 2001

Xavier Pick

As part of my commission to illustrate the working life of Rochdale Infirmary, I spent a few days observing the Maternity Unit. Initially, I was a bit daunted, and the staff were somewhat bemused by the presence of an artist in their midst. After the formalities and introductions were over, I got to work, looking at all aspects of the department.

I started by meeting a young couple who were awaiting the arrival of their baby in the next few hours. I thought they were surprisingly relaxed (the husband was watching The Weakest Link on the box!) but labour had only just begun. Out of respect, I didn't witness the birth itself – I had an appointment to witness a Caesarean section being carried out, but I felt that such an image might be inappropriate to decorate the walls of the hospital. The midwives were very helpful, though, and I was shown the water birthing room. Though there was no birth actually scheduled, the staff explained the procedure to me, and one obliging midwife very kindly posed for me in the dry bath, much to the amusement of everybody watching.

Next, I spent some time in the Special Care Baby Unit. Judith, the nurse assigned to 'look after' me, was very helpful and hospitable, and she explained her daily tasks, demonstrating with one of the tiny babies – bathing, weighing and feeding. I asked whether she became attached to the babies – she replied 'Of course!', but added that she had her hands full with her own children at home. I explained that I wanted to portray images of caring and nurturing – she understood and

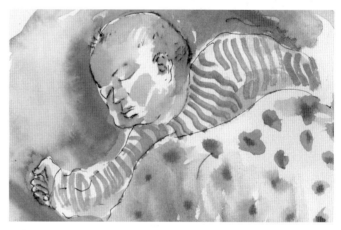

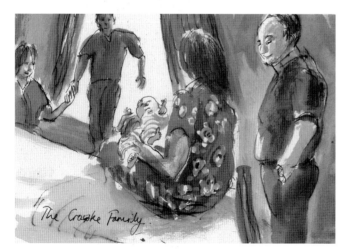

The Craske Family

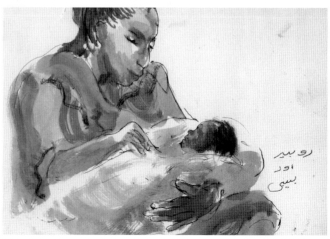

replied, 'You mean like Mother Earth'.

The subject of mother and child has fuelled artistic expression throughout history. For an artist, it is a fascinating subject, and one which is fundamental to human nature. In fact, the earliest primitive sculptures are of maternity figures, and the subject has dominated the visual arts in every culture ever since then.

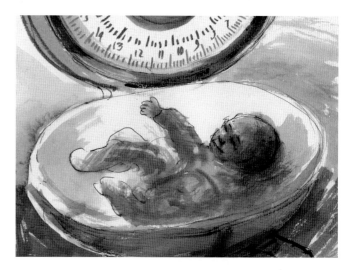

To see the joy and happiness of families welcoming a new baby into the world was wonderful to witness. I spent a day with one particular family as streams of well-wishers came in to see them, bearing gifts of toys, flowers and football scarves! Next door, there was an Asian family, and the mother thanked Allah for his miraculous gift.

Hospitals are not always places we like to visit, for obvious reasons, but it genuinely was an honour to depict this aspect of the Infirmary, and to witness the love, joy and amazement associated with one of life's most precious moments.

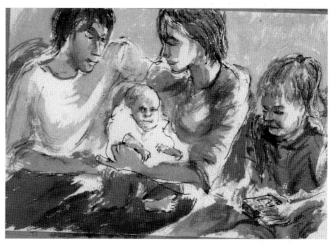

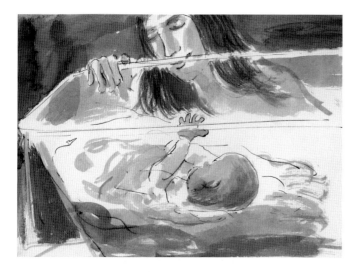

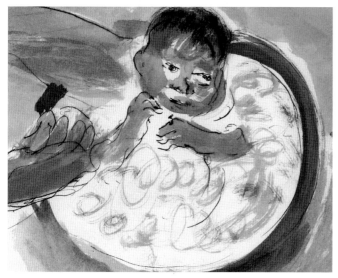

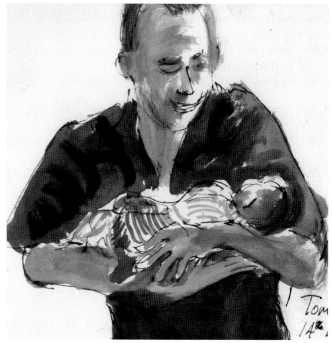

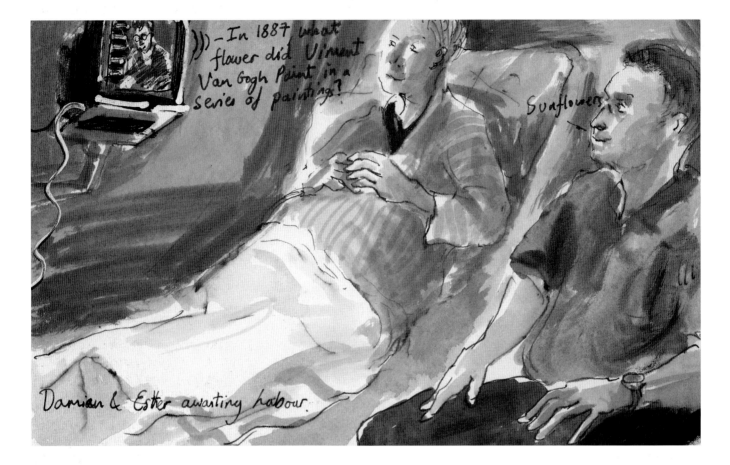

Damian & Esther awaiting labour.

Xavier's work as shown here is now decorating the walls of Rochdale Infirmary; prints are available. For more information visit www.xavierpick.com

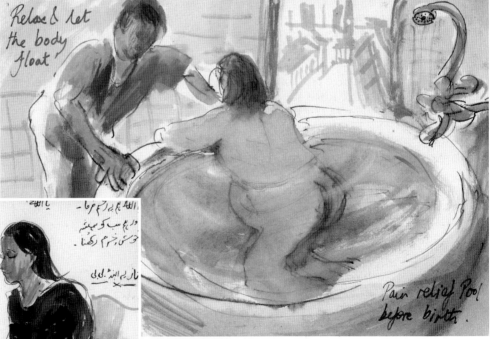

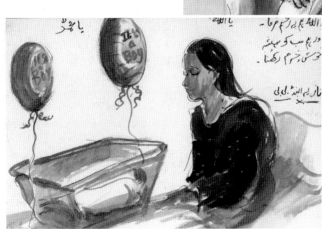

Let's make room for this baby

Karen Dunlop

I was working a routine shift on delivery floor when Hannah, a primigravida, was transferred in established labour. I took over from the ward midwife who told me that Hannah's cervix was 4cms dilated with intact membranes, contracting strongly 1:3 and that she was requesting some pain relief. Hannah was accompanied by her husband Jordan and her sister Rose.

Initially Hannah was comfortable sitting in a rocking chair and she was soon using Entonox effectively. She was well supported: Rose was giving massage during her contractions while Jordan provided verbal support. I maintained a quiet but watchful presence whilst writing my notes. As the contractions became more painful Hannah asked where I was and Jordan reassured Hannah that I was in the room. I rejoined the 'group' and quietly explained to Hannah that as Jordan and Rose were doing such a good job I was keeping a low profile.

Hannah wanted to change position, and chose to lie on the bed on her left side. Rose sat on the bed. Jordan pulled up a chair so he w as in an intimate position with Hannah and could maintain eye contact. Hannah was contracting strongly now 1:2 and was coping well with the Entonox and lots of encouragement.

After an hour and a half a sudden spontaneous rupture of membranes occurred, soaking Rose – much to everyone's amusement.

Shortly after this Hannah began involuntary pushing. She asked if I could examine her. Her cervix was fully dilated, as expected from her body language, and she began actively pushing her baby out. Jordan held her hand and gave physical support, while Rose and I offered encouragement about the effectiveness of her efforts, from the end of the bed. Rose's enthusiastic progress reports were helping Hannah. The vertex was visible and advancing.

At this point another midwife, Sally, came into the room, went to the opposite side of the bed to me, between Jordan and Rose and began physically changing Hannah's position, saying 'Put your leg up here. Let's make room for this baby.' She went on to instruct Hannah how to push and to show Jordan how to hold Hannah.

Rose slipped away and sat on a stool in the corner of the room saying nothing while Jordan did as he was instructed. I quietly told Sally that Hannah had tried pushing, in such a way and didn't like it, in fact she was pushing brilliantly in her own way and didn't need any instructons. Sally ignored me and carried on instructing Hannah and Jordan. I called Rose back into the 'group' saying that Hannah couldn't hear her encouragement, which was a shame as Rose's progress reports had really helped. As each contraction passed she would look to Rose for verbal confirmation that the baby really was coming.

Sally was called away from the room, and once she'd left the 'group' reformed to support Hannah. As her daughter was born onto her tummy Hannah said 'We did it'.

Jordan and Rose had been excellent at supporting Hannah through her labour and birth with just touch, encouraging words and their physical presence - so much so that I felt cross when a colleague came into the room and by her actions destroyed the atmosphere. I particularly felt cross that I did not feel able to stand up to Sally at this point and be a true advocate for Hannah. I would never interfere with another midwive's clinical skills/professional judgement to such a degree if called to assist at their birth.

I wonder how Hannah felt, no longer having support from Jordan and Rose at such a crucial time. When Hannah was at her most vulnerable (the vertex was almost crowning) she had a complete stranger 'manhandling' her and telling her how to push her baby out. Jordan and Rose were made to feel that their efforts at the birth were inadequate.

Rose had joked about Hannah having 'three'

midwives but I think she was right. Between us we had encompassed the art and science of midwifery using my knowledge base and their intuitive actions. Sally displayed none of these qualities.

I would like to think that this short reflective piece might make midwives stop, look and listen when entering a labouring woman's room, in order to add to the atmosphere, rather than destroy it.

The Practising Midwife 2002; 5(1): 49

A tale of two births

Rosalind Holland

It was the third week of my midwifery elective at a mission hospital in rural Kenya, I had just finished assisting at the birth of a gorgeous little girl. Miraculously in an area where there is very little antenatal care and the practice of female genital mutilation is widespread, Mary, the mother, had not needed an episiotomy and the girl's cry was as lusty as I could have wished for at birth. After a week in which most of the babies' Apgar scores were below 7 at delivery, I had resorted to holding my breath, crossing my fingers and willing everything to be all right. Not a recognised midwifery technique but it worked for me: hope-based practice.

Glowing with our achievements, I wandered through to the corridor to see it any other women were waiting for admission to the labour ward. Alice was dressed in the brightly coloured strips of cloth that Kenyan women wrap around themselves called Kangas. Using a mixture of pidgin Swahili, English, mime and a few words of Meru (the local dialect), I asked if she would lie on the bed in the examination room as all women were expected to have a VE before admission to the labour ward. I turned away to look at her notes, turned back and the whole of the sheet was bright red; crimson blood spreading in all directions. A massive APH. I had just completed an obstetric emergency exam chanting all the procedures I needed to know but Alice's haemorrhage was way beyond my skills. There were no buzzers or bells in the room, so with a word to Alice I ran to find my mentor, Gladys, on her tea break across the hospital courtyard. She looked as if about to tease me for my constant haste but instead, seeing my expression, immediately came running. I could not have been longer than two minutes but the blood had begun to pool between Alice's legs.

Gladys issued a string of orders whilst she reassured Alice, inserted a venflon and put up IV fluid. She listened with her pinard moving the instrument to different places on Alice's abdomen and looking at me shook her head slightly. I stroked Alice's hand: breath-holding and finger-crossing had no place here. The theatre was prepared and the missionary doctor arrived, a retired abdominal surgeon, and, before Gladys or I could stop him, did a vaginal examination. Blood gushed between his fingers like tap water and Alice's colour visibly paled. Placenta praevia, he diagnosed, sheepishly aware of his mistake. The theatre smelt of ether that made my head spin. On the oxygen monitor, Alice's SATs dropped to 48% as she continued to bleed and the surgeon's hands shook. The baby was delivered, greenish from thick meconium; a perfectly formed little girl who had died, Gladys thought, a few hours earlier.

The surgeon stabilised Alice's bleeding and I helped the Kenyan nurses squeeze IV fluids back into her body. There was no blood bank at the hospital. Blood was donated by relatives: a mixed blessing in a country where AIDS infects one in every six adults. Alice was lucky, the Kenyan nurses said, because she had been brought to the hospital by her brothers who would be able to donate blood for her. Still unconscious, pale and without her baby, Alice was wheeled off to the surgical ward. The surgeon estimated that she had lost half the blood in her body but she was alive and would, he thought, recover well.

Back on the labour ward, I glanced around a curtain and there was Mary, still breastfeeding her little girl. After a bit of smiling and mime, I offered to wheel her round to the post-natal ward before my shift finished. An easy task for the end of a long day except that there were no free beds. It was up to me to pick a mother at random from the long row of beds to share with Mary and her new baby. The 'lucky' mother moved over without comment and the two women were sitting up together in their bed equally feeding their babies as I left. The wealth of differences between this hospital and my English teaching hospital made me smile, albeit ruefully, as I went to boil for 20 minutes then filter the water I needed, before I could make myself a much deserved cup of Kenyan tea.

Creating reflections

Reflective practice and the expressive arts

Charlotte Walker

When I entered my midwifery education, my background as an antenatal teacher meant that I was already well acquainted with the concept of 'reflective practice'. Whilst training and teaching with the NCT, I became comfortable with using reflective tools such as diary keeping, and conversations with peers, clients and tutors, as a means of evaluating my practice and identifying areas for improvement.

During my first year as a student midwife, however, I have evolved an additional tool for reflection: using creative writing, which I have always pursued as a hobby, to illustrate and inform my practice. Many of my clinical experiences, particularly in intrapartum care, have been emotionally resonant as well as significant for my development of practical skills and judgement, and I now use writing, in particular poetry, to explore the under-addressed affective components of my experiential learning.

Writing fictional stories can also give great insight to midwives (Kirkham, 1997a, 1997b), but poetry is a particularly valuable means of addressing the emotions of practice, as it constitutes 'an exploration of the deepest and most intimate experiences, thoughts, ideas: distilled, pared to succinctness' (Bolton, 2001, 173).

As Douglas (1999) points out, as healthcare workers we perform certain clinical tasks with such frequency that they become routine, but for clients they are likely to be new and unique events. When tasks have become so commonplace to us that we no longer view their impact from the client's perspective, we run the risk of ceasing to question the value of the 'care' we give. Midwives who had the benefit of a poet in residence found that bringing the arts into health helped them to reflect on their clients' lives and experiences (Rigler, 1998), and I have found poetry a useful medium for reintegrating the voice of the client into the 'amalgam of deductive theory with observation, interpretation and experimentation by the practitioner' (Bryar, 1995) which forms the basis for

Time of birth

> *If words are power, how immense*
> *The strength of those first few to reach*
> *The neonatal ear.*
>
> *How significant the light*
> *Her pupils first contract against,*
> *Her retinae receive.*
>
> *One shocking and reflexive gasp*
> *Fills pristine passageways with air,*
> *Spurring independence.*
>
> *Nostrils emptied, primal smells*
> *Insinuate themselves, begin*
> *Imprinting neural seams.*
>
> *Digits splay and limbs extend.*
> *Initial touch of latex glove*
> *Creates a self in space.*

midwifery decision-making. In order to practise effectively, the midwife must make use of theory, research evidence and reason, but must also employ intuition, memory and empathy. Using reflective triggers from the expressive arts requires 'right brain' activity, which is associated with sensitivity, aesthetics and creativity, rather than 'left brain' logic and rationality (Johns, 2000; Bolton, 2001), attributes which can be seen to be core elements in providing woman-centred care. Kirkham (1997b) feels that midwives lack an appropriate vocabulary for discussing the affective and creative elements of midwifery, and that a means of developing reflection is needed which assists us in seeing these aspects. Arts-based reflection may therefore be a means of emphasising and valuing the 'art' of midwifery, and re-affirming its distinctness from the pure science of medicine (Jackson and Sullivan, 1999).

The poems: two examples

'Time of birth' was written having completed my first Delivery Suite placement, and combines my growing awareness of underpinning theory (onset of neonatal respirations and newborn reflexes have managed to work their way in) with an empathic identification with the baby. As Bolton (2001) asserts, poetry can offer startling insights to the busy practitioner, and during the writing of this poem, I became aware that when I am conducting a delivery, I tend to focus on the mechanical rather than the personal, seeing the baby as 'the fetal skull' and the mother as 'the perineum'. My attention has become so concentrated upon assisting the one to leave the other without mishap, that I am less aware of the birthing environment. Looking at the birth from the baby's perspective makes me ask new, sometimes uncomfortable, questions about my practice. Do I really require such bright lights 'to see what I am doing'? How much trust does this display in the ability of women's bodies to birth their own babies? How much thought do I give to the fact that my 'competent' handling of the newborn is a first and alien experience of touch? These insights are points to plough back into the development of my personal practice when I am next giving intrapartum care.

The events depicted in 'Twin Dignities' took place during my first ever shift in the hospital Delivery Suite.

Twin dignities

'Do doctor's gown up, please.' I have to stretch,
On tip-toe in my nursey lace-up shoes.
Around the registrar, the midwives fetch
The metal poles and sinister ventouse,
Wheel their trolleys, deftly lay out sets
Of instruments he may decide to use.
My one task now fulfilled, I move to stand
Beside the bed-head, offering my hand.

Senior students harmonise, suspend
Numbed legs into loops with fluid speed.
Spreading drapes allows us to pretend
It's only flesh: on that we're all agreed.
Scissors flash, we hear the tissues rend,
Although the Sister speaks to question need.
Interloping fingers dig inside
Anaesthetic-deadened parts spread wide.

Figure 9.6.1 Creative exercises to aid reflection

Bolton (2001) offers an exploration of reflection using creative writing, including practical suggestions

Capacchione and Bardsley (1994) suggest a variety of useful journalling, art therapy and creative writing techniques. The exercises are aimed at pregnant women, but may be valuable for the midwife wishing to focus on her antenatal clients' experiences

Sellers' (1991) collection of guidance by and for women writers is a rich seam of exercises for anyone beginning or developing creative writing

Taylor (2000) has put together a 'kit-bag of strategies' for creative reflection

Response to the creative works of others:

The paintings of Jonathon Waller (James, 1998)

Mamatoto (The Body Shop, 1991), a collection of birth photographs and folklore

Birth (Dubost, 1998) contains photographs of pregnancy, birth and babyhood in many cultures

The Virago Book of Birth Poetry (Otten, 1993) and In the Gold of the Flesh (Palmiera, 1990) are two anthologies of useful poems

Welcome to the World (Siegen-Smith, 1996) is an anthology of both poems and photographs about birth and babies from around the world

Cosslett (1994) analyses women's writing about birth, and is a good starting place for locating short stories and novels which deal with labour and delivery.

There is a descending hierarchy at work here, with the doctor at the top, and the labouring woman at the bottom, which is mirrored in the rigid rhythm and rhyme scheme (ottava rima). Evidently, I had far more dignity in this situation than the client whose vulva was on display to the room; as a very new student midwife, however, I felt shocked and faint at my first experience of assisted delivery, and had insufficient knowledge or skill to have a useful and identifiable role. Above me in the hierarchy, therefore, were the senior students and the qualified midwives, who were better able to minister to the doctor's needs. Becoming habituated to this hierarchy robs us of our empathy with the client asked to assume undignified positions such as lithotomy, and as qualified midwives, our empathy with students.

Reflective stimuli from the arts

While the process of writing creatively is one I feel comfortable with, evidently it will not suit all who wish to address the 'right brain' aspects of clinical experience. Reflection, in fact, can be achieved through any number of means, including writing, creative audio-visual work, dance, the visual and sculptural arts, music and needlework (Taylor, 2000). Nor does one need to be the 'creator' to make use of the arts: responding to the work of others, for example reading literature and poetry, can also help the healthcare professional to achieve empathy with other people, and to increase self-awareness and awareness of the situation of others (Grant, 1998). Baker (2000) describes a successful approach to midwifery education which assists final-year students in their analysis of practice situations by presenting them with dramatisations. Opportunities for creative reflection are limitless, and potentially richly rewarding.

REFERENCES

Baker K. 2000. Acting the part: using drama to empower student midwives. Practising Midwife, 3(1), 20-21

The Body Shop. 1991. Mamatoto: a celebration of birth. London: Virago

Bolton G. 2001. Reflective Practice: writing and professional development. London: Paul Chapman

Bryar R. 1995. Theory for Midwifery Practice. Basingstoke: Macmillan

Capacchione C, Bardsley S. 1994. Creating A Joyful Birth Experience. New York: Fireside

Cosslett T. 1994. Women Writing Childbirth: modern discourses of motherhood. Manchester: Manchester University Press

Douglas I. 1999. Reflective practice. In: Hogston R and Simpson P (eds). Foundations of Nursing Practice. Basingstoke: Macmillan

Dubost J (ed). 1998. Birth: photographs of Magnum Photos. Paris: Magnum Photos

Jackson D, Sullivan J. 1999. Integrating the creative arts into a midwifery curriculum: a teaching innovation report. Nurse Education Today, 19(7), 527-32

James J. 1998. The shock of creation. New Generation, 17(1), 4-6

Johns C. 2000. Becoming a Reflective Practitioner. Oxford: Blackwell Science

Grant J. 1998. The humanities and midwifery. Practising Midwife, 1(11), 41

Kirkham M. 1997a. Stories and childbirth. Reflections on Midwifery. London: Balliere Tindall

Kirkham M. 1997b. Reflection in midwifery: professional narcissism or seeing with women?. British Journal of Midwifery, 5(5), 259-62

Otten C (ed). 1993. The Virago Book of Birth Poetry. London: Virago

Palmiera R (ed). 1990. In the Gold of the Flesh: poems and birth and motherhood. London: Women's Press

Rigler M. 1998. Arts in health. Changing Childbirth Update, 11, 9

Sellers S (ed). 1991. Taking Reality by Surprise: writing for pleasure and publication. London: Women's Press

Siegen-Smith S (ed). 1996. Welcome to the World: a celebration of birth and babies from many cultures. Bath: Barefoot Books

Taylor B. 2000. Reflective Practice: a guide for nurses and midwives. Buckingham: Open University Press

The Practising Midwife 2002; 5(7): 30-31

Normal until proved otherwise

Jill Parker

My midwifery philosophy incorporates a belief that birth is normal until proved otherwise. When I was training, my care of a specific client (we'll call her Rebecca) involved antenatal appointments, parenting sessions, her birth and postnatal visits. During parent education, we discussed positions in labour, mobilising and a low intervention preference. Subsequently, Rebecca asked me if I could care for her in labour. I discussed this request with my community mentor and agreed to be 'on-call' for Rebecca. I did hope that the midwife in charge on the day she went into labour would agree to provide a mentor for me. The following is an account from my journal.

Rebecca telephoned this morning. She was term and in labour, coping with her contractions at home. She had already contacted CDS and was told it was OK for her to remain at home for as long as she felt able. She was determined to complete her early labour at home with her partner. She bathed, used TENS and mobilised throughout the morning.

By midday she was experiencing stronger and more frequent contractions and rang me to say she would be going into hospital within the hour. I telephoned CDS, the midwife in charge agreed to my attendance and agreed that someone would mentor me. I made my way to CDS in order to prepare the room for Rebecca, who had specifically requested in her birth plan a mattress on the floor if possible as she hoped to labour on 'all-fours'.

She was aware of hospital policy for a 20 min CTG on arrival and had agreed to this. I began to prepare the room, all that we had discussed during classes, a beanbag, a mattress, a pinard stethoscope for intermittent auscultation and a sonic aid. I was aware of being watched by the midwife in charge, who in a loud voice said to two midwives sitting at the desk: 'What is SHE doing?' On hearing this, I replied: 'I'm getting the room ready for Rebecca, she has specifically asked for a mattress on the floor.' She replied: 'Put it back until we

have ruled out the abnormal.' I felt embarrassed in front of the other midwives and annoyed that I had been made to feel so inexperienced and naïve in hoping for a normal birth.

However, I did say that I believed in birth being normal unless proved otherwise. I immediately thought of the theory-practice gap I had read about, and the paradigm of childbirth as normal only in retrospect. There is some evidence to suggest differing philosophies do exist between midwives. Some hospital midwives may focus on the clinical events of childbirth, considering 'real' midwifery as the management of a medical diagnosis. I believe that my training in both community and hospital has given me a different focus, having not spent too long thus far in hospital. I focus on supporting women and their partners through their experience. Obviously, should deviation from the 'norm' occur, I want to be able to deal with any emergency situation. I did remove the mattress from the floor, but left it visibly outside the room so that Rebecca on her arrival could see that it was there to use if necessary. Fortunately, by the time Rebecca's labour had progressed sufficiently for her to be on 'all-fours', I had acquired another mentor. She appeared to hold the same philosophy of care and despite the presence of thick meconium, and eventually an FSE, Rebecca laboured upright and gave birth to a healthy daughter with spontaneous pushes and had an intact perineum. Interestingly, following her request for syntometrine for third stage, and explanations of possible side effects, Rebecca vomited ++ on her way to the ward and we accepted that the syntometrine was the likely cause.

I felt very satisfied with my participation in this birth experience. I was assertive in that despite removing the mattress from the room I left it visibly outside. I also articulated to the midwife in charge that my philosophy was one of normal until proven otherwise. I would not have done either of those things earlier in my training. I now know what it feels like to be a woman's advocate despite the seeming lack of support from some other midwives. Caroline Flint has observed this lack of support between midwives, particularly in hierarchical organisations. The professional midwife is essentially orientated towards being part of an obstetric team in hospital, but she also hopes to meet the needs of the woman she cares for within (the confines of) the practice of the obstetric team. This can cause stress and confusion for a student midwife and midwives currently practising. They may struggle to reconcile their own developing philosophy of what a midwife is. I believe as a pragmatist that I will have to work for several years in the hospital before I might be considered for a community-based post, and learn how to survive in the increasingly busy hospital environment. I know that some midwives thrive in the high-tech atmosphere. Others leave. Recent work on burnout shows how crucial the first five years post-qualification are in terms of retention of staff – midwives whose expectations of professional autonomy are not met leave within five years. My own objective for my future is to develop autonomous midwifery practice that assists women and their families through the 'bio-social' birth process and not to become a 'nurse-midwife'. In order to do this, I must be strong and assertive, challenging routine practices accepted in hospitals by some midwives who may have become inflexible and unresponsive to clients' and the services changing needs. It might be easier to accept old routines, and not attempt to update and improve our practice. In fact, practising within a patriarchal organisation tends to lead to centralised decision making. Important decisions are often taken several layers away from where those decisions become actions. The further removed practitioners are from the decision-making process the less responsible they feel for their actions. This can lead to a culture of dependency where many practitioners take fewer decisions for themselves, escalating decisions up through the structure.

I feel that I am currently motivated enough to attempt autonomous practice. I believe in debate and discussion and I am keen to share my learning with others. The poster I produced in relation to ensuring a safe physiological third stage for my term seven assessments has recently been shared with other students at the request of my tutor and current mentor. Personal experiences in practice were also shared, and a questioning approach to 'blanket' policies was highlighted. Routine practices are gradually being challenged. One example, following the publication of National Institute for Clinical Excellence guidelines on CTG monitoring has recommended cessation of the 'blanket' policy for an admission trace, with recommendations for intermittent monitoring for the low-risk woman. Much discussion has been prompted amongst midwives. Those who believe in 'normal' until proved otherwise are happy to implement them. Those midwives comfortable with the 'old' practice may feel uneasy.

The Practising Midwife 2002; 5(10): 42

A winter homebirth

Jenny Fraser

It was a cold and windy wet November night. Karen was expecting her third baby and had planned to give birth at home. It was half past nine in the evening and she had just contacted her midwives to say that her contractions were infrequent but gradually increasing in strength, that she was happy on her own for the time being but that she felt that she would need to be in contact again shortly.

Karen had had a forceps delivery in hospital for her first baby, Joshua, 10 years earlier. She had found the whole experience traumatic and upsetting. Because of this she planned to have her second baby at home. She knew her community midwife, Lyn, well, as not only was she cared for antenatally and postnatally by her for the first baby, Lyn lived in the same small village. Lyn told Karen that she was concerned about delivering a baby at home, so far away from the hospital and regularly shared her concerns with Karen about what she would do if the labour became complicated, as she did not feel very confident about coping in such circumstances.

Karen commenced labour with her second baby at term but the labour started to slow when her cervix was about 4 centimetres dilated. Lyn became concerned about the 'lack of progress' and transferred Karen into the maternity unit. Karen was cared for in the unit by a sensitive, intuitive and insightful midwife. This midwife managed to forge a positive and caring relationship with Karen very quickly enabling Karen to feel well supported by this midwife. With no intervention Karen, with additional support from her partner, had a straightforward normal birth. Karen described this experience as being empowering and a life-changing event. Karen had been exceptionally disappointed that this life-changing event had not happened at home and felt that she had been pressurised into hospital at a vulnerable moment. She was immensely grateful that she had been cared for in the hospital by a respectful, kind and considerate midwife, and someone with the qualities to enable this birth.

During this third pregnancy Karen's partner left her. She was bewildered and upset and had to plan for a new baby and deal with her two other children's distress because their father had left the home. Karen chose two midwives to care for her during this pregnancy and, because of the system in place, the midwives would be able to be with her for the birth. Karen and the midwives built up a strong bond, which included emotional support as well as physical, and Karen found the resources to cope with the impending future. By the time Karen reached the point of being in labour she knew her midwives well and trusted them. Karen knew that she was fortunate to be able to access this type of care.

Karen called again at eleven o clock in the evening to say that her contractions were increasing to a point where she felt that she would welcome some support. The two midwives duly arrived at the house and Joshua and Flora were in bed. Karen had a friend there in case the children needed caring for. Having made all these arrangements Karen was free to labour in peace, knowing that the children were fine and that she had familiarity with her two midwives who knew all her wishes and concerns.

Karen had a birthing pool in the kitchen. This had previously been filled. The midwives were unobtrusive during the labour. At intervals the well being of both Karen and the baby were monitored. Some time later the electricity failed and the house was plunged into darkness. Karen remained calm and in control, she made her own decisions as to when she wanted to be in the pool and when she wanted to get out and pace around. It was her home, her territory and she knew her way around even though it was dark. At intervals she went upstairs and could be heard pounding the floorboards. Very little was said.

In the early hours of the morning Karen got into the pool to give birth. In the absence of any other lighting some candles were lit. Karen gave birth to her new daughter whilst on all fours in the birthing pool, in the kitchen only lit by candles. Karen caught the baby herself in the water and raised her to the surface. It was a cementing and beautiful moment. The baby did not cry loudly but a gentle meowing sound could be heard. At this point the lights came back on and Joshua and Flora woke up and came down stairs. They were fascinated by their new sister and after a few minutes promptly took themselves back to bed.

This short but true story has sought to show the complex interplay between the physical and psychological aspects of giving birth. It is more complex than the place of birth or whether the woman knows the midwife. Karen had her second baby in hospital with a midwife whom she had never previously met, yet this midwife managed to create an environment whereby Karen felt free and safe to give birth in the way that she desired. If Karen had been unfortunate and not had the care of such a midwife then she could have felt undermined and subsequently could have failed to have given birth in the way that she had hoped. This could have spilled over into the third baby and the outcome could have been so different. She knew her community midwife but the interaction was not fitting, maybe Karen felt the anxiety within the midwife culminating in the need to be transferred. Who knows, but it is worth the speculation.

For this third and final baby, the ingredients were in place, the midwives were known and trusted carers, Karen felt empowered and in control; she was in her home, which was her choice for birthing her baby. Every midwife needs to reflect on every single contact between her and a woman, no matter how short the contact, as it can have major repercussions on the woman should the midwife get it wrong. Each and every contact a midwife has with a woman can possibly affect and influence the physical outcome of birth.

The Practising Midwife 2002; 5(11): 42

Index

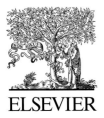

ELSEVIER

 Books *for* Midwives

CHURCHILL LIVINGSTONE   Mosby   THE PRACTISING MIDWIFE   ✤ Baillière Tindall

MIDWIFERY PUBLISHERS OF CHOICE FOR GENERATIONS

For many years and through several identities we have catered for professional needs in midwifery education and practice. Leading publishers of major textbooks such as *Myles Textbook for Midwives* and *Mayes' Midwifery: a Textbook for Midwives*, our expertise spreads across both books and journals to offer a comprehensive resource for midwives at all stages of their careers.

Find out how we can provide you with the right book at the right time by exploring our website, **www.elsevierhealth.com/midwifery** or requesting a midwifery catalogue from Health Professions Marketing, Elsevier, 32 Jamestown Road, Camden, London, NW1 7BY, UK Tel: 020 7424 4200; Fax: 020 7424 4420.

We are always keen to expand our midwifery list so if you have an idea for a new book please contact Mary Seager, Senior Commissioning Editor at Elsevier, The Boulevard, Langford Lane, Kidlington, Oxford, OX5 1GB, UK (m.seager@elsevier.com).

Have you joined yet?
Sign up for e-Alert to get the latest news and information.

Register for eAlert at www.elsevierhealth.com/eAlert Information direct to your Inbox

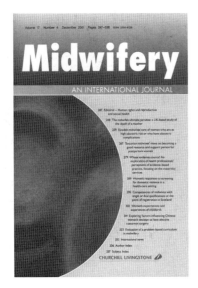

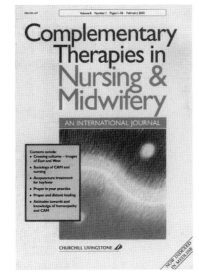

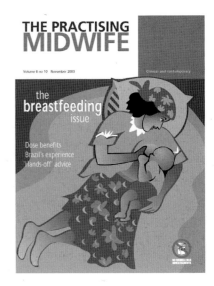